PANDEMIC INDIA

DAVID ARNOLD

Pandemic India

From Cholera to Covid-19

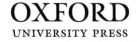
OXFORD
UNIVERSITY PRESS

OXFORD

UNIVERSITY PRESS

Oxford University Press is a department of the
University of Oxford. It furthers the University's objective
of excellence in research, scholarship, and education
by publishing worldwide.

Oxford New York

Auckland   Cape Town   Dar es Salaam   Hong Kong   Karachi
Kuala Lumpur   Madrid   Melbourne   Mexico City   Nairobi
New Delhi   Shanghai   Taipei   Toronto

With offices in

Argentina   Austria   Brazil   Chile   Czech Republic   France   Greece
Guatemala   Hungary   Italy   Japan   Poland   Portugal   Singapore
South Korea   Switzerland   Thailand   Turkey   Ukraine   Vietnam

Oxford is a registered trade mark of Oxford University Press
in the UK and certain other countries.

Published in the United States of America by
Oxford University Press
198 Madison Avenue, New York, NY 10016

Library of Congress Cataloging-in-Publication Data is available

ISBN: 9780197659625

Printed in Great Britain by Bell and Bain Ltd, Glasgow

CONTENTS

LIST OF FIGURES AND TABLES

Figures

Section 1: Plague

Section 2: Covid-19

Tables

LIST OF ABBREVIATIONS

ABP	*Amrit Bazar Patrika*
AIDS	Acquired Immune Deficiency Syndrome
ARDPH	*Annual Report of the Director of Public Health*
ARMAC	*Annual Report on the Municipal Administration of Calcutta*
ARMCB	*Annual Report of the Municipal Commissioner for the City of Bombay*
ARSC	*Annual Report of the Sanitary Commissioner*
AYUSH	Ayurveda, Yoga and Naturopathy, Unani, Siddha, and Homoeopathy
BJP	Bharatiya Janata Party
BMJ	*British Medical Journal*
HIV	Human Immunodeficiency Virus
IJMR	*Indian Journal of Medical Research*
IMG	*Indian Medical Gazette*
IMS	Indian Medical Service
IOR	India Office Records
MERS	Middle East Respiratory Syndrome
NAI	National Archives of India
RAMC	Royal Army Medical Corps
RNP	*Reports on the Native Press*

LIST OF ABBREVIATIONS

SARS	Severe Acute Respiratory Syndrome
ToI	*Times of India*
WHO	World Health Organization

ACKNOWLEDGMENTS

We live, think, and so write in catastrophic times. The coronavirus pandemic of 2020–1 has been the provocation and driver behind this work, but writing a book during a series of pandemic alarms and lockdowns has presented its own challenges, including lack of access to libraries and archives and the absence of live, face-to-face interaction with other scholars. It has made reliance on the internet and online communication immeasurably greater. But, at the same time, I have greatly benefited from the stimulus and camaraderie of scholarship through a series of collaborations, most of which have been hatched and delivered electronically.

Among those who greatly helped me by involving me in their projects and agenda, I owe particular thanks to several conference or roundtable organizers and volume editors, namely: Vinayak Chaturvedi, whose kind invitation was an initial point of departure for the writing of this present volume, for organizing a special issue, to which I contributed 'Pandemic India: Coronavirus and the Uses of History,' *Journal of Asian Studies*, 79 (2020) and which was republished in Vinayak Chaturvedi, ed., *The Pandemic: Perspectives on Asia* (2020); Clare Anderson for convening 'Epidemics in the Past and Now: A Roundtable on Colonial and Postcolonial History,' which was published in the *Journal of Colonialism and Colonial History*, 22 (2021); Guy Beiner for inviting me to contribute an essay on 'Representation and Remembrance: The 1918–19 Influenza Epidemic in India' to Guy Beiner, ed., *Pandemic Re-Awakenings: The Forgotten and Un-forgotten*

'*Spanish Flu*' *of 1918–19* (2022); to Christos Lynteris for the 'Visual Plague' conference at St. Andrews University, held pre-Covid in 2018, and for including my essay 'Picturing Plague: Photography, Pestilence and Cremation in Late Nineteenth- and Early Twentieth-Century India' in his edited volume *Plague Image and Imagination from Medieval to Modern Times* (2021); and Mark Bradley for the invitation to join in the pandemic conversation for the *American Historical Review*, scheduled for publication in 2022. I am further beholden to the organizers at Birkbeck in London for inviting me to join in an online seminar on 'Covid-19 in Historical Perspective' in November 2020; and to Jahnavi Phalkey and her associates at the Science Gallery, Bengaluru, for hosting my online talk on 'Science and Seeing: The Visual Technology of Contagion in 19th-Century India' in May 2021. Still further back, I am most grateful to Margot Finn for inviting me to speak at the Royal Historical Society meeting at Strathclyde University in October 2018: the occasion and feedback helped revive my interest in pandemics and resulted in my exploratory essay 'Death and the Modern Empire: The 1918–19 Influenza Epidemic in India,' published in *Transactions of the Royal Historical Society*, 29 (2019).

I especially want to thank Michael Dwyer at Hurst for so readily agreeing to take on this project, his editorial team at Hurst for seeing it through to publication so efficiently and supportively, and the two anonymous reviewers for their helpful comments and suggestions. Also to Warwick Anderson, Guy Attewell, Rustom Bharucha, Nandini Bhattacharya, Jane Buckingham, Ian Catanach, Raj Chandavarkar, Pratik Chakrabarti, Samuel Cohn, Rohan Deb Roy, Tim Dyson, Deepak Kumar, Myron Echenberg, Harald Fischer-Tiné, David Hardiman, Mark Harrison, Stephen Legg, Projit Mukharji, Robert Peckham, Mridula Ramanna, Madhu Singh, Michael Worboys, and the members, past and present, of the Global History and History of Medicine centers at Warwick. As the notes and bibliography to this book will show, I owe them all a debt of gratitude for help and generosity and for, over many years, having helped shape my ideas about medicine, disease, empire, and postcoloniality.

Additional thanks go to the British Library, the Africa, Asia and Pacific reading room and its obliging staff; and the Wellcome Library in London; Warwick University Library (its invaluable online facilities) and the National Archives of India. Also, more personally, to Juliet Miller, who made possible this book (and several more before it), but who also, in the nicest possible way, reminded me that there is more to life than books.

London
December 2021

INTRODUCTION

Pandemics matter. They matter to our lives and to our histories. They matter, in an increasingly globalized world, to how we see the past, present, and future; how we view ourselves and appraise those around us. Pandemics shape—sometimes shatter—our everyday lives. They threaten our livelihoods and challenge our modes of governance. They question the values by which we live; all too often in modern times, they determine the causes from which we die. As the devastating Covid-19 pandemic of 2020–1 brutally reminded so many people around the world, they imperil our fragile existence on this troubled earth.

The pandemic, in all its awful magnitude, was still ongoing as this book was being written, with no clear sign of when and how it might end. As a history, however, this book is only concerned with events up to the end of 2021, and the pandemic is accordingly referred to here as occurring in 2020-1. However, even by early September 2021, as the deadly second wave of the pandemic began to recede, Covid—the coronavirus SARS-CoV-2—had left an estimated 4.6 million people dead and caused 20 million cases worldwide. Of this mortality more than a tenth—535,732—was attributed to South Asia, from Afghanistan to Myanmar, and in this region 439,895 deaths and 37.5 million cases were recorded in India alone. At the time this placed India third, behind only the United States and Brazil, in the global reckoning of Covid deaths. And these were only the official statistics. Through poor reporting, misdiagnosis, and data

1

denial, the figures for India were likely to have been many times higher than the official record indicated. A calculation made by researchers at the Center for Global Development in the United States in July 2021, based on the number of excess deaths rather than reported Covid deaths, suggested that to date more than 4 million people had possibly died from the virus in India. The claim was hotly contested, but even the 414,000 deaths officially registered at the time still amounted to a massive mortality.[1] Statistics only ever form part of the pandemic equation, and their accuracy can always be questioned, but they signal a greater loss—of family and friends, of health and livelihood, of personal well-being and national prosperity. Whatever criteria we employ, Covid was a catastrophe of immense and terrifying proportions, one that, in terms of cases and deaths, of geographical reach and social dislocation, put the coronavirus of 2020–21 on a par with many earlier pandemics. We may never know for certain how many died in the Covid pandemic in India and around the world, any more than we can say with any exactitude the number who perished in the great influenza pandemic of 1918–19, when India, too, suffered an almost unimaginable death toll, now estimated at between 12 and 20 million deaths, or half of all fatalities worldwide. Not without justice has India been described as having been in recent centuries 'the home of great epidemics.'[2]

Why did India suffer so much? Why did it figure so largely, and so repeatedly, in the pandemic experience of modern times? It is not just the scale of India's mortality that matters and the complex reasons for it, important though they undoubtedly are. It is also the form that mass mortality has taken and the manner of its representation. As with comparable disease episodes over the two centuries preceding Covid, what happens in India—or emanates from India— resonates around the globe, defining the very nature and significance of pandemics as global phenomena. At times, India has almost been ignored on the world stage: the extent of its suffering discounted or downplayed as being no more than natural or inevitable in a country so poor and yet so populous. At other times the reverse has been the case, and India's misery has been blazoned across the planet. As Covid mortality soared in India in April 2021, images circulated around the world of blazing funeral pyres, of bodies abandoned or only half buried along the banks of the Ganges. Here, at least in Western eyes, was the horrific spectacle of uncontrolled mortality, of deaths too numerous to be counted, and of corpses too plentiful to be buried or burned. Here was not just the visible specter of mass mortality, but also, many commentators suggested, a lurch backwards into a resurgent medievalism, the Black Death revisited. India is central to the discussion that follows because it is pivotal to understanding the pandemic past and how we carry the ponderous burden of that past forward into the present and future.

Pandemic India offers both a regional perspective and a 'long history' of the 2020–1 coronavirus pandemic. It examines a sequence of epidemic diseases that affected India from the early nineteenth century onwards, diseases that, as they moved into or passed out of the subcontinent, became pandemics as we now understand that heavily freighted term. Although in the lee of Covid-19 it may seem that pandemics have always been with us, the idea of a pandemic, as an epidemic of exceptional magnitude, near-global reach, and explosive destructiveness, is historically relatively recent. It was a term rarely used before the 1860s, and for decades thereafter it struggled to find professional recognition among epidemiologists and sanitarians, still more acceptance among the general public. As this book argues, India, through its seminal experiences of cholera and plague, and the threat these diseases were taken to pose to the security and well-being of the entire world, was foundational to the emergence of the pandemic idea. As a seat of empire, India provided a platform from which pandemic disease might be observed and investigated, its origins methodically examined, its dissemination closely tracked and meticulously documented. Perceptually as much as epidemiologically, India came to be seen as one of the principal distribution points for the spread of 'world diseases,' a site of international risk and global insecurity. But India was also a potential site of redress—a laboratory where new measures could be devised, whether in practice successfully or not, for the containment of pandemics and their future prevention. While histories of the great pandemics of the nineteenth and early twentieth centuries—cholera, plague, influenza—commonly elaborate on the experience of Western countries, making these eruptions episodes in the travails and achievements of the modern West, it was in India, not in Europe or America, that by far the greatest mortality from these world-traveling diseases occurred. It has been calculated that of 72 million deaths worldwide from pandemics of cholera, plague, and influenza between 1817 and 1920, 40 million fatalities occurred in India. One country bore half the disease burden of the entire planet.[3] And there, too, as across the Global South, such diseases tended to remain as resident infections, long after the rest of the world had forgotten about them or had liberated itself from their enslavement. India has a unique historical relationship with pandemics: of this, Covid-19 was but the most recent reminder.

Unsettling the Past

In moments of crisis we tend to turn to the past, in search of lessons perhaps or in quest of origins, meanings, and consequences. In history we hear echoes of our own despair, discern glimmerings of hope for our future. The past, we know, is not simply recycled and mechanically repeated. However, by returning to history we also empower the present to educate our understanding of the past, to pose questions and invite answers that, but for present-day issues and circumstances, might never have been raised or addressed. *Pandemic India* is in this sense a presentist history. By this I do not mean an anachronistic imposition of the language and values of the present onto a compliant past, a narrative of predetermination in which past events simply serve to point the way purposefully and inevitably forward to the present. Rather, I intend a critical revisiting of the past, an unsettling of the sediments of previous pandemics. In India the highly infectious coronavirus Covid-19 that emerged in China in late 2019 generated intense interest in, and speculation about, the pandemic past. History took on a new urgency, agency, and relevance. The press and social media, as well as historians, sought parallels between Covid and earlier pandemics, especially those embedded in the nation's colonial past. For some commentators it was a case of 'pandemic déjà vu,' with the retrieved and reimagined experiences of plague and influenza looming large over the present. Others strove to extract more precise lessons from that history, refining them for contemporary consumption. Fascinated by past horrors or seeking a route through the current catastrophe, critics quarried history for instructive parallels and worrying analogies. History was mobilized to shed light on a helter-skelter present.

Pandemics have normally staid and sober historians reaching for superlatives, straining for apocalyptic effect. This book offers a more measured interpretative overview of Covid's antecedents in the history of pandemics in South Asia from the early nineteenth century onward. It does not claim the insights of a trained epidemiologist but seeks to present a historian's critical view of what pandemics have meant to India before and since independence in 1947. It aims to raise questions, particularly in the light of Covid-19, about the political and social significance of what happens when global disease is enacted on a regional stage. Pandemics do not exist conceptually or experientially in isolation from a wider historical context, but neither do they function only at an elevated and abstracted global level. They derive their meaning, too, from local histories and regional narratives, from the intensity of human experience, from statements of difference as much as from professions of universality.

There are perhaps four or five ways in which one can structure an epidemic or pandemic narrative. One is to write the biography of a contagious disease, to trace its life history from birth, through maturity, to death, situating its epidemiological career within the specificities of time, place, and environment, of cultural world and social milieu. Another is to adopt a more mathematical model, one which traces the rise and fall of a disease, its social impact, its demographic and political consequences, essentially in terms of what statistics tell us. A third approach is to look to policy, the assessment of disease in terms of risk and the adjustments and countermeasures taken by states or by those, domestically and internationally, who advise them on matters of medical science and public health. A fourth possibility is to locate the pandemic narrative within a history of concepts and ideas—how certain ideas about disease have come into being, gained social traction and scientific authority, become hegemonic or reshaped the theoretical underpinnings of society and governance. And, finally, pandemic narratives can be located in relation to the human experience of disease itself, the subjective fears and expectations such episodes arouse, their articulation through visual culture and artistic creativity, and their preservation in memory and memorialization. There are elements of all these narrative strategies in the book that follows but also, I believe, a critical appreciation of their relative strengths and weaknesses, for part of the argument of this work is to demonstrate that pandemics are far too complex—in their nature, impact, and consequences—to be answerable to one narrative form to the exclusion of others.

There are many possible pandemic histories, even for South Asia; this book can only address some of them. But alongside pandemics themselves, this is also a book about time, about history understood through divergent, overlapping, or stalled temporalities, what Dipesh Chakrabarty characterized as hetero-temporalities or 'time-knots.'[4] One of the complicating characteristics of pandemics is the way in which they play upon our notions of time. They exist, as Covid-19 has done, in the 'now' time we inhabit, and often occur everywhere, across countries and continents, at the same, or almost the same, moment in time. That is part of their terror. In fact, that simultaneity, now so worryingly apparent to us as we watch our television screens, read our emails, or trawl social media, was less apparent in earlier pandemics; those of the nineteenth century—cholera, for instance—took far longer to unfold. They required months, even years, in the case of the first cholera pandemics, to travel from one part of the world to another, or for news of their fatal advance to be broadcast around the globe. There is a history as to how those pandemic episodes then speeded up, moving faster, being seen sooner, being reacted to more quickly. With modern means of transport and communication, with the global rise of mass media, it has been possible, as with Covid in the twenty-first century, to track pandemic waves and surges on a daily, almost hourly basis, with the same disease (even allowing for mutations and variants) erupting and returning worldwide at more or less the same time and eliciting similar responses in countries geographically, culturally, and politically distant from one another. This simultaneity might be an illusion, but we could know, if we needed or cared to, day by day, with varying degrees of reliability, how many people have died in Delhi, London, or New York, how many cases there have been in Italy, Brazil, or Bangladesh. Social media and online journalism could keep us informed of epidemiological trends, social reactions, and official pronouncements almost as they happened. This sense of global immediacy, of universal nowness, is one of the ways in which contemporary pandemics exert their hypnotic hold over us.

But, from a historian's perspective, pandemics do not simply exist in now time. Even as they unfold, they are caught up with the debris of past times, layered over with former events and resurgent traumas, laced with future fears and dystopian prognoses. They have a dynamic that is asynchronic. The past—real or imagined—moves in parallel with our present, arguing with us, shapeshifting itself to accommodate or reformulate the present, feeding back to us an evolving understanding of what happened in earlier pandemics or might happen in future pandemic times. Pandemics unsettle the cozy sediments of time. The temporal geology of our world is not composed of neatly layered, uniform strata but is a jumble of tangled and contorted strata, fractured planes, and abrupt unconformities. Given the plenitude of our historical awareness and the twenty-first-century abundance of memories, archives, and online resources, we inevitably think of the Covid pandemic in relation to the influenza of 1918–19, or, from an Indian perspective, we find ourselves revisiting the bubonic plague of the 1890s and 1900s. The past doesn't leave us alone.

To take one example of this temporal confusion: the historical and even the epidemiological understanding of the Black Death of fourteenth-century Europe has owed much to the scientific observation of bubonic plague undertaken in late nineteenth- and early twentieth-century India. This recent knowledge has then been redeployed to make assumptions about earlier plague pandemics. Diseases, however, are no more fixed and changeless entities than the societies they inhabit. They change with time and circumstance; they mutate, sometimes they disappear or are reborn in a different form, and so retrospective diagnosis, extended over centuries of intervening change, can be grossly misleading. And yet the observed plague of 1890s India became the yardstick for assessing what may (or may not) have been the same disease in 1340s Europe, just as, in a further entangling of this pandemic time-knot, contemporary opinion in 1890s India feared the return of the Black Death or the London plague of the 1660s. The very idea of the Black Death as an 'Oriental' disease, issuing from Asia, devastating Europe, owed much to the comparison made from the 1830s onward with the eruptions of a latter-day plague—namely, 'Asiatic' cholera. The pandemic present becomes heavily laden with real or imagined pasts and sometimes several pasts simultaneously.

Cholera, plague, and influenza pandemics might surface almost simultaneously in several different, widely dispersed places—London, Hamburg, Buenos Aires, Bombay—and so prove integral to a highly interconnected modern world of trade, transport, communications, and medical science. Yet these pandemics also served, in Western minds, to delineate the temporality of the modern, 'civilized' world from the imagined medievalism of Indian minds and bodies, from the supposedly ancient superstitions and timeless routines of village India. Itself a representative product of nineteenth- and twentieth-century globalization, the modern pandemic created or accentuated a visceral sense of other times and of other places yet to heed the call of modernity. In pandemics multiple temporalities converged and collided: they did so once again in Covid-19.

Decolonizing Contagion

There is one specific temporality this book seeks to engage with. Pandemics, as far as India is concerned, exist not only now but also in the time of empire. Until the arrival of Covid-19 most of the pandemics India experienced—cholera, plague, influenza—occurred during the long years of British rule from the mid-eighteenth century until 1947. The manner in which those disease events impacted on India, how they were responded to by people, state, and medical science, and became entwined with the country's social, political, and demographic history, all bore the deep impress of foreign domination. Like the famines with which they were so frequently enmeshed, India's pandemics, their human cost and governmental mismanagement, constitute part of the indictment of colonialism itself, part of its ethical accountability, and an ingredient in what many scholars now see as the bitter legacy and recurrent trauma of colonial rule. This is a history grounded in the past, yet still alive and without apparent closure. Given that India's pandemic past and its historical sensibilities were (and are) so intricately bound up with the time of empire, it was unsurprising that Covid-19, despite falling more than seventy years after the end of the British occupation, revivified colonialism as a vital reference point for the pandemic present and as an ongoing reminder of the injustices (but also, in some quarters, the achievements) of the colonial era.

This unfinished history of empire gives rise to a contradictory impulse—one from which neither this book nor its author can claim to be immune. On the one hand, it remains essential to recognize the constituent role of empire and the West in the way in which India was centrally implanted within the evolving pandemic idea and how epidemics—and pandemics, their monstrous kin—arose, were represented, responded to, neglected, contained, historicized, and (all too often) marginalized in historical memory. Not only did empire appear as lead actor in this pandemic drama; it was also the self-authorized chronicler of its own actions. So central was its material, ideological, and archival presence, such have been its impact and its legacies, that it is hard (and surely futile) to try to conceive how such a history of pandemics might have unfolded in the absence of empire. There is a second tier to the empire question. If the time of empire is, in some respects, still not over, where does that leave post-independence India and its nation-state? Did the history of India's pandemics undergo a sea change with independence, or do we still see the same pandemic patterns persist, the same vulnerabilities reenacted, the same reactions of society and state played out once again, only now in the time of the nation?

At the same time there is, in the academic community and beyond, an intense desire to escape the suffocating fumes of the past, to topple empire from its pedagogic pedestal, to decolonize history and the writing of history. That weighty phrase—decolonizing history—can encompass a wealth of different agendas, from radical curriculum reform in schools and universities to demands for apologies and reparations from the ex-colonial power. But in the midst of this there is a wholly legitimate determination to recuperate and restore non-Western testimony, agency, and experience, and to construct a history in which, in our case, Indians and Indian civil society count at least as much as the nagging voice of empire or in which an insurgent narrative of postimperial India serves to counter and recontextualize a pandemic history that doesn't abruptly and conveniently end in 1947. In an article published early on in India's Covid emergency, Arundhati Roy remarked that historically 'pandemics have forced humans to break with the past and imagine their world anew. This one is no different. It is a portal, a gateway between one world and the next.'[5] It was a bold statement of possibilities, an expression of hope that adversity could be turned prospectively to advantage. Roy's idea of pandemic as portal was widely criticized, as sounding too optimistic at a time of overwhelming chaos and suffering. But it can be understood as a legitimate attempt to break with the past, to look to the future rather than dwelling yet again on a jaded past.

There are several ways in which, while acknowledging the indelibility of empire, India's pandemic history may be decolonized. This requires us, first of all, as an exercise in the history of epidemiological ideas and social concepts, to interrogate the very notion of a pandemic, to understand when and where that term originated, how it was deployed to differentiate and divide as much as to construct connectivity and posit universality, and to examine how that conceptual lineage has been carried forward into the present. Moving on to statistical and policy analysis, a decolonizing history involves recognizing, critiquing, and seeking to explain the extraordinary extent of pandemic mortality and morbidity on the subcontinent. This lethality is particularly apparent when compared with the Western experience of precisely the same diseases, diseases which have until recently been written up as if they were primarily the historical property of the West. Decolonizing past pandemics entails viewing critically how local experience in Asia, Africa, and across the Global South departed from, or became subordinated to, a disease chronology created by and for the West.

Why did India suffer so disproportionately—because it was so populous or poor, because it was ecologically vulnerable or singularly exposed to outside influences, because it was colonized and so denied autonomy, even with respect to managing or imagining its own diseases? Decolonizing India's pandemic history requires us to try to write a history of disease that questions empire's truth claims, a history that empire itself did not (or could not) write, a history written not in denial of colonialism's material strength and hegemonic power but which gives due weight to other subjectivities, agencies, and narratives. So far as it is possible, such a history needs to broaden its categories of evidence, to seek sources that retrieve an Indian voice, a vernacular authority that hosts other kinds of conversations, that speaks apart from, yet repeatedly interrupts, colonialism's domineering discourse.

That revisionist agenda might be framed in two other ways, too. One is by asking who sought or exercised ownership over India's pandemic portfolio. It is, of course, not possible to own a pandemic in the same legal or consumerist sense in which one might buy a house or acquire an automobile. But it can be owned in a wider cultural, political, and epistemological sense. Ownership—or claims to ownership—can be established over disease as over any other calamitous resource. Who owns—who takes or denies responsibility for—a famine, an epidemic, a drought, a cyclone, a flood? Who manages disaster or is blamed for failing to act and resolve the crisis? Who provides the science, the technical solutions, the human infrastructure? Who invests political time and administrative effort in identifying causes or seeking solutions? A regime, an organization, an identifiable set of social actors, can be seen to take responsibility for a pandemic, for its origin, containment, and suppression, or, shirking responsibility, point the finger of blame at others. Someone can claim a superior knowledge of a contagion that renders other possible ways of knowing defunct and dangerous; someone can appropriate disease in such a way as to annex it to their political agenda, their scientific mission or civilizational creed, while denying that legitimacy to others. And, over time, ownership might be transferred from one set of individuals to another, from one hegemonic regime to another.

Ownership might, in a literal sense, be instrumental, through the commercialization of contagion, the capitalism of curing, the profit-making business of manufacturing, selling, and patenting the drugs and vaccines that treat or prevent disease. Or, again, it might be manifested through the diplomatic advantage and 'soft power' gains to be gleaned from seeming to be in command of a pandemic or able to control and reallocate the means of its prevention and containment. Diseases, especially those we call pandemic, can be owned in the sense that someone makes them their own, appropriates them to their own power, authority, and profit, or denies someone else the right or ability to own them. How, at what point, and in what ways did empire assume or repudiate that ownership or India assert its own claims to ownership?

An additional, and in part complementary, way of addressing the relationship between pandemics, empire, and its postcolonial legacy is through a discussion of violence. Epidemics—still more, pandemics—are inherently violent. There is violence in what contagious disease inflicts on the human body, how cells are attacked, the respiratory tract infected, the gut sent into violent spasms. It is not surprising that such diseases are often described in the language of invasion and conquest. But the violence of pandemics is evident in the way in which they tear at the social fabric, unleash the coercive and punitive power of the state or the violence of internecine social conflict. Who speaks for or against the violence of the pandemic? Who seeks to profit from its vicious anger or assuage its violent rage?

Violence has also become a central issue for those who write about empire. Indeed, for many who write or speak about empire, violence is its epitome, the essential means and manner of its authority and control. Do pandemics, therefore, present colonial violence in yet another form? Do they assist, allow, or legitimate the violence of colonialism and its use of coercive power? Or do they, on the other hand, show up the duality of a colonial regime in which hegemony sits alongside coercion, or in which other forms of non-colonial hegemony also find a platform and a home? How far do we travel in pandemics through physical and epistemic violence to an alternative world in which care and compassion have a place? And if violence is the hallmark of the colonial pandemic, where does that leave its postcolonial successor? There are no easy answers, but it is the task of this book to seek clues and explore possibilities.

1

WHAT IS A PANDEMIC?

Pandemic is a word we all now use—freely, perhaps unquestioningly. It has entered our daily lives and the vocabulary of everyday speech. But what exactly *is* a pandemic? One recent writer notes that a pandemic 'is best thought of as a very large epidemic.'[1] Another writes, more informatively: 'An epidemic is the rapid spread of infectious disease to a large number of people in a given population within a short period of time,' while a pandemic 'is an epidemic that has spread across a large region, for instance, multiple countries and continents.'[2] The term may signify a new or rapidly emerging infection—like Severe Acute Respiratory Syndrome (SARS) in 2002, Middle East Respiratory Syndrome (MERS) in 2012, Ebola in 2014, Zika virus in 2016, and Covid, the novel coronavirus, in 2019–20— but one that has either spread worldwide or shown the potential to do so. But, even in terms of mortality, the range of possibilities is remarkably wide. SARS, first reported in China in November 2002, remained confined to a handful of countries and, by the time the World Health Organization (WHO) declared the threat from the virus over in July 2003, had caused fewer than 800 deaths, roughly the same as with MERS in 2012. SARS's successor, Covid-19, by contrast, rapidly exceeded that death-toll and within months caused tens of thousands of deaths. It left no country untouched.

By another definition, as well as crossing national and regional boundaries, a pandemic has four distinguishing marks: it is a novel pathogen; there is a general lack of public immunity to it; the disease has an efficient mode of transmission and so is able to spread rapidly; and it results in a high level of morbidity.[3] Epidemiologically, all of these factors (and possibly others) play a part in defining a pandemic, though historically many of the disease episodes identified in the past as pandemics were not the eruption of new pathogens but (like cholera, plague, or influenza) recurring eruptions or mutated versions of an already known and established contagion. Another way of presenting pandemics epidemiologically is to argue that many pathogens have a natural reservoir within animal, bird, or insect populations: what transforms them from animal diseases into human pandemics is anthropogenic environmental change and increased contact between animals and humans.[4] But these technical definitions only address the epidemiology of contagious diseases, not the manner in which they are socially received and culturally constructed.

In an article first published during the 1980s AIDS crisis—a crisis we might now, given its global dimensions and the estimated 32 million deaths that followed, better describe as a pandemic—Charles Rosenberg asked: 'What is an epidemic?' He posed the question because the term was used 'so casually and metaphorically' that it called for the formulation of 'an ideal-type picture of an epidemic based on repetitive patterns of past events.'[5] His response was to argue that an epidemic was not simply a biological event but also a social and cultural performance. An epidemic was a drama: it assumed a dramaturgic form. 'Epidemics start at a moment in time,' Rosenberg wrote, 'proceed on a stage limited in space and duration, following a plot line of increasing and revelatory tension, move to a crisis of individual and collective character, then drift toward closure.' An epidemic further took on the properties of a pageant, 'mobilizing communities to act out propitiatory rituals that incorporate and reaffirm fundamental social values and modes of understanding.' It was this 'public character and dramatic intensity,' coupled with the unities of place and time, that made epidemics 'as well suited to the concerns of moralists as to the research of scholars seeking an understanding of the relationship among ideology, social structure, and the construction of particular selves.'[6]

There is much of undoubted utility in Rosenberg's approach in thinking about pandemics rather than the epidemics his essay addresses. But there are also limits to his 'dramaturgic' model. What happens, for instance, when there is no obvious unity of time or place, when time (or the perception of time) is knotted up, and when the 'place' on which the drama is played out is empire-wide or global in its dimensions? (Rosenberg does add, in a footnote, that 'even worldwide epidemics are experienced and responded to at the local level as a series of discrete incidents,' but this seems to me to be only partly true.)[7] And what happens when—as in many a colonial situation—society is itself deeply divided and can reach no lasting consensus as to why epidemic (or pandemic) diseases are caused and how they spread? And what follows when diseases don't obligingly die away, when the problems they create or expose remain intractable? Who is to decide, and by what criteria, when the final curtain is to fall on the pathogens' play?[8] Rosenberg's model seems too neat and orderly to meet the sprawling, messy reality and ideological overlays of the modern pandemic. As Covid-19 demonstrated, the conceptual difficulty of defining a pandemic is accentuated by the fact that precisely the same disease attaches itself in singularly different ways to different social systems and political structures and to different pasts—real or reconstructed. Even within a single imperial and postimperial system, like that of the British Empire and its successor states, the baroque architecture of a single pandemic might be very differently memorialized and reimagined.[9]

The apparent universality of a pandemic may be objectively grounded in its biology (the same, or nearly the same, pathogen occurring in places distant from one another), but its bewildering diversity of impact and meaning issues from a host of different local circumstances. The idea of a global pandemic almost defies the imagination. How can we imagine, let alone adequately comprehend, things happening in such diverse ways and in so many different places and time zones all at once? Far from possessing a simple unity of place, time, and emplotment, a pandemic has to be understood as being both expansively global (or nearly so) and, simultaneously, profoundly local.

Like epidemics, pandemics are historical constructions as much as epidemiological events or social performances, but pandemics are more than epidemics writ large. As Mark Harrison observed 'Labelling a disease "pandemic" endows it with a potency lacked by other [diseases], even when those are considered to be epidemic.'[10] By using the term 'pandemicity' in this work, I seek to encompass both the objective nature of a given disease and the pathogens that cause it *and* the social activities, the cultural meanings, and the political associations with which that disease entity is historically imbued. Erica Charters and Richard McKay put it thus: 'Epidemics are not solely a function of pathogens; they are also a function of how society is structured, how political power is wielded in the name of public health, how quantitative data is collected, how diseases are categorized and modelled, and how histories of disease are narrated.' And, they add, 'Each of these activities has its own history.'[11] As I once proposed in discussing one of the most emblematic of pandemic diseases, 'cholera in itself has no meaning: it is only a microorganism. It acquires meaning and significance from its human context, from the ways in which it infiltrates the lives of the people, from the reactions it provokes, and from the manner in which it gives expression to cultural and political values.'[12] That assertion, it seems to me, remains as valid for Covid-19 in the twenty-first century as it was for cholera, plague, and influenza in earlier times.

Pandemic Propositions

By discussing each of the four major pandemics that affected India over the past two hundred years, this book aims to trace the lineage of the modern pandemic phenomenon and its changing meaning and significance. For the moment, though, it may be helpful to consider some core propositions of that now normalized knowledge since, in one form or another, they underpin the discussion that follows.

1. *Pandemics are recurring historical phenomena.* We know from the historical record (and increasingly from archeological evidence

and genome sequencing) that pandemics occurred in the past, even though questions remain about the precise nature and origin of the pathogens involved, and the duration and lethality of the pandemic episodes they unleashed. Pandemics even of the same disease do not repeat themselves in exactly the same form, but they are understood to be a recurring feature of human history. It is, however, widely argued that pandemics have become more prevalent over the last two hundred years, and even in recent decades, as human populations have expanded, as anthropogenic environmental change has accelerated, and as the world has become more socially and economically integrated. By their geographical extent and the scale of their mortality, we can distinguish pandemics from ordinary epidemics. We can place them in chronological sequence, make comparisons and contrasts between different pandemic episodes, use them as a source of reference for contemporary outbreaks, and deploy them to predict the likely nature and impact of future pandemic events.

2. *Pandemics have a distinctive spatial as well as temporal presence.* They are thought of as extending far beyond epidemics in their geographical range: they are, or have the perceived capacity to be, global in their reach and so depend upon a concept of the globe as a shared site of human habitation and of social, economic, and political interconnectedness. As spatial phenomena, they have historically been tracked, mapped, and measured in ways that demonstrate their geographical exceptionality and mark them off from ordinary epidemics. Pandemics are assigned a specific place of origin. This has almost invariably been understood as lying outside the Western world—in Asia, Africa, Latin America, and the Caribbean. In this respect, pandemics and epidemics invoke an imaginative geography in which alien places are assigned characteristics that distinguish and differentiate them from the 'home' norm. Pandemics are construed as a threat to global security and Western hegemony, even though their actual demographic impact may be (and generally has been) far greater in the colonial or developing world than in the West, and the

diseases that cause them have tended to remain there in endemic or epidemic form long after their pandemic phase has passed.

3. *Pandemics are exceptional events.* They result in (or threaten to cause) mortality on a massive and wholly abnormal scale, often with exceptional virulence or violence in a remarkably short space of time. Crudely put, pandemics are a game we play with numbers. Counting the dead (still more than numbering the sick, a far more problematic proposition) serves as a primary means by which to judge the lethality of the disease, and to assess the susceptibility or resilience of the recipient society or of specific social groups within it, and as an instrument for measuring their otherwise incalculable horror. As exceptional events, pandemics have the capacity to disturb or displace existing social norms and challenge current state practices. They provoke (if only in anticipation or in their initial phase) extreme reactions from societies and governments; they pose new, possibly quite unforeseen, risks. They can threaten, and sometimes transform, established political structures, economic processes, and dominant beliefs. They can impel or accelerate significant changes in science and medicine and create new sites of international cooperation and global governance. But, on the other hand, they can also reaffirm and entrench existing social values and prevalent worldviews. Pandemics can be cataclysmic but not necessarily transformative. They might not be so momentous after all.

4. *Pandemics are subjective events as well as epidemiological phenomena.* Pandemics transmit more than pathogens. They provoke fear and incite panic; they generate a powerful sense of victimhood and vulnerability that may precede the arrival of a pandemic but also extend well beyond its actual occurrence. They become profound cultural episodes, as reflected in literature and visual imagery, and also as sites of memory and affect, triggers for reimagining or revisiting past traumas. In occasioning a quest for meaning, purpose, and accountability, pandemics can produce a proliferation of rumors and conspiracy theories, and result in scapegoating,

blaming, and a deepened sense of social and political injustice. Pandemics serve as a means by which to typify or castigate entire societies or specific social entities. They accentuate or reinforce prejudicial understandings of how others live and die, and they create or intensify the individual or collective sense of danger, risk, and insecurity.

Metaphor and Myth

There is another way to establish what makes a pandemic such a potent social phenomenon and such a powerful historical and cultural marker. In an essay first published in 1988, Susan Sontag explored what she saw as the 'metaphors' arising from the then emerging epidemic of HIV/AIDS in the United States. She argued that certain illness (like leprosy and syphilis) had long been subject to moralistic explanations, with epidemics interpreted as metaphors for evil, as 'plagues' and curses, inflicted as punishment for some imagined transgression or supposed wrongdoing. Commonly, she noted, disease was seen to come from somewhere else, from some 'primitive' or exotic location, some distant but dangerous place. In particular, the denizens of the Western world, that 'privileged cultural entity,' regarded themselves as under threat from outsiders, 'colonized by lethal diseases coming from elsewhere.'[13]

Sontag wrote of epidemics, but much of what she described could be applied, even more emphatically, to pandemics. She wrote of metaphors; one might equally speak of myths. For the historian, the story of pandemics is a not a neutral narrative, built solely upon objective fact, but a complex, multi-layered discourse laced with subjectivities. And, apart from invoking metaphor, another way of saying this is to observe that pandemics are a fecund source of myth and mythologizing. However, the use here of 'myth' calls for some explication. The idea of a sharp distinction between historical time and mythic time can easily be exaggerated,[14] but, as momentous events in the lives of those who suffer them or seek their meaning, pandemics become, like barnacle-covered sea wrecks, encrusted with myths, fables, parables, and prophecies—myths of imagined causation and putative origin, fables of heroic intervention and magical cures, parables and prophecies as to how the world might end or yet be saved.

No two pandemics are identical, and yet they exude a mythic essence, evoking the possibility of underlying and eternal truths or resuscitating atavistic fears and atemporal anxieties. By their vastness and the violent destruction they wreak, by the epic struggles against evil they entail and the magnitude of the suffering, grief, and death they occasion, pandemics speak beyond the immediacy of individual events and experience to deeper meanings, to a profounder psychological and social significance. Pandemics are not just linear events—moving sedately through time, linking one place or time to another—they are abrupt, revelatory moments that expose or reiterate fundamental beliefs about how societies act and function. Myths do not stand outside history; they frequently help to make it, or to make it even halfway intelligible. Myths are part of a pandemic's structure, integral to its architecture. Myth was a word much used during the Covid pandemic, mostly critically to identify and refute what were seen to be irrational claims, 'misinformation,' 'fake news,' and bogus science. We might see this irrational attachment to untruth as an inherent, if paradoxical, feature of our modern age, but many of these modern myths closely resembled the dark and disturbing rumors that swirled around pandemics in the past and were no more securely founded in any established truth.

Historians are taught to be wary of myth. As Richard Evans argued: 'History has always been seen by historians as a destroyer of myths more than a creator of them … In destroying myths, historians have often sought to substitute for them narratives which are more closely grounded in the sources.'[15] But while myths deserve to be interrogated and, where necessary, rebutted, they are also an ineluctable part of history-making and history-writing. Drawing on her extensive study of Hindu mythology, Wendy Doniger defined a myth as 'a story that a group of people believe for a long time despite massive evidence that it is not actually true'—that word 'actually' consciously or unconsciously echoing the nineteenth-century German historian Leopold von Ranke's belief that historians should study history as it 'actually happened' (or how it 'essentially was').[16] But, Doniger continued, we need to use history to understand myth;

myth does not in itself constitute history or yield evidence that things actually (Ranke again) happened in the way that myths imply. Myths summon up an imaginary world, the better to enable us to understand good or evil. They provide metaphors and meaning; they don't represent actual events. 'Such myths reveal to us the history of sentiments rather than events, motivations rather than movements.' But myths are still able to influence history and affect its outcomes. Referring to one of the causes of the Indian Mutiny and Rebellion of 1857–8, Doniger remarked: 'Ideas are facts too; the belief, whether true or false, that the British were greasing cartridges with animal fat started a revolution in India. For we are what we imagine, as much as what we do.'[17]

By invoking myth, I am not trying to suggest that such pandemic explanations and narratives were necessarily false: some were grounded in indisputable fact; others were not. But they provide one means of challenging dominant knowledges and exploring established truth claims, including those presented by or on behalf of the colonial order, a way of recognizing alternative mindsets and other worldviews. Myths represent ways in which, in formal historical writing as much as in popular journalism and the mass media, in public remembrance and retelling, certain fundamental ideas and resonant themes constantly resurface. Myths may contain a kernel of evidence-based truth: that may be part of their ancestry and authority. But they also serve as super-truths. They rely on much more than a narrowly academic notion of factuality, touch on deeper meanings and a socially and culturally constructed network of aspirations and fears. Myths become part of the academic agenda as well—the hypotheses and assumptions scholars toil over, the theories and refutations they weave into their own narratives. Pandemics are mythic because they are larger than life, larger than individual lives, and because they are often inexplicable or unacceptable at the level of normal human experience. They are *modern* myths because, while they speak to ancient fears and beliefs, they also express anxieties uniquely born of the modern age. And while, like pandemics themselves, myths contain elements of the universal, they also gain traction from the particular culture in which they reside.

Pandemics as History

On 11 March 2020, the director-general of the World Health Organization, Dr. Tedros Adhanom Ghebreyesus, made a long-anticipated announcement: the outbreak of the coronavirus known as Covid-19 had become a pandemic. He explained that since initial reporting of the disease at Wuhan in central China in December 2019, the WHO had been monitoring the situation closely and was 'deeply concerned' by the spread and severity of the disease and by the inactivity of many governments. Earlier, on 30 January 2020, the WHO had recognized the coronavirus outbreak as a 'public-health emergency of international concern,' and on 11 February it named the disease SARS-CoV-2 or, more simply, Covid-19, but still avoided calling it a pandemic.[18] Not until 11 March did the WHO openly declare that Covid could now be 'characterized as a pandemic.' Against a background of criticism of the WHO's ill-judged or hasty responses to the previous crises caused by SARS in 2002–3, Swine Flu in 2009–10, MERS in 2012, Ebola in 2014–16, and Zika virus in 2016, Dr. Tedros went on to say that 'pandemic' was not a word to be used 'lightly or carelessly.' If 'misused,' the term could cause 'unreasonable fear, or unjustified acceptance that the fight is over, leading to unnecessary suffering and death.'[19] But by early March 2020 it was clear that the coronavirus had a foothold in several countries: the likelihood of a global pandemic had become real. News agencies around the world confirmed that the coronavirus was spreading quickly and the death-toll rapidly mounting.

Grim confirmation of its spread was given by the Coronavirus Resource Center website at Johns Hopkins University, which, through constant updates, tracked the growth in Covid-19 cases and deaths—from East Asia and Southeast Asia, to Iran, India, and Pakistan, to western Europe and the United States, to Latin America, and sub-Saharan Africa. The red dots on the map representing deaths, daily increasing in size and numbers, began to proliferate and converge, resembling a rash—measles, perhaps, or the eruptions of smallpox—spreading out across the stricken body of the globe. Even before this, and without waiting for WHO endorsement, 'pandemic' was a word already in hectic circulation, sped, faster even than the virus, by newspapers, television, and radio, by word of mouth and social media. Precedents were hastily drawn from other pandemics, both recent and more distant in time—was this new coronavirus like SARS or Ebola or, more scarily still, the Spanish Flu of 1918–19, with its 40 million deaths worldwide? If Covid could escalate so rapidly even in affluent countries with well-resourced healthcare systems, what might be the cost in human lives and economic dislocation to the poorer, developing countries of the Global South where, even in ordinary times, hospitals and medical personnel struggled to cope? 'Pandemic,' the word Dr. Tedros had been loath to utter, summoned up a nightmare of dystopian possibilities, a landscape of escalating fear and looming catastrophe.

For a term now in such common use, 'pandemic' has had a remarkably short and slippery existence. It was rarely used before the 1860s, even by the emerging community of epidemiologists (there never have been pandemiologists), and then often only to mean a disease that traveled more widely than any normal epidemic. The *pan* (the Greek prefix meaning 'all') in pandemic has always been open to confusion. Is a pandemic a disease that is widespread across a single *demos* (people), or is it only pandemic when multiple countries, and perhaps several continents, are affected? Is pandemic a statement of risk, of potential danger, or a measure of the known distribution and quantifiable fatality of a disease? Not until the so-called Russian Flu of 1889–92 did the term gain wide circulation and begin to signify to the public a disease that literally spread worldwide and did so with disconcerting rapidity. Even in 1918–19, when the Spanish Flu devastated societies around the globe, epidemic was the preferred description and the term that was at least as commonly used even among epidemiologists to describe what we would now unhesitatingly label a pandemic or even with hindsight regard as the 'classic' pandemic of modern times. In India, which lost between 12 and 20 million people to the 1918–19 influenza, greatly in excess of any other country, the disease was almost invariably described as an epidemic, rarely as a pandemic.[20] Indeed, when the p-word was used it was often quarantined within inverted commas and treated as a suspect or unfamiliar expression. Why were even medical professionals reluctant to use a term that has now become so commonplace? The growing convention has been to refer to epidemics when speaking of only one country or region and pandemics when many countries and regions are involved (a practice broadly followed in this book). But sometimes, by way of extra emphasis, we speak of 'global pandemics,' though there has been no consistency even in this. What imaginaries, what epidemiological arithmetic, does that half-redundant 'global' bring into play? How global is 'global' and by what criteria do we measure it?

Many historians have been wary of the pandemic idea. In 1976, when William H. McNeill published *Plagues and Peoples*, a seminal work in the historical study of disease as a global phenomenon, he presented a wide-ranging overview of human contagions, from the 'plagues' of ancient China and Rome, via the 'transoceanic exchanges' of the European age of exploration and discovery, to the global 'peregrinations' of cholera in the nineteenth century. 'Plague' and 'pestilence' occurred repeatedly in his book; 'pandemic' appeared only once. This was when McNeill disputed the 'grand theory' of three 'great pandemics' of bubonic plague, as cataclysmic but isolated and short-lived events, an interpretation which he saw as purely a European invention or based solely on Eurocentric perceptions. In his view—and it is one that accords with much recent historical scholarship—plague never disappeared after the Black Death of the 1340s but continued for centuries thereafter in the Middle East and large parts of Eurasia.[21] Only Europe understood it as occurring in three separate and clearly defined pandemic episodes. In McNeill's vast prospectus epidemic diseases issued from those parts of Eurasia where they had long been resident, and came, especially after the European voyages and conquests of the fifteenth and sixteenth centuries, to target hitherto untouched and highly susceptible populations, like those of Mexico and Peru at the time of the Spanish invasions. Smallpox and other contagions exploited the immunological difference between peoples who belonged to 'the civilized disease pools of Eurasia' and those that did not. These, then, were not pandemics in the sense that people everywhere were equally susceptible and simultaneously affected. They were the diseases that immunologically secure conquerors visited upon the vulnerable and the vanquished.[22]

Contrast that skepticism about the meaningful existence of pandemics with the work of another American historian, Alfred W. Crosby. In 1976, the same year as McNeill's *Plagues and Peoples*, Crosby published a book on the influenza of 1918–19 (a catastrophe McNeill barely even mentions).[23] First entitled *Epidemic and Peace: 1918*, Crosby's study was republished in 1989 with the more provocative title *America's Forgotten Pandemic: The Influenza of 1918*. In this book, a historiographical landmark in its description of influenza as a 'forgotten' historical episode, Crosby used the word 'pandemic' repeatedly, often arbitrarily interchangeable with 'epidemic,' and with the adjective 'pandemic' applied alike to the disease and its victims. It was thus both America's pandemic and the world's, spiraling out from the United States to war-torn Europe, and beyond to ravage Africa, Asia, and the Pacific. Although Crosby's book stimulated other historians of disease and medicine to adopt the term for themselves and contributed to the fashion for its scholarly use, pandemic here bore no special meaning except to communicate the enormity of the event and its unprecedentedly wide extent and lethal tally.[24]

World Disease and Global Pestilence

If we spool back from the Spanish Flu of 1918–19 to the year 1911, we can begin to see why the idea of pandemics had such an equivocal history. On 8 March that year Dr. James Cantlie addressed the Royal Society of Arts in London on the subject of 'Plague and Its Spread.' Despite its name, the Royal Society of Arts often hosted discussions about disease and attracted speakers and audiences well versed in current epidemiology. Cantlie was a highly qualified public health expert, having worked in Hong Kong as a member of the local sanitary board during the outbreak of bubonic plague there in 1894, and he had watched with alarm the onward career of the disease in the seventeen years since. 'The prevalence of plague in the world in epidemic form since 1894,' he began by saying, 'is a matter of supreme interest and importance to people of every nation.' In the course of his lecture, Cantlie spoke of the endemicity of plague, resident in the Mongolian steppes and possibly also in northern India and East Africa, and he referred, some twenty times, to plague as an epidemic. Only twice did he call plague pandemic, even when discussing the Black Death of the fourteenth century 'with all its horrors.' On the two occasions when he labeled plague a pandemic it was in looking to the future, in hoping for its speedy disappearance, and to contrast the periodic eruptions of the disease with its normal state of endemicity among the burrowing marmots of Central Asia. Since endemic and epidemic adequately defined the two principal phases of plague's existence, the one local and quiescent, the other expansive and aggressive, pandemic must have seemed to Cantlie a largely redundant or unedifying term.[25]

When Cantlie finished, several other distinguished epidemiologists rose to comment. Professor W. J. R. Simpson, formerly of Hong Kong and Calcutta,[26] spoke first, remarking how of late plague 'had spread in a very short time over a considerable part of the world.' He drew attention to its enormous impact on India where more than 7 million deaths from the disease had already been recorded. But he made no reference to plague as a pandemic, whether currently or in former times. When another expert, Dr. L. W. Sambon, spoke, he too described as an epidemic the plague that 'overran the world in the fourteenth century'—the world, that is, as known to late-medieval Europe. He did, though, go on to say: 'The present pandemic of plague was the widest that had ever been known in history, because for the first time Australia, South Africa, and America had been attacked.'[27] Here, then, was recognition that the dissemination of plague to every inhabited continent might merit the pandemic label: there was an alarming novelty, post-1492, about the newfound ability of this ancient contagion to cross oceans and infect every inhabited landmass. But pandemic was still not a term that the experts—at least those gathered in London in 1911—saw much value in using, except as an occasional alternative to epidemic, a term that clearly for them had far greater substance. Why?

Any physician raised in the Hippocratic tradition, as most doctors still were in the West in the early and mid-nineteenth century, was accustomed to the language of epidemics. Ancient but still influential texts like *The Epidemics* and Thucydides' account of 'the plague of Athens' in 430 BCE gave vivid testimony as to how epidemics arose, spread, and impacted on society.[28] But the idea of a pandemic had no established place in the Western medical canon—nor perhaps in the medical literature of any other civilization. Its awkwardness was often apparent. On the afternoon of 19 April 1873, at a meeting of the Royal Dublin Society, the Reverend Samuel Houghton, MD, FRS, gave a lecture on 'The Contagion Theory of Epidemics.' His main topic was the cholera epidemic of 1866. He explained that the discussion entailed the use of three 'hard Greek words'—epidemic, endemic, and pandemic—'words,' he added, to the amusement of his audience, 'which were not infrequently used by men to hide their ignorance.' By epidemic 'was generally understood a disease which was a foreign visitor—a disease introduced into another country,' as cholera had been into Britain from India. An endemic disease was one, by contrast, that was 'native to the place where it was found,' such as cholera on the banks of the Ganges in India. But Houghton had to confess that he did not know exactly what 'pandemic' meant or where it fitted in.[29] He may not have been alone in his confusion, even among the scientists of his day. What could such an awkward expression add to the authoritative notion of an epidemic?

In posing this question we might see in the emergence of the pandemic idea something akin to Michel Foucault's theory of the genealogy of knowledge.[30] A concept such as that of a pandemic might lack a single clear point of origin, a sole author, to whom it could be traced back, or on whose pronouncements it solidly relied. But somehow, despite all the contradictions it might entail and the resistance it might provoke, a certain way of thinking became established—in this case in medical thought and, more gradually, in public discourse from the mid-nineteenth century onward—acquired authority and familiarity, to the extent that one might now wonder whether it had a history at all.[31]

Into a world of epidemiological thought in which established notions of endemic and epidemic disease were firmly entrenched—in the canonical literature, in medical training, in professional practice—the idea of pandemics introduced a further conceptual tier to the existing understanding of disease, to the history and geography of disease, and to the strategies and means needed for disease containment. Pandemic gave a name to an emerging idea; it provided a conceptual framework for a growing volume of recorded data, even if closer scrutiny might suggest (as with bubonic plague) a mismatch between the way in which pandemics came to be identified as discrete phenomena and the messy, lived reality of how epidemic diseases actually rose and fell but never quite disappeared. One of the routes by which the pandemic idea came to be implanted—was given ownership—in the West was through authoritative works of medical history that sought to synthesize history, geography, and medical science. Among the earliest of these was J. F. C. Hecker's pioneering account of the Black Death, first published in German in 1832 and subsequently translated into English. Although Hecker did not use the term pandemic, he did describe plague as a global phenomenon. Writing at the very moment when cholera—the ur-pandemic of the modern age—was making its first destructive inroads into Europe, he made a direct connection between that earlier 'Oriental plague' and the 'new pestilence' arriving in seemingly similar fashion from Asia. Here was fertile ground for the idea of pandemics as 'general pestilences ... affecting the whole world,' of Asia as the principal source of such 'universal pestilences,' and for the intricate interplay between the temporality of cholera in contemporary Europe and the time of the Black Death almost five hundred years earlier.[32]

Central, too, to this genealogical progression was August Hirsch's magisterial account of infectious diseases, first published in Germany in 1859 and appearing in an expanded English edition in 1883. Significantly, despite the importance of data culled from British Empire sources, this was a Western, and by no means exclusively anglophone, endeavor. Hirsch (and his translator) made repeated use of the term pandemic, especially in relation to two diseases—influenza and 'Asiatic cholera'—both of which were conceived of as encompassing 'almost every part of the inhabitable globe.'[33] In encyclopedic fashion Hirsch was tidying up and attempting to bring system to the anarchic disorder of human disease across time and space by identifying, as in the case of cholera (the pre-eminent *weltkrankheit*, or 'world disease,' of his day), a series of clearly definable epidemic and pandemic episodes, principally as they affected Europe or were recorded (as in India) by European observers overseas. Epidemiological events, scattered across the centuries and from around the world, were thus compressed into an orderly narrative of recurring pandemics, elevated from isolated, localized incidents into a governing idea of transglobal significance.[34] While cholera and influenza were becoming established as paradigms of pandemicity, smallpox too made an appearance. Although this was a disease often associated with India in the nineteenth century, and the Muslim pilgrim traffic from South Asia through the Red Sea to Jeddah and Mecca, it was also widely present in contemporary Europe. Particularly influential here was an outbreak of smallpox that began in western and central Europe in the late 1860s but whose spread was then intensified by the troop movements and social disruption caused by the Franco-Prussian War of 1870. Despite the increasing use of vaccination, the disease not only raged in Europe, causing many fatalities there, but also reached the Americas and Australasia. Some contemporaries and later commentators spoke with alarm of the 'smallpox pandemic' of the 1870s.[35]

The emergence of the pandemic idea between the 1830s and the late nineteenth century required a combination of factors for its successful maturation. It called for a definition of the world that extended beyond Eurasia, a vision of globality impossible before the fifteenth and sixteenth centuries and only fulfilled by the European expeditions and conquests of the eighteenth and nineteenth centuries. It required the continuing, and indeed expanding, inflow of data from the extra-European world, and more especially from those imperial sites of medical observation and statistical record-keeping that made such a systematizing, globalizing effort meaningful and possible. It needed the professionalization of history and geography to provide the temporal framework and spatial parameters for detailed analysis and for making contrasts, comparisons, and analogies. It was reliant on an array of innovative technologies—among them modern means of transport and communication, global postal services, and mass circulation newspapers—to explain how disease could now spread so far and so fast and to provide updated accounts of the geographical progress of disease. It had to be fueled by advances in the understanding and observation of infectious diseases, the rise of epidemiology, bacteriology, and tropical medicine, and by the creation of the institutional sites, the rise of mobile medical personnel, and the specialist journals and monographs by means of which data could be collected, processed, and disseminated, within empires and between colonial and metropolitan centers.

The pandemic idea had, too, to overcome resistance to such an innovative concept. To speak of pandemics was to represent the world—and not just the world of contagion—in a new and menacing light. In an age in which time and space appeared to be contracting, in which knowledge of the past and speculation about the future were fast accelerating, the idea of contagion on a global scale might be seen to threaten the security of civilization, the serenity of progress, and the wholesome pursuit of profit. Covid-19 demonstrated anew the dilemmas governments experience when faced with disease on a pandemic scale. On the one hand, they want to protect the health of citizens by isolating suspect cases, imposing quarantines, closing borders, and restricting the flow of people and goods. On the other, they want to restore economic growth and financial stability by removing those barriers as quickly as possible. Perhaps they are slow and reluctant even to create such constraints in the first place, knowing how economically—and perhaps politically—damaging they are likely to be.

This was a dilemma the nineteenth century also faced. While most continental powers in Europe favored quarantines and cordons sanitaires as a long-practiced means of checking the progress of diseases like bubonic plague, Britain, as the first industrial nation, as the main beneficiary of burgeoning international trade, was resolutely wedded to liberalism and the philosophical principle as well as the economic advantage of free trade. Besides, as the rulers of an expanding empire in India, and with vital commercial and strategic interests across the Middle East and the Indian Ocean, the British were hostile to measures directed against their Eastern possessions and the diseases that emanated, or were alleged to emanate, from them.[36] Skeptical of the very idea of contagion, of the free passage of disease from place to place, from people to people, the British preferred to doubt the pandemic idea and to insist on the primacy of the local conditions—environmental, social, governmental— that fostered and facilitated disease, and so stressed the need to focus on local (rather than transnational) measures of amelioration and containment.

Pandemics had an alarming aura of universality. They suggested the frightening ability of a disease not just to advance inexorably within a given society, but also to leap from one country or even continent to another, unchecked by political borders, unconstrained by medical expertise and sanitary knowhow, and in apparent disregard for those differences of race, climate, and culture that were so central to the Victorian worldview and the imperial mindset. That all races and all places were alike in their vulnerability, that plague for instance might travel unhindered from China to India to Australia and California, was an idea that challenged many preconceptions of the imperial age. In a world predicated on difference, how could disease have the freedom to roam as if those essential differences didn't really matter? The period in which pandemics began to be discussed was precisely the era in which ideas of racial and geographical difference were at their most commanding. It was the time when tropical medicine as a new and distinctive medical specialism, emphasizing the singularity of tropical climates, of tropical parasites and disease vectors, of tropical races, their physiology, their social behavior and material being, was gaining unprecedented authority within the medical profession, in home and colonial governments, and among the metropolitan public.[37] Pandemics, in the globalizing sense that term increasingly implied, might be possible, and should certainly be feared and guarded against; but in the Western world they ran counter to cherished notions of superiority and difference.

Allied to this was the question of origin and direction. Where did pandemics begin? What was their geographical genesis and what did this say about the nature of a disease and its powers of contagion? In what kinds of social conditions and physical environments did plagues and pestilences first arise and then proliferate? Where did they wreak most havoc? In the premodern past, such origins might be unfathomably obscure, lost in some semi-mythical corner of Asia or Africa; but in the nineteenth and early twentieth centuries they could be identified with some precision and the geographical progression of a disease tracked in worrying detail. In his 1911 lecture, James Cantlie spoke of the particular dangers presented by the pneumonic form of bubonic plague and the ease with which it could be spread from person to person (rather than through infected rats and their fleas, as was by then understood to be the more common route). Severe as bubonic plague had already been in China and India, he observed, 'yet a worse form might develop' with pneumonic plague. 'China and India may have been but the fostering beds in the development of the [plague] bacillus' which had now 'attained its highest development in Manchuria.' But, from these epidemic epicenters, plague in its dreaded pneumonic incarnation might 'pass over the world, as it has frequently done before, in the form of the Black Death.'[38] 'Fostering beds' was a weighty, prejudicial phrase, suggesting that, even if a contagion like plague did not actually originate in China or India, those were the places, the host societies, that did most to incubate the disease and to send it forth on its global career.

Four years earlier, in June 1907, W. J. R. Simpson, one of those who spoke at Cantlie's talk, had himself given a series of lectures at the Royal College of Physicians in London on the same subject, plague. Here he did make some use of the pandemic idea both to refer to the current outbreak and to sketch comparable past episodes—the 'Justinian pandemic' of the sixth century (541–2 CE) and the Black Death of the fourteenth century (1346–53).[39] Simpson had also used the pandemic terminology and this sequencing of plague pandemics in his *Treatise on Plague* (1905), and it is striking how often India's colonial physicians and health officials framed their contemporary observations of disease within a historical narrative, one which both magnified their own achievements as researchers and administrators and laid down temporal markers and epidemiological templates that many historians of medicine have subsequently adopted.[40]

In his 1907 lectures Simpson's principal focus was on India, where, since its first arrival in Bombay ten years earlier, plague had caused more than 5 million deaths. 'At present,' he remarked, 'the chief interest of this pandemic lies in India.' Maps and statistics for the province of Punjab revealed to his audience just how devastating the Indian epidemic had been; but, he argued, more shocking still would have been a comparable death-toll in Europe. While India's 5 million plague deaths had garnered remarkably little international attention, an equivalent number of fatalities in Europe would be considered 'appalling ... a catastrophe of the first magnitude.' Three million people in Great Britain and Ireland would have died if plague had struck with the same severity as it had in Punjab. Clearly, to Western eyes, deaths in India, however great their number, mattered substantially less than deaths in the West or were an expected outcome. And yet, while concerned to highlight developments in India, Simpson was still more intent on showing what might happen if plague were to move, as it had threatened to do, from Asia to Europe. India's suffering was Europe's warning. The West, he urged, should not complacently assume that plague was a disease of the past and would 'not prevail in epidemic [or, as we would now put it, pandemic] form again.' The 'dying millions in India' constituted 'a problem of the greatest urgency and danger,' Simpson cautioned. But plague 'if left as it has been within recent years to take its own course bids fair in such circumstances to overwhelm not only India but also to be a danger to the world.'[41] Tackling plague in India, taking responsibility for its containment there, was less a necessity in itself than a prerequisite for protecting Europe and saving the Western world from a return to scenes of mortality not seen since the Black Death.[42]

Conversely, once the immediate threat of bubonic plague to the West had receded, it could be safely characterized as no more than a 'pseudo-tropical' disease. It was, according to Erwin Ackerknecht in 1965, now a disease largely confined to the tropics 'not because of the climate nor because of any greater susceptibility of some races, but because it is a disease that breeds in poverty and the tropics in our times are the poor countries.'[43] Like some exotic and venomous viper, plague had been put back in its tropical box.

Divided by Disease

Historians have written of the unification of the globe by disease, identifying plague, smallpox, cholera, and other epidemics as among the essential agents of that unificatory process.[44] But, as Covid-19 again demonstrated, we should be aware of the differential impact of the disease itself as well as the differing abilities of rich and poor nations to contain the coronavirus, to afford effective prophylactics, and employ appropriate remedial measures. One might, therefore, speak with equal merit of the division or *dis*-unification of the globe by disease. The world is, and has long been, divided in terms of where pandemic diseases come from (or are seen to originate) and by their varied impact on different parts of the globe. Pandemics may suggest the real or potential universality of infectious disease; they do not connote a uniformity of affliction, expertise, and resource.

The direction in which a disease traveled clearly mattered to contemporaries and endowed the modern pandemic idea with much of its potency. If diseases like bubonic plague or cholera or influenza arose from China, India, or elsewhere in the ill-defined but ever-threatening 'East,' then those societies, or those regimes (like the British in India) that ruled over them, had a responsibility to contain or eliminate the disease as close to its source as possible and prevent its remorseless, westward spread. China and India were repeatedly targeted as both the authors of their own epidemic misery and the source of the pandemic afflictions that menaced the 'civilized' West. What would it mean in an age of high imperialism, for the much-vaunted moral, social, medical, and technological superiority of the West, if an arcane disease like plague could cause as much havoc in modern Britain or France as in supposedly feudal China or quasi-medieval India? The unsettling idea of a pandemic, roaming the globe, was inimical to the West's collective notion of its superior standing in the world.

We might perhaps argue that the evidence of the nineteenth and early twentieth centuries ran counter to these Western pretensions. After all, cholera, while originating in India, did invade Europe and North America several times over the course of the nineteenth century, causing panic and inflicting heavy mortality: during an outbreak in the German city of Hamburg as late as 1892, 10,000 people perished in a matter of weeks. Influenza in 1889–92 and more especially in 1918–19 left a huge death-toll. Bubonic plague in the 1900s reached (but did not widely infect) London; it made limited inroads into Australia and the Americas. And yet, as the nineteenth century progressed, Western societies grew more confident of their ability to deploy their advanced sanitary skills and evolving medical knowledge to contain or repel epidemics, while what happened in Asia—on a far greater scale—was all too often shrugged off as regrettable but unavoidable or unstoppable.

We can see this geographical and racial bias at work if we turn to the pages of the *Manchester Guardian*, one of Britain's more liberal newspapers, for the months and years after the 1918–19 influenza pandemic had passed its peak and at a time when mortality figures for India were being revised upward from an initial estimate of 6 million to over 12 million. In May 1919 the paper reported the 'staggering statement' of the secretary of state for India, Edwin Montagu, that 'no less than two-thirds of the entire population of India had suffered from the influenza.' This fact, 'if well established,' the paper remarked, put 'the recent epidemic on a hideous eminence alongside the black plagues of the centuries we are apt to condemn as the age before sanitation.'[45] The suffering may have been horrific, but, so the paper implied, this great mortality (and the India in which it happened) belonged more properly to an earlier time, not to the modern age of sanitary science.

Four years later, in February 1923, under the headline 'An Appalling Death-Rate,' the same newspaper noted the 'astonishing figure' of 12.5 million influenza deaths now given by India's census commissioner. But, the article's author observed, 'When the latest of the epidemics to scourge mankind swept round the globe in a fatal cycle, it was, *of course*, among the unaccustomed peoples that it proved most deadly.' The 'native' populations of Africa, India, China, and the Pacific inevitably suffered most, 'who had not through generations of experience gained the relative immunity that the more sophisticated races enjoy'—thereby making race the central explanation for such huge (but, it would seem, entirely predictable) mortalities as well as ignoring the fact that the Russian Flu of 1889–92 had also circulated in China and India and might thereby have brought those countries 'experience' and some degree of immunity as well.[46] This was, too, a vaccine story, albeit, in India's case, a negative one. The *Manchester Guardian*'s correspondent hoped that a prophylactic vaccine would soon be available for use against influenza, just as vaccination had already been successfully deployed in India against smallpox. But, the article added, a flu vaccine might actually be of little use there, since Indians had recently shown strong opposition to the taking of the census in 1921 (at a time of intense anticolonial resistance) and so would presumably refuse a state-sponsored vaccine as well. 'The medical man, even with a vaccine for influenza almost within his grasp, may well be discouraged for similar reason from hoping easily to stop its spread in such a country as India. A people so resentful of questioning [in the census operations] is not easily persuaded to accept vaccination.'[47]

In other words, India's enormous and unparalleled mortality from influenza was seen to be a consequence of its inherent racial susceptibility and its perverse hostility to colonial rule and medical progress. Influenza might have been worldwide, an unstoppable tide, but in India specific reasons explained why one (non-Western) country had suffered most and might do so again in future. The human tragedy of influenza in India was inevitable, self-inflicted, or both. The *Manchester Guardian*'s views on this subject may have been extreme, but they were not unlike those voiced in other British newspapers and other commentaries which, in one fashion or another, blamed India, in Malthusian terms, for having such a large population (approximately 320 million at the time), for its lack of modern hygiene and sanitary awareness, and for its widespread and persistent poverty—as if British rule had had no part in that impoverishment.[48]

A brief coda. In October and November 1919, as influenza was in retreat in India and the West, a series of press reports drew readers' attention to the threat of a 'new epidemic.' This concerned cases of influenza on troopships carrying British soldiers back from India to British ports. One ship recorded 100 cases of influenza, another 63 cases and 2 deaths. In fact, the resulting mortality was slight, and the troops were effectively quarantined on disembarkation.[49] Nonetheless, the impression was created (as with the Bombay plague of 1896 or the Surat plague of 1994) that India was the great incubator and disseminator of epidemic and pandemic disease and, even though influenza had not originated in India, it still threatened to reignite a global conflagration.

2

THE TIME OF CHOLERA

Love in the Time of Cholera by Gabriel García Márquez is set in an unnamed city in an unidentified country (presumed to be Cartagena in Colombia), and ranges with the freedom of fiction over a long, if rather indeterminate, period between about the 1850s and the 1930s. Cholera, a haunting presence rather than statistical fact, frames the lives of the book's characters; it presides over the shifting temporalities in which they play out their existence. The time of cholera is a time of suffering and death, but also paradoxically, for such a violent disease, one of hope. It distinguishes a somnambulant past, a world of crumbling palaces and imperial reverie, obscure rites and arcane superstitions, from the forward-facing time of steamboats, telegraphs, movie houses, and modern medicine. Cholera conjures up a mythic past; it lurks in the darkened antechamber to 'bold modernity,' and yet, if only in memory, it still stalks the present. In a drama performed on the northern coast of South America, cholera connects Márquez's unnamed land to Europe, the epicenter of modern medicine, but also, in the opposite direction, to the fabled Orient. Cholera, even here, is 'Asiatic.'[1]

Love in the Time of Cholera is a work of fiction, not of medical history, but it has many resonances in contemporary life. Cholera returned to Colombia in the early 1990s, shortly after the novel was published, and a severe epidemic erupted not far away in Haiti in 2010–11, resulting in more than 9,000 deaths. As much for its title as for its contents, the novel attracted a wide readership and took on a new significance during the Covid pandemic: by a simple substitution it became possible to write, even in scientific and medical journals, of 'love in the time of coronavirus,' or, more simply, love having been jettisoned 'in the time of coronavirus.'[2] Márquez's fiction conveniently frames the historical quest: What *is* the time (and the place) of cholera? To what or whose history does cholera belong? What entangled or regressive temporalities does its pandemic history express?

Historically, cholera is at the heart of the pandemic narrative. Beginning in the early nineteenth century, it built a platform for subsequent thinking about what a pandemic is and does, how it erupts and travels, how it behaves and perhaps (eventually) fades into obscurity. Cholera does more than denote a particular disease. It defines a relationship (evident even in Márquez's late-twentieth-century novel) between 'Oriental' India and an Occident that identified itself as both victim and savior.

Making Cholera Pandemic

Cholera was the first modern pandemic, ravaging India and encompassing the globe. Indeed, in the view of many medical historians, from 1817 and into 1920s the history of cholera *was* 'the history of pandemics.'[3] The earliest outbreak for which we have detailed information began in eastern India in 1817 and lasted until 1823: this is now designated the first pandemic. Five further pandemics followed in 1826–38, 1839–52, 1863–74, 1881–96, and 1899–1923, though the actual dates given to these episodes vary considerably.[4] Since these dates represent a largely European perspective on the disease, they do not easily map onto the experience of India where cholera remained endemic and intermittently epidemic for a large part of the nineteenth and twentieth centuries.

Cholera first manifested itself pandemically in Bengal in the early nineteenth century, but it is clear from a range of sources that the disease was present in South Asia well before 1817. British India's nineteenth-century epidemiologists, combining current medical knowledge with a quest for historical antecedents, recognized that epidemic cholera was not an entirely new phenomenon, and they constructed a shadowy lineage for the disease that projected the time of cholera back into previous centuries. A major outbreak at a Hindu bathing festival at Hardwar on the upper Ganges in 1783 alone was said to have caused 20,000 deaths. As India's pandemic narrative has repeatedly shown, it was not the last time that Hardwar figured thus. Evidence for a cholera-like contagion, with severe stomach cramps and fatal diarrhea, was traced further back to the seventeenth century, though seemingly without the rapid transmission and mass mortality for which cholera subsequently became notorious.[5] And yet both the location and the timing of the 1817 epidemic appeared then, and still more with hindsight, to be of epochal significance. The disease is known to have erupted first in deltaic Bengal: reports of its progress came from Jessore district (now in Bangladesh) in August 1817 though it had probably been circulating in the vicinity for months before that.[6] In this ecologically fluid zone, where the intermingling Ganges and Brahmaputra periodically changed course, the low-lying deltaic terrain lay scarred with abandoned river channels, littered with stagnant pools, shifting sandbanks, and sodden marshes. Monsoon rains, swollen rivers, and violent cyclones wrought their watery havoc. Significantly in the career of cholera, an essentially waterborne disease, 1817 was a year of heavy rainfall and widespread flooding.[7]

Thickly forested and thinly populated, for centuries the delta had been remote from the main centers of political power and economic activity in South Asia. Then, with the Mughal conquest of the region in the 1570s, these marginal tracts were integrated into a wider system of administrative control and agrarian exploitation. On this ecological frontier, 'Incessant, strenuous human effort transformed the wild wetlands and tropical forests of the delta into domesticated wetlands of paddies and palms.'[8] For the Mughals and then for the British, Bengal became one of the most agriculturally productive, revenue-rich provinces of India. The Mughals built their regional capital at Dacca in the eastern delta in 1602; in 1690 the British established Calcutta, the 'city in the swamp' that became their own commercial hub and administrative capital.[9] As Bombay, India's western metropolis, later became the epicenter for plague and influenza, so from the early nineteenth century Calcutta in the east served as cholera's nursery. What had once been a relatively isolated and, in terms of human settlement, marginal zone was transformed into a nexus of regional and global trade, its maritime connections spanning the Indian Ocean and the seas beyond. An opportunist pathogen, cholera now had a route by which to invade and ravage the world.

The cholera-causing bacterium, a comma-shaped vibrio, originates as a marine microorganism that can survive in a semi-dormant state in water that is too salty or too cold for it to actively thrive. The vibrios reside in brackish streams and estuarine waters in the intestines of minute crustaceans called copepods, and possibly also in the gut or on the surface of other marine creatures. In the right environmental conditions, the vibrios emerge from their dormancy, multiply rapidly, and infect human hosts.[10] That cholera epidemics have such an ecological ancestry, as animal-borne pathogens that then cross into humans, makes them highly relevant to the story of present-day pandemicity. We have become accustomed to the idea of new diseases, from AIDS and SARS to Ebola and Covid-19, as resulting from radical shifts in the relationship between people and environments. Deforestation, climate change, surging populations, and an inexorable demand for food and other resources have pushed against environmental limits or overturned existing ecologies, so that infections previously confined to birds, bats, pigs, monkeys— or marine invertebrates—have spilled over into humans, who then pass them on among themselves through person-to-person transmission.[11] Cholera was an earlier iteration of this now familiar story. In deltaic Bengal an ecological frontier had been breached, a watery ecology transformed to suit human needs, a city with tens of thousands (ultimately millions) of inhabitants sited in an uncongenial swamp. A disease that for centuries may have been locally present, or sporadically epidemic across the subcontinent, now found the conditions in which to thrive and the freedom to crisscross the globe. 'Pandemics,' it has been said, 'appear for a reason. And that reason is the size of the host population and the degree to which it has disturbed its environment. Upsetting the balance of nature is something the human species has done rather well.'[12]

In 1817 lower Bengal experienced 'probably the most terrible of all Indian cholera epidemics.'[13] Consternation and confusion marked the arrival of this 'most alarming and fatal disorder.'[14] In Jessore in the summer of 1817 an estimated 10,000 people died within two months. The disease spread to Calcutta, where 4,000 deaths were reported; then, traveling via Patna, Benares, and Allahabad, cholera pushed into northern and central India, attacking Bombay in August 1818 and Madras in October. In 1819 it began journeying overseas, crossing to Ceylon, before moving on to Mauritius, Southeast Asia, China, and, by 1822, Japan.[15] A short respite followed. Then a second, more truly global pandemic erupted in eastern India in 1826, passed along caravan routes into Central Asia and southern Russia before arriving in Moscow in 1830. From there cholera marched on into eastern Europe, reaching Britain in 1831, and crossing to Canada and the United States in 1832. By the standard of later pandemics, the movement of these first two cholera pandemics was fitful and slow, taking months to unfold, but it still seemed to contemporaries that cholera's terrifying advance and alarming death-toll put the whole world at risk.

Cholera laid a foundation for subsequent thinking about pandemics. Even the shocking scale of mortality attributed to the disease—wildly overestimated at 50 million worldwide by 1832—has a more contemporary ring about it, as if anticipating the influenza of 1918–19 with its more reliable estimates of 40 million dead.[16] And yet no two pandemics are alike. For all its foundational characteristics, there was much that marked out cholera as distinctive and at variance with the pattern of more recent pandemics. First, unlike many later pandemics (plague apart), cholera was caused by a bacillus, not by a virus. Its entry into the human body was via water and food, through the mouth and the digestive system, rather than through the upper respiratory tract like influenza or Covid-19. Second, with the partial exception of smallpox, for which South Asia was also a significant source of contagion, of all the modern pandemics cholera was the only one to have an indisputable origin in India, as opposed to India serving (as with plague) as a site of reception, incubation, and onward dispatch. All but the latest of the several cholera pandemics—caused by the El Tor biotype first observed on the Indonesian island of Sulawesi in 1961—can be traced back to Bengal, though by the end of the nineteenth century cholera was intermittently endemic across a wide arc of Asia, from India to Japan. Outbreaks could occur almost anywhere.[17]

Third, although its origins as a 'world disease' can be traced to Bengal in 1817, cholera took far longer than many modern pandemics to reveal itself as a global threat: it was the cumulative effect of repeated eruptions rather than one single cataclysmic event that gave cholera its pandemic profile. Unlike the Spanish Flu of 1918–19, the time of cholera spanned generations. Further, what India experienced differed from what the West knew of cholera. By far the greatest number of cholera deaths in the nineteenth century occurred on Indian soil. Britain lost an estimated 130,000 lives to cholera over the course of the nineteenth century; over the same period and into the first quarter of the twentieth century, the same disease cost India in excess of 25 million lives.[18] For Western societies cholera took the form of a series of short, shocking, but relatively well-defined 'invasions,' spread over eighty years from the late 1820s to the early 1890s. But in India after 1817 cholera was seldom absent from one part of the subcontinent or another, a resident disease periodically exploding into deadly epidemics, only some of which became pandemic.

Cholera was a colonial contagion, a disease of empire as much as a global pandemic. Empire not only facilitated the spread of the disease: it also made it possible for European observers to witness the initial outbreak in Jessore, to identify cholera almost from the outset as an exceptionally dangerous disease rather than a routine recurrence of the many fevers and fluxes that afflicted the region. For Europe thus to witness this epidemiological event, to be midwife at its birth, was central to the idea, now so familiar to us, that new and lethal pathogens periodically arise to endanger the world and that such diseases can then be tracked and mapped from their place of origin—deltaic Bengal in the case of nineteenth-century cholera— and from there throughout their global dissemination. Before cholera no disease in history had ever been traced in such detail and across such vast distances. Here was unprecedented material for the modern pandemic idea.

Cholera and the 'Civilized World'

In the early nineteenth century cholera was invariably described as an epidemic, and not a pandemic, disease. But, in deference to its increasingly global career, it was commonly identified as 'Asiatic cholera' or 'Indian cholera,' an indication of its ultimate source, even when the immediate locus of infection lay much closer to hand. We have become wary in the twenty-first century of using specific peoples or places to identify pandemic diseases: hence, the more neutral designation Covid-19 rather than 'Wuhan' or 'Chinese' fever and the rapid substitution of 'Delta variant' for what was at first called its 'Indian' strain. The nineteenth century had no such qualms, and its stigmatizing name firmly imprinted on cholera its identity as an alien disease, a menace from beyond Europe's borders. As Richard Evans observed in summarizing Western views, 'the disease was widely understood as Asia's revenge: a deadly invasion from the supposedly backward and uncivilized East, launched just as Western civilization, in the eyes of many Europeans, was reaching the height of its progress and achievements.'[19] Cholera was civilization's spoiler. It seemed perversely to exploit the very lines of trade and communication, even the conquering armies, that made the West modern, powerful, and proud. It was Europe's own emblematic technologies—telegraphs, railroads, and steamships, the excavation of the Suez Canal—that facilitated the westward migration of the 'Asiatic' contagion or carried news of its westward incursions.

Cholera brought Europe 'dangerously close to India.'[20] So close that the recurrent explosions of pandemic cholera felt like a repeated assault not just on Western civilization at large but also on those whom the West held in high regard. In his history of Orissa in 1872, the colonial administrator and historian W. W. Hunter laid the ultimate blame for cholera epidemics on Hindu pilgrimage to the temple of Jagannath in Puri and the annual Ratha Yatra (Car Festival). This, as he saw it, was the epicenter from which the disease 'radiates to the great manufacturing towns of France and England.' The Indian pilgrim might 'care little for life or death,' he declared, but 'such carelessness imperils lives far more valuable than their own.' The 'squalid pilgrim army of Jagannath, ... impregnated with infection,' could at any time 'slay thousands of the most talented and beautiful of our age in Vienna, London, or Washington.'[21] Was there no one 'talented' or 'beautiful' among India's own cholera dead?

The mechanism by which Western countries sought to address the cholera problem underscored their perception of the disease as a transnational menace, rather than a merely local or regional threat. Starting in 1851, a series of international sanitary conferences were held, attended mostly by representatives of the main European powers, as well as from the Ottoman Empire and the United States. In almost all of the twelve meetings held by 1914, cholera topped the agenda.[22] It is striking that many other deadly diseases prevalent at the time in the non-West, such as yellow fever, provoked nothing like the degree of international consternation and cooperation that cholera did, largely because they were regarded as more specifically tropical afflictions and so less likely to land on Europe's shores. It was cholera that 'more than all the others combined, stimulated the nations [of Europe] to persist in their efforts to reach agreement on the measures to be taken to limit the spread of epidemic diseases.'[23] The conference held at Constantinople in 1866 went further than previous meetings in focusing on the need to prevent 'further incursions of this Asiatic scourge,' and it also categorically identified India as cholera's epidemic source. Delegates approved a resolution which stated: 'Asiatic cholera, which on various occasions has travelled throughout the world, has its origin in India, where it arises and where it exists in a permanent endemic state.'[24] Once established, the India connection was seldom forgotten, even late in the century. The British epidemiologist John Burdon-Sanderson remarked in 1892: 'every epidemic of cholera which reaches Europe has its starting point in the house of some Hindoo on the banks of the Ganges.'[25] 'House' or 'home'—there was a perverse domesticity about the way the West imagined India's cholera. Or as the French sanitarian Henri Monod put it that same year: 'there is only one cradle for cholera on the face of the earth—and this is India.'[26] India's cradle, Europe's grave.

It was primarily (though not exclusively) in relation to cholera that the term 'pandemic' entered international sanitary discourse. India might experience epidemics of the disease, with all that that implied about local causation and intraregional transmission. But, more widely, epidemiologists were starting by the 1850s and 1860s to refer to *pandemic* cholera and to identify a series of pandemics, each originating in India. In the first edition of his *Handbook* on the history and geography of infectious diseases in 1859, August Hirsch described 'Indian cholera' as a 'world-disease' and chronicled the pandemic career of this contagion from 1817 onwards.[27] An editorial in *The Lancet* in 1867, having similarly traced the disease back to 1817, listed each subsequent cholera eruption leading up to 1866 and as they affected the West. Cholera was thus construed as a recurring threat, each time starting in Bengal and invading Europe overland through Russia or, more commonly, via Egypt and the Red Sea. Past knowledge informed present urgency and drove the need for future action. Given 'the lessons of previous pandemics,' a turn of phrase again familiar in the time of Covid-19, *The Lancet* urged precautions be taken in the clear expectation that there would soon be another outbreak.[28]

An article in the same journal in 1873 by Dr. William E. Smart, inspector-general of the Royal Navy, likewise described three 'westward invasions of cholera' in 1827, 1843, and 1864. The author tracked their movement across Europe and into the Americas, labeling these the first, second, and third pandemics. Although he and his contemporaries struggled to explain the 'morbific principles' behind the disease and 'their modes and means of extension and progress,' he had no doubt that 'the phenomenon of Asiatic cholera' owed its ultimate origin to one or two possible 'Asian homes,' of which the Ganges–Brahmaputra delta was the most likely.[29] And yet, even in the 1860s and 1870s, the status of the term 'pandemic' was not entirely assured. The author of an article in the *British Medical Journal* in 1868, reporting on a discussion at London's Epidemiological Society, seemed to struggle with the word, referring to the cholera 'epidemic' of 1865 before adding 'or rather pandemic,' as if still unfamiliar with the idea.[30]

The notion that pandemics characteristically came in 'waves' also had its birth in this period and again particularly in relation to cholera. The term began by being applied to the annual occurrence of infectious diseases like smallpox and scarlet fever in Europe in the 1880s, with a seasonal peak in spring and summer being followed by a trough in autumn and winter.[31] But controversy arose over one specific use of the 'wave' metaphor, in such a way as to inhibit acceptance of the wider pandemic idea. From the 1860s, Robert Lawson of the Army Medical Service argued that 'pandemic waves' of disease periodically advanced across the globe, from the tropics to the northern temperate zone, carried by high-level winds.[32] Lawson based this claim on his personal observations of disease in the West Indies and West Africa and on the voluminous data from around the world by then available to metropolitan epidemiologists. Lawson was an authoritative figure, and continuing uncertainty about the etiology and transmission of cholera gave his ideas some traction.

However, by the 1880s and 1890s, at the dawning of the age of bacteriology, such ideas seemed to many epidemiologists highly speculative, even mystical. Could disease really be spread globally by something as remote as high-level winds? Moreover, the 'wave theory' was caught up in attacks on the British medical establishment in India for clinging to outmoded and unsubstantiated beliefs about the aerial transmission of cholera at a time when the waterborne theory and the bacillary cause of cholera were gaining wide international acceptance.[33] There was a fundamental ambiguity about Britain's position on cholera, for it was both the ruler of India, and so responsible for its health, and part of the Western world that viewed with alarm India's recurring epidemics. Among the most acerbic of metropolitan critics was Ernest Hart, editor of the *British Medical Journal*, who visited India in 1894–5 and contemptuously dismissed all theories based on 'air currents' and 'pandemic waves.' On returning to Britain, Hart observed: 'We are told that the influence is not yet extinct of the old spirit which subjected to persecution medical officers [in the Indian Medical Service, or IMS] who did not follow their superiors in attributing cholera to telluric influences, pandemic waves, epidemic constitutions, cholera mists, blue clouds, and so on.'[34] To Hart such bizarre claims were pure obfuscation, or, as we might say, mere myth. To him there was nothing mysterious about cholera: it was a lethal disease spread by person-to-person transmission and through contaminated water, a 'filth disease carried by dirty people to dirty places.' Obscure aerial pathways had nothing to do with it. 'It is not,' he insisted, 'by wilfully closing its eye to the evil, or by fatalistic resignation to what is conveniently assumed to be inevitable, or by talking of "air currents" and "pandemic waves," that India can be purged of this foul stain on its good name and made no longer a standing menace to the health of the civilised world.'[35]

In Hart's view, the British government in India was 'directly responsible to the world for the recurring epidemics of cholera. As long as they shut their eyes to the fact that impure water was the cause of cholera in India, so long would they continue to bear the heavy responsibility of the recurrence of cholera in epidemic form.'[36] He might scorn the very idea of 'pandemic waves,' but, in emphasizing the responsibility of India's colonial government for allowing cholera to persist in the subcontinent and so periodically to roam the globe, he was still arguing for the idea of pandemics as a menace to the 'civilized world,' and one that needed to be tackled at source, in India itself. Pandemics were real, even if 'waves' were not.

The Many Lives of Water

Cholera was, and is, a largely waterborne disease. The victim ingests the cholera vibrio, which multiplies in the small bowel and generates an intestinal toxin. The small bowel then secretes isotonic fluid in greater quantities than the colon can absorb so that a watery diarrhea is ejected. Intense purging and vomiting results, then rapid dehydration: unless effectively treated, death can ensue within twenty-four hours.[37] Cholera encapsulated the violence of a pandemic disorder; indeed, so ferocious were its symptoms that it was sometimes mistaken for arsenic poisoning. Victims could be alive and in apparent good health one day and dead the next. To onlookers and carers, cholera was a singularly distressing disease. Apart from the uncontrollable vomiting and diarrhea, the victim's skin became wrinkled, the face took on a ghastly bluish hue, the eyes looked sunken, the voice faded to a whisper, and death quickly ensued. Today cholera can be successfully treated by rehydration therapy, but previously, given the sudden onset of the disease and its rapid progression, medical intervention was seldom effective.

In South Asia water—and the bacillus it harbored—had many lives. Cholera was an accomplice to many an aqueous disaster, as when cyclones barreled in from the Bay of Bengal, bringing mass destruction in their wake. In one of the greatest catastrophes to hit late-nineteenth-century India, a cyclone struck coastal Bengal on 31 October 1876: in the cholera epidemic that followed, officials numbered 75,000 dead; the true figure may have been closer to 100,000.[38] A scarcity of water, as much as its catastrophic excess, might also trigger high cholera death-rates. While no direct correlation between cholera and malnutrition has been established, poverty, hardship, and hunger created conditions in which the disease thrived.[39] The drought and famine that so frequently in the nineteenth century followed food shortages and the failure of the monsoon resulted in desperate villagers drifting away from their homes and crowding onto relief works or into insanitary cities, where they drank polluted water, ate contaminated food, and so contracted cholera. This exposure to the disease was so common after 1817 that cholera became an invariable accompaniment to famine as two streams of mortality—one from disease, the other from hunger and social dislocation—converged.[40] A large percentage of those who perished in India from cholera over the course of the nineteenth century, as many as 15 million people by 1865 and a further 23 million more between then and 1947, died during or in the immediate aftermath of famines.[41] In a single year, 1877, at a time of acute drought, food shortages, and mass hunger, more than 357,000 people died of cholera in the Madras Presidency alone, equivalent to 12.2 deaths for every 1,000 of the population; in the worst-hit districts, that figure nearly doubled. Even among those who received treatment, the death-rate could reach 60 percent.[42] A further 200,000 people died of cholera in the Madras famine of 1897–8.[43] From 1908, the decline of epidemic cholera in India broadly correlated with the dwindling incidence of famines, a connection tragically resurrected with the Bengal famine of 1943. Even after 1947, floods, cyclones, droughts, and famines, in India and neighboring Bangladesh, brought fresh, often deadly outbreaks of the disease.

Cholera thrived in a social ecology that closely connected people with water. This was true around the world, especially where the inhabitants of cities and slums were dependent on impure drinking water.[44] In India the association between water and cholera was compounded by religious practice. Among Hindus water has powerful associations with purity, with the requirement for ritual washing and bathing, and the drinking of holy water from the Ganges and other sacred rivers to wash away sins and free the worshipper from the cycle of rebirth. Although the original source of the infection might lie elsewhere, the onward transmission and mass dissemination of cholera were closely identified with the periodic Hindu bathing festivals held at Hardwar, Allahabad, and Benares on the Ganges, and at Nashik on the Godavari. These festivals had ancient origins, but their increased accessibility and the growing number of pilgrims attending them by the second half of the nineteenth century owed much to modern road and, more especially, rail construction.[45] At these sacred sites pilgrims from different disease environments congregated in their tens of thousands: they bathed; they sipped water from the sacred stream, then carried it back with them to their homes and families, thereby facilitating the onward spread of cholera. Hindu gatherings of this kind came to be seen in the nineteenth century as being primarily responsible for seeding several devastating epidemics. They became, in today's pandemic jargon, 'super-spreader' events. The Hardwar Kumbh Mela of 1867 was a prime example. As an official report put it: 'That cholera went with the pilgrims from Hurdwar and accompanied them to a greater or lesser distance in every direction from it is a fact which admits of no dispute.'[46] Other Hindu fairs and festivals were similarly implicated, especially (as Hunter had claimed) the annual pilgrimage to Puri.[47] According to a committee in 1868, 'pilgrimages are in India the most powerful of all the causes which conduce to the development and to the propagation of epidemics of cholera.'[48] But then, as now, governments, colonial and postcolonial alike, found it hard, or politically difficult, to ban such mass gatherings or even, in sanitary terms, effectively to police them.

By the 1860s pilgrimages, fairs, and festivals had become a primary focus of colonial public health intervention and concern in

India, echoing a deeper Western preoccupation with India as a land in which epidemic disease and arcane religion conjoined. The factuality of contagion bled into a colonial myth of Indian irrationality and irresponsibility. In reality, India's cholera problem had many more causes than religious observance alone. However, such observances annexed India's cholera to a different temporality from that of the international pandemics, a chronology governed by annual pilgrimages (like that to Puri) and by longer-term cyclical events like the twelve-yearly Kumbh Melas at Allahabad and Hardwar. But pilgrims, whether Hindus traveling to the Ganges, or Muslims on *hajj* from Bombay to Mecca, were only one of the many means by which cholera became mobile.

Cholera's Terrors

For much of the nineteenth century cholera remained a baffling and enigmatic disease. Theories abounded as to its causes and the best way to prevent and treat it. As late as 1869 one survey of medical evidence from Britain and India concluded that little more was understood about cholera than fifty years earlier when it first burst onto the world stage. It had kept its 'secret history'; it still roamed the earth, free to practice (in a phrase that uncannily anticipated talk of a 'corona jihad' in 2020) its 'cholera terrorism.'[49] And yet, pandemic though it repeatedly was, cholera was far from demonstrating, in India as elsewhere, that everyone and everywhere was equally at risk. Cholera belied the egalitarian myth, the ungrounded claim that, when it came to pandemics, 'we are all in this together.' Impure water was not the only hazard. So, too, were poverty and the way in which contagion capitalized on the vulnerability of the poor. India's poverty took many forms. As early as the 1817 epidemic in Calcutta, cholera was found to be most prevalent among the impoverished residents of the 'native town' or those living in 'wretched hovels' on the city's margins. 'The higher classes of Native, and Europeans generally, inhabiting the better raised and more airy parts of the town, suffered proportionally less than the lower ranks.'[50]

Indians who lived and worked close to water, who drank, bathed, or toiled in contaminated water, who lacked proper shelter, and subsisted on a meager diet, were among the most susceptible. These included boatmen and fishermen in Bengal and pearl divers at Tuticorin on the Coromandel coast, where 443 people were attacked and 187 died in a single outbreak in 1822.[51] From the 1850s onward railroads helped disseminate cholera as they did other infections; but cholera was present, too, in their very construction. The workers who built India's railroads lived in makeshift, insanitary camps: they endured exposure to the elements, had scant access to water fit to drink, and, when they fell sick, lacked medical attention. In 1859 a third of the 4,000 or so 'coolies' (laborers) on Bengal's East Indian Railway perished from cholera in the space of six weeks.[52] Worse still was the fate of workers on the sixteen-mile stretch of the Bhore Ghat incline, where a route was blasted through the Western Ghats from Bombay to Poona. In the course of construction between 1856 and 1863 more than 40,000 laborers were employed there at any one time, in monsoon rain and summer sun. Cholera was rife, with as many as ten deaths a day between late 1859 and May 1860.[53] Over the eight years of work on the Bhore Ghat 25,000 Indians died, most of them victims to cholera, making it 'the deadliest railway project ever undertaken anywhere in the world.'[54]

In an age of increasing labor mobility and expanding regional and global networks of migration and trade, cholera had become by the mid-nineteenth century a characteristic affliction of the mobile poor, a sign and symptom of an India, driven by capitalism and empire, relentlessly on the move. Cholera erupted among migrant workers in crowded indentured labor depots in Calcutta and Madras, awaiting ships to take them to tea and coffee estates in Ceylon, and to sugar plantations in Mauritius, Natal, the Caribbean, and Fiji. Cholera ravaged workers huddled into steamers and ferried up the Brahmaputra to the tea estates of Assam. The migrant poor died in their thousands, and yet in the scornful eyes of European employers and sanitary officers the blame lay with the workers themselves and their 'dirty habits,' not the system that engaged and transported them. Only gradually did estate managers and doctors take partial ownership of this foul disease and recognize a responsibility to maintain at least minimal health standards among employees.[55] Less immediately visible to the outside world, and still less amenable to sanitary control, were sickness and mortality among field laborers, many of whom moved around rural India during the sowing or rice-transplanting season and again during the harvesting months, often at times when cholera was most rampant. They camped in fields, washed in sluggish streams, defecated in the dried-up watercourses that became 'elongated latrines,' and drew their water from polluted tanks and irrigation channels, infecting themselves and spreading disease in the locality. Cholera thereby became endemic in the Cauvery and Kistna–Godavari deltas in the Madras Presidency, where seasonal labor migration, intensive rice cultivation, and a watery terrain of rivers and canals partly replicated the disease ecology of lower Bengal.[56]

Cholera exploited analogous conditions, too, in the army. Just as migrant labor was one of the mainstays of the colonial economy, so was military manpower essential to the expansion and consolidation of British rule. The army first appeared in this pandemic story not as the agency of disease control and sanitary regulation that it became during the 1890s plague but in the role of victims and super-spreaders. One of the ways in which cholera traveled across India or erupted in local pockets of infection was through the army. An estimated 1,500 Indian and European soldiers and camp followers died of the disease within a week while campaigning against the Marathas in central India in November 1817.[57] During route marches, especially before the railroads came to their rescue, soldiers and their numerous camp followers suffered hardship, hunger, and thirst; they fell sick, passed cholera on to their comrades, or bequeathed it to the towns and villages through which they passed. Elaborate but not always effective measures were devised by which soldiers on the march or in camp might evade cholera. They were ordered to quit their barracks or camping ground as soon as cholera appeared, 'instant removal from an infected spot' being 'the best safeguard.'[58] That was seldom sufficient to save lives.

Crowded and insanitary, and in close proximity to insalubrious bazaars, army barracks became deathtraps, with some of the most severe epidemics of the nineteenth century occurring in barracks among European soldiers, their wives, and children. In an outbreak in the North-Western Provinces and Punjab in August 1861 there were 1,929 cases of cholera: 1,231 European soldiers and their family members died, almost two-thirds of those infected. In Mian Mir cantonment on the outskirts of Lahore, 880 men, women, and children were attacked and 535 died in a month.[59] As cholera spread, so did fear, panic, exhaustion, and demoralization. At Mian Mir, in what might almost be a scene from Covid in India in 2020–1, hospital surgeons were reported to be 'worn out and breaking down from fatigue and consequent sickness, and the medical subordinates [were] too few in number to attend properly to the numerous patients who require[d] to be looked after.' Soldiers' morale was crushed by 'a devastating plague which the hand of man is unable to stay.'[60] Forty years into its long reign, cholera was still the 'king of terrors.'[61]

As in Britain, cholera spurred recognition of the need for sanitary reform. A royal commission, appointed before the Mian Mir outbreak to examine the health of the army in India, published its report in 1863. It made repeated reference to cholera, the loss of army lives, and the urgent need for improvement. But soldiers were not the only institutional casualties. So, too, were prisoners, and in the nineteenth and early twentieth centuries the army and the jails in India provided essential sites for the observation of disease, the acquisition of medical statistics, and early experiments in contagion control (a role they had largely forfeited by the 1920s). In conditions comparable to those in the army barracks—unhealthy confinement, poor ventilation, deficient hygiene, impure food and water—prisoners suffered a similar fate to soldiers. With death-rates at times exceeding 50 percent, to be a prisoner in a time of cholera could prove tantamount to a sentence of death: only gradually, over several decades, did cholera morbidity and mortality in jails come under more effective control.[62] Army and jail statistics help pose a further issue—gender. Whether men were more or less susceptible to cholera (and other epidemics) than women—and why—is unclear. Men might be more exposed in places where they formed the great majority of inmates and laborers, such as jails, barracks, and workcamps; but women, too, went on pilgrimages, and some (in far smaller numbers than men) were committed to overcrowded prisons. They worked in paddy fields transplanting rice, up to their calves in muddy water; they, too, toiled on plantations, washed clothes, drew water from contaminated wells and streams, and, of necessity, drank from polluted tanks and rivers. They might, for cultural reasons, be less likely than men to receive timely medical attention or be cared for when sick. Pregnancy, childbirth, and nursing an infant child further increased their risk of contracting cholera or succumbing to its fatal embrace.

Cholera could potentially affect all strata of society, just as it could, in theory, attack any country where analogous conditions prevailed. It could infect and kill Europeans as well as Indians, the rich and powerful as well as the migrant laborer and the famine poor. Individual cases can be cited to show this: Sir Thomas Munro, governor of Madras, died of cholera in 1827; as did General George Anson, commander-in-chief of the Indian Army, early on in the Rebellion of 1857. For Europeans, cholera was one of the diseases that made India a place of anxiety and dread. And yet, among Europeans and Indians alike, the poor, the hungry, and the ill-housed suffered disproportionately. Statistics on the British Army in India and on Europeans in the Indian Army showed a wide discrepancy between the officer class and rank-and-file soldiers, the latter being far more likely to sicken and die from cholera.[63] Officers were better paid and better nourished, had superior access to clean water and uncontaminated food, lived in spacious bungalows rather than crowded barracks, and might have greater sanitary awareness. If they fell sick, officers were more likely to receive prompt medical treatment and have the means to recover. They were not immune, just better able to protect themselves.

It was not uncommon for Europeans to regard cholera as a disease of Indian poverty and 'filth.' Julia Maitland, a civil servant's wife living in relative comfort at Rajahmundry in the Madras Presidency, wrote in 1837 that there was 'little fear of cholera among Europeans,' except while traveling. 'It is caused among the poor natives by bad feeding, dirt, and exposure to the climate.' She and her husband kept cholera medicines in the house, not for themselves but 'in case any of the servants should be attacked.' That, she thought, 'very unlikely,' as they were 'well fed and sheltered.'[64] Anecdotal evidence suggests, too, that by the late nineteenth century Europeans in general felt increasingly safe from this disease of 'poor natives.' Writing in 1892, the year when more than 10,000 people died from cholera in the German city of Hamburg, a correspondent of the *Times of India* voiced some complacency about the disease. 'In India,' the writer observed, cholera 'is always with us.' It was 'perpetually present in the village round the corner,' but the 'sahebs and memsahebs' who lived nearby felt little more than 'a mild kind of regret that it should be working its mischief there.' It did not make them fear for their own safety, nor did it interrupt their recreational round of tennis, dances, and picnics.[65] Likewise, in 1911, two colonial health experts, writing mainly for European readers, described cholera as 'the outcome of filth and filthy habits and easily preventable by a due recognition of this fact.'[66]

Cholera Mata

In *The Faces of Injustice*, the philosopher and political theorist Judith Shklar asked: 'When is a disaster a misfortune and when is it an injustice?' The answer, she suggested, might intuitively appear obvious. 'If the dreadful event is caused by the external forces of nature, it is a misfortune and we must resign ourselves to our suffering.' Conversely, if the disaster was attributable to 'some ill-intentioned agent, human or supernatural,' then it was an injustice 'and we may express indignation and outrage.'[67] In practice, Shklar acknowledged, the distinction was seldom so clear-cut. Perceptions shifted over time; no clear dividing line might be drawn between divine or natural causation and human culpability or negligent inaction. She did, though, suggest that there might be a discernible trajectory over time as, over centuries, societies transitioned away from divine explanations and belief in 'natural disasters' and increasingly sought out human responsibility and accountability. Famines, for instance, 'are not what they used to be' and, like many 'no-longer pure misfortunes,' were now far more likely to be attributed to 'human injustice or folly or both.' Famine had become 'a politically avoidable disaster.' And when little was done to prevent it, a compelling sense of injustice arose.[68]

Shklar's discussion is highly pertinent to India's epidemic and pandemic experience. At what point, if at all, was there a shift from seeing such episodes as 'natural disasters' to regarding them as something for which there was at least a degree of human responsibility or for which specific groups or individuals could be held morally or empirically to blame. As she admitted, this is no easy distinction to draw. But, as noted earlier, cholera was seen internationally in the nineteenth century as a contagion for which India and its rulers were explicitly responsible. Cholera was not some inexplicable event or manifestation of divine wrath, especially so once, late in the century, its causative pathogen had been identified. It was a consequence of human folly and (as Ernest Hart insisted in the early 1890s) government neglect, a recurring calamity for which the authorities in India needed to take proper responsibility.

However, on the ground in India this sense of human culpability and imperial mismanagement was far less apparent. Despite its global notoriety, cholera in India remained a disease largely experienced and understood locally, and this was reflected as much in the attitudes and responses of the Indian public as in those of the colonial administration. Even if cholera was, pandemically speaking, a new disease in 1817, it still slotted into established cultural patterns and existing coping mechanisms. Whatever international sanitary conferences might decree, Indians authored their own understanding of cholera and sought what for them appeared to be appropriate means for its containment. Thus, in a return to mythical time rather than in accordance with the West's notions of pandemic causation and chronology, among Hindus (and, given the eclecticism of Indian religious beliefs and practices, some Muslims) disease was conceived of as the work of specific deities, almost invariably identified as a goddess, the 'Mata' or mother of the disease. The goddess embodied *shakti*, the principle of female power: socially, and in this respect ritually, women stood in closer proximity to disease than men did.

The deity might unleash disease as a punishment for human neglect or wrongdoing, but conversely her veneration provided a conduit through which her human devotees might have some role in preventing or assuaging that affliction. Disease deities could protect as well as punish, much as, in a very different cultural idiom, modern immunology employed a modified or attenuated form of a deadly virus to buy protection against the virus itself. Smallpox was the most widely observed expression of this duality. Fiery Sitala, in taking possession of a human body, manifested her presence through the victim's raging fever and eruptive pustules; but her wrath could be appeased. Through songs sung in her praise and through 'cooling' rites, the capricious goddess might be mollified, coaxed into quitting her human host without causing death or the disfiguring pockmarks and blindness that made her visitations so feared.[69]

The response to many other diseases followed a broadly similar pattern, if seldom so elaborately as with Sitala. Thus, there was a cholera deity, identified by Hindus in Bengal as Ola Chandi and among Muslims as Olabibi. As goddess of the fluxes, she was worshipped, mainly by women, who prayed and made offerings at shrines erected in her honor.[70] The very existence of such a deity and of places dedicated to her worship attested to the fact that cholera had long been known in Bengal. Her veneration, taken up with fresh fervor when the 1817 epidemic struck, served as an archive of past experience of the disease and a reminder of the likelihood of future episodes. Rather than nurturing a sense of injustice against human actors, the propitiation of Ola Chandi suggested that responsibility rested with a divine agency: if deities were capricious, their motives inscrutable, they could still perhaps be appeased, their wrath averted. Sitala and Ola Chandi provided a rationale as to why epidemics occurred, why some individuals fell sick while others were spared. They articulated an essentially local practice of disease cognition. Such deities bore local names and were worshipped in small, local shrines: they were not the grand gods and goddesses of the Hindu pantheon. Moreover, the idea of disease deities established a highly versatile cultural idiom, one that could be reworked to meet new dangers—like bubonic plague in the 1890s—and the image of the disease goddess, benevolent or destructive, vividly resurfaced in the iconography of the coronavirus, as the 'Corona Mata' of 2020–1.[71]

India's disease deities presented the possibility of an alternative and indigenous disease narrative to that represented by colonial medical and sanitary discourse, and yet Sitala and her sisters were not immune to hostile incorporation into that increasingly dominant epistemology. Belief in 'disease godlings' was used in colonial ethnography as evidence of the irrational and superstitious nature of

Indian ideas about disease and a deep-seated opposition to modern medicine and progressive public health. By implicating cholera in Hindu religious practices and the obscurantism of village life, colonial critics deflected responsibility away from the deficiencies of their own sanitary regime and onto Indian 'others.' 'The peasant is too ignorant to understand the necessity of sanitation,' wrote anthropologist-administrator William Crooke, 'too indifferent and suspicious to seek medical relief. He [sic] regards disease from a fatalistic point of view.'[72] The fact that Indians were seen as resistant to change or unmindful of epidemic danger provided a convenient excuse for the state's lack of the political will and financial commitment needed to eliminate rather than contain cholera. Although this criticism was directed mainly at Indian villagers, it was levied against the more affluent elements of urban society as well. Why, demanded Bombay's health officer during the plague epidemic of 1896, were middle-class Indians 'willing to do everything to appease the gods' while doing very little 'to cleanse the over-crowded houses or chauls [slum tenements]'?[73]

Apart from disease deities, cholera took on other identifiable manifestations of the demonic or the divine. Women, hair loosened and dress disheveled, began a frenzied dance or entered a prophetic trance, claiming possession by the disease deity; others, adorned and enthroned, were revered as avatars of the cholera goddess. These living goddesses attracted large crowds until they were stopped or arrested by magistrates as 'imposters' or for threatening disorder. Other individuals, again mainly women, identified not as gods but as cholera-causing 'demons,' were mobbed and beaten to death.[74] A further response, one in which an assignment of blame was still more evident, was scapegoating. Cholera was seen as an invasion—not in this instance of Europe by an 'Asiatic' disease but by some human agency from outside the village or town, an affliction for which something or somebody needed to be beaten or expelled. This was far from being a uniquely Indian response: attributing responsibility for misfortune to others has commonly characterized the social reaction to epidemic and pandemic disease. 'Blaming,' as Dorothy Nelkin and Sander Gilman wrote with respect to AIDS in the 1980s, 'has always been a means to make mysterious and devastating diseases comprehensible and therefore possibly controllable.'[75]

In village India an offering of food or an animal sacrifice was made to the cholera deity or the evil spirit from which the disease arose, taken to the village boundary, and there dumped: in some cases, a painted buffalo or human 'scapegoat' was chosen and forcibly driven off, in the hope that the disease would also leave and not return.[76] Widows (stigmatized as 'witches') or Dalits ('untouchables') were the most likely targets for expulsion. In 1865 the British political agent at Rajkot in Kathiawar was so incensed by high-caste attacks and the 'sanguinary persecutions' of the untouchable Bhangis blamed for outbreaks of cholera that he offered 50 rupees for the best essay in Gujarati explaining the true nature of the disease.[77] Scapegoating was—and remains—an immensely powerful idea, one that can be rationalized as 'a quest for order and certainty in an anxious and disruptive situation.'[78] But it entails discrimination, violence, and often rampant xenophobia. In the sense of blaming and targeting a victim—in the era of Covid, more likely to be from an ethnic or religious minority—this practice has had a long and vicious life in India since the first cholera epidemics. It has not gone away.

Local Disease in a Globalized World

Of all the diseases subject to scientific scrutiny in nineteenth-century India cholera was perhaps the most closely observed. The 1817 epidemic coincided with a period in India when the English East India Company was engaged in an intensive process of mapping, surveying, and compiling inventories of its newly acquired territories. If the outbreak had occurred a century earlier, say in 1717, as the Mughal Empire entered its long decline, not only might the material and social means have been missing for its pandemic dissemination (Mughal India lacked the kind of epidemic information order and monitoring structure that had emerged in early modern Europe), but cholera in a distant corner of the globe would surely have provoked far less consternation in the West. It might never have become, or been perceived as, a 'world disease.' To figure fully in the global imagination pandemics needed to be seen, not just suffered. They required the apparatus of modern scientific observation and enquiry, and this colonial India was able to provide. The disease narratives and topographical surveys compiled and conducted by Company servants were part of the authoring of the pandemic, allotting cholera a place within the expanding annals of colonial science, medicine, historiography, and governance.

At the same time, cholera demanded close attention to the diseased body and the cadaverous dead. Medical observation in India grew up around cholera more than any other disease. Some of colonial India's earliest and most detailed medical texts pertained to cholera or devoted large sections to a subject of such compelling local and international interest. Charts, graphs, and statistical tables detailed the progress, more often the rapid deterioration, of cases hourly observed, the effects of largely ineffective treatments, and the differences assigned to race, age, occupation, and gender; post-mortems scrutinized the victim's diseased inner state. This morbid interior landscape of the body complemented the exterior terrain envisaged by medical topography.[79] Even if the ultimate aim was to use the singular corpse to generate universal meaning, cholera took on the attributes of a profoundly local disease.

There was a further sense in which, for British India, the problem of cholera was, as Mark Harrison described it, a 'question of locality.'[80] From the outset, observers linked cholera to local climatic conditions—heavy rain, high humidity, 'changeable weather,' 'atmospheric vicissitudes.'[81] While cholera's etiology continued to perplex, speculation was rife that it was due to 'some noxious quality in the atmosphere, affecting in a peculiar manner the functions of the stomach and intestines.'[82] The violence of the disease seemed inextricably linked to the intemperate nature of the Indian climate. Over the fifty years following the 1817 outbreak, environmental explanations for cholera morphed into a complex and idiosyncratic epidemiology. To many medical writers, armed with data from dozens of meteorological stations across India, seasonality seemed the dominant factor in explaining why and how epidemics occurred. What could be seen in the skies or measured in a rain gauge outweighed anything that might be observable under a microscope.

How cholera ever became pandemic was hard for India's sanitarians to explain except perhaps through the existence of broadly analogous climatic conditions. According to the statistician James Bryden in 1869, 'an invading cholera' was 'never ... spread ... by human intercourse alone.' 'The highways by which cholera travels are, *in this country*, aerial highways, and not routes of human communication.'[83] Cholera was tied to what his colleague H. W. Bellew termed India's 'special climatic conditions,' meaning primarily the monsoon. Such an assertion ran directly counter to the idea, endorsed as recently as the 1861 international sanitary conference, that cholera was spread by person-to-person contagion.[84]

In blaming the climate, and hence omnipotent, unalterable nature, the British in India were shrugging off their own responsibility for cholera. They could hardly be expected to outlaw the monsoon. But, apart from the attribution of disease to climatic peculiarities, the accumulating literature on Indian cholera created a confusing melange of local causes and intimate contagions, a mosaic of marshes, jungles, soils, and winds that seemed by their very complexity to disempower science while at the same time to insist that India was distinctive and dangerous. While in India into the 1870s and 1880s climatic determinism still bore the authority of indisputable orthodoxy, in the West it was increasingly contested, culminating in the identification of the cholera bacillus by the German bacteriologist Robert Koch in 1883–4. In this epic discovery, metropolitan microscopy seemed to triumph over colonial meteorology and to create for cholera a new universality, for the same microscopic pathogen could be detected anywhere in the world, from cosmopolitan Calcutta to sleepy Cartagena.

And yet in India the arguments in favor of climate and season did not meekly bow out. The bacteriological explanation for cholera was grudgingly accepted by many in India's medical establishment, but the discovery of the bacillus seemed only partly to account for the timing and location of actual outbreaks of the disease. Indian environmentalism survived to qualify and incorporate the universality of Koch's bacteriology. Statistical data compiled by the 1920s revealed for instance for the Madras Presidency 'a definite relationship between the incidence of cholera and the prevalence of rainfall or the degree of humidity.' The disease showed 'great exacerbations shortly after the onset of the rains, and decline[d] more or less rapidly when the monsoons die[d] away.'[85] In North India, there was a predictability about the westward movement of cholera epidemics along what Bryden had earlier called the 'northern epidemic highway.' Starting in Bengal in November, they entered Bihar and eastern districts of the United Provinces in March, the rest of the United Provinces in April, and Punjab in May.[86] This local epidemic sequencing was of greater practical value than the broad pandemic chronology by which Europe knew cholera, making it possible to predict when (even, to a degree, where) cholera outbreaks were likely to occur and allow time for countermeasures to be taken. By the same token, this made it harder for British India to conceive of cholera as pandemic rather than a disease answering to specific causes and local circumstances.

Building the Sanitary Empire

In an imperial setting cholera entailed both denial and appropriation. In building their sanitary empire in India, the British repeatedly asserted the superiority of their medical practice and public health expertise. Indigenous healers proffered their own remedies: some of these were tried or, for want of effective alternatives, were provisionally accepted, but in general the colonial regime denied them a legitimate role. Making cholera pandemic involved blaming India for being its recurrent source while simultaneously denying its *vaids* and *hakims*, its traditional physicians, a substantial say in managing the very disease for which their country had become notorious. Medical pluralism did not come easily to the colonial health authorities, especially when European health—in India or in the West—was at stake. Nor could Ayurveda and Unani (the systems, respectively, of Hindus and Muslims) easily speak the new language of state medicine and public health. For much of the nineteenth century Indians' attempts to own cholera, to comprehend it in terms of local beliefs and customary therapeutic strategies, to participate freely and through their own agency in measures for its treatment and containment, were largely spurned.

The shocking loss of European troops at Mian Mir, the criticism voiced internationally about India as the undisputed source of pandemic cholera, the continuing spate of epidemics that erupted during famines or following religious pilgrimages or melas—all these failed to revolutionize India's public health. But they did oblige the Government of India to recognize a need for improved hygiene and enhanced sanitary policing, most immediately with respect to the army and jails but also more widely across Indian society. The appointment in 1868 of sanitary commissioners for each province and a sanitary commissioner accountable to the central government signaled a partial shift in state policy, though it took decades for more effective and comprehensive measures to be adopted. Gradualism prevailed.

India's sanitary state, such as it was, grew to slow maturity with, and through, cholera. Although the British in India were loath to defer to international pressure, if only from fear of provoking resistance from their Indian subjects, a raft of piecemeal measures was slowly assembled. The British believed that, whatever its precise etiology, cholera could be most effectively controlled by local means. While cholera's reach was global, epidemics of the disease 'were local events affecting the population of a circumscribed space, usually a village, town, city or region but rarely an entire country.'[87] Apart from prisons and cantonments, the authorities targeted the fairs, festivals, and pilgrim haunts that were seen to be the primary disseminators of disease. A Madras report of 1868 listed seven headings under which sanitary action should be undertaken, ranging from the construction of temporary camping grounds, the erection of latrines, and the provision of clean drinking water, through to waste removal, medical supervision, and the sanitary duties of the police.[88]

The perceived nature of the disease as much as the manner of its transmission made it impossible to devise a single solution to the cholera problem. As in many Western countries, cholera was associated with urban sewage disposal and a clean water supply. John Snow's investigation of cholera in London in the 1850s, centering on the Broad Street pump, indicated how the disease might spread through contaminated water to infect an entire community. In

India the provision of clean water remained problematic. The rivers and tanks from which many people drew water for cooking and drinking readily became infected with cholera, and botched attempts to improve the water supply might even increase the risk of contamination. For a host of financial, political, and technical reasons, many water and drainage schemes, relegated to underequipped and tax-averse municipalities, remained incomplete, even decades after they were first proposed. In India local government was often part of the problem rather than the solution. The introduction of a potable water supply in Calcutta in 1870 slashed the death-rate from cholera by two-thirds, but that still left a third of the population, including slum dwellers, reliant on unsafe water sources and exposed to infection. The high cost of installing drainage and sewerage works, of providing clean water not just for a resident population but also, as in the case of Puri, for the many thousands of pilgrims who flocked to fairs and festivals, was viewed as prohibitive or, at best, required years for sufficient funds to be found.[89] As British India's representatives informed the international sanitary conferences, in arguing against quarantines and other unwanted measures, improvements to urban water supplies and sewerage *were* having a positive effect. And yet they cut cholera mortality without eradicating the disease or preventing its periodic recurrence. Increasingly, to colonial health officials, cholera was 'a disease of the villages,' places largely untouched by sanitary improvement.[90]

If the 1860s marked one tentative advance in colonial cholera policy, the 1890s signaled another. The British in India were faced with mounting international pressure from the international sanitary conferences to act more decisively against cholera, especially following Koch's discovery of the cholera bacillus.[91] Domestic considerations were also involved, including the continuing economic cost of cholera in terms of Indian lives lost and the impact on productive labor, not least plantation and factory workers. However, the colonial government also believed it necessary, in its own interests, to weigh up the political risks of greater intervention: creating sanitary subjects was not without risk. Such measures might provoke occasional complaints, but they gradually gained acceptance or support, especially when Indians were actively involved as sanitary officers or influencers of local opinion.[92] However, the political and religious mood of India was changing, and when in March 1892 the Government of the North-Western Provinces ordered the dispersal of pilgrims gathered for a bathing festival at Hardwar (once again the touchstone) because of a feared cholera epidemic, there was an outcry. Police and health officials were accused of physically mistreating pilgrims and of violating the terms of Queen Victoria's proclamation of 1858, which had promised religious toleration. The central government grew nervous, fearing that in a time of Hindu revivalism and mounting nationalist fervor the incident might spark a backlash: 1857 had not been forgotten.[93] The episode was seen as a timely warning against excessive sanitary zeal. But it underscores how dramatic was the passing, only five years later, of the Epidemic Diseases Act of 1897 in which political caution was cast aside in a draconian attempt to curb bubonic plague. In India cholera was never as heavily politicized an issue as plague, perhaps because it was primarily seen as a disease of the poor. And yet the authorities feared that cholera might *become* an anticolonial cause and so proceeded warily, rejecting proposals that the Epidemic Diseases Act be used against cholera as well as plague.[94]

If pandemics can be weaponized, so can the means and methods of their containment. Throughout this story, from cholera to Covid-19, the pandemic narrative is closely entwined with the history of vaccine prophylaxis. Vaccination has become a vehicle for exemplary tales of resistance and progress, of colonial beneficence and international risk, of national pride and postcolonial self-reliance. Today, the rapid development of a vaccine as well as its deployment to millions is seen as the most effective, even the only viable, means of checking a novel pandemic like Covid; a great deal of scientific expertise and political capital is invested in its discovery and delivery, and in claims for national ownership. But in the cautious world of colonial pragmatism and medical conservatism, the quest for a vaccine against cholera was not even on the agenda until the 1890s, almost a century after Edward Jenner had pioneered vaccination against smallpox. And yet arguably the greatest single advance in cholera control in India came not with Koch's discovery of the bacillus in 1883–4 but a decade later with the anticholera vaccine devised by the Russian-born, Paris-trained bacteriologist Waldemar Haffkine. Working in Bombay in 1893–4, Haffkine pioneered a prophylactic vaccine using attenuated cholera vibrios. At the time many senior medical officers in India were deeply skeptical about the efficacy of the vaccine and doubted the value—or practicality—of inoculation compared with more conventional measures. The government was anxious to avoid being too closely identified with the vaccine for fear of inciting popular opposition, insisting that only volunteers be inoculated and coercion strictly eschewed.[95] It was years before anticholera inoculation became officially accepted as a front-line weapon against cholera.

With time, however, Haffkine's vaccine came to be extensively used in India's public health campaigns and particularly to protect at-risk groups such as soldiers, prisoners, and pilgrims. Among the first to be inoculated—by Haffkine himself—were 11,000 tea-estate workers in Assam in 1894–5.[96] The sustained decline in cholera in India dated, however, only from the mid-1920s, a decline in which inoculation surely played as momentous a role as the dwindling risk of wholesale famine. In 1893 in the North-Western Provinces, which had recorded over 363,000 cholera deaths only a year before, Haffkine's prophylactic was administered to a thousand volunteers. By the 1920s the scale of operations had greatly increased—with 32,500 individuals inoculated in 1927, 60,900 in 1928, and 93,000 in 1929. In 1935, when the Magh Mela fair was held at Allahabad, more than 207,000 people received the vaccine.[97] Compulsory inoculation followed at other mass religious gatherings, such as Pandharpur in western India in 1936 and at Hardwar and Ayodhya in the United Provinces after 1945.[98] Although the value of inoculation was limited in the sense of being effective for only a few months and conferring no long-term immunity, this was enough to protect pilgrims while attending a bathing festival. With hindsight, Haffkine's prophylactic was hailed as a major breakthrough in cholera control in India.[99]

* * *

The time of cholera is not over. Cholera still lives in the present tense, still inhabits our modern world. And yet today the disease seldom attracts the kind of pandemic fears and epidemic anxieties that it did in the nineteenth century: since the 1970s oral rehydration therapy has proved a relatively cheap and effective means of combating the disease. Fewer than 100,000 cholera cases are currently reported worldwide each year, with relatively few deaths. Even so, outbreaks continue to occur in eastern India, in West Bengal and Odisha, close to the disease's old endemic site: they persist because a large part of the population remains without clean water and effective sanitation. Over the ten-year period 1997–2006 India reported to the World Health Organization a total of 37,783 cases of cholera and 84 deaths, though analysts suggest that the incidence of the disease was 'hugely under-reported' and that the actual number of infections and fatalities may have been up to ten times higher.[100] Serious outbreaks happen periodically in other parts of the world, as in Haiti in 2010–11 and during the civil war in Yemen in 2016–20. But the world no longer fears cholera as it once did; the pandemic threat has receded. Epidemics, it has been suggested, only 'end' through 'widespread acceptance of a newly endemic state,' more especially when that endemic state lies outside Europe and North America.[101]

From the outset cholera was seen as having a unique and troubling relationship with India. This was not unjustified. Between 1817 and 1920, as many as 80 percent of all cholera deaths recorded worldwide occurred in India, a pattern of disproportionate mortality later matched by India's experience of bubonic plague and influenza.[102] But 'Asiatic cholera' was also a concept, a pioneering articulation of what, in medical and political terms, pandemicity might mean, quite as much as it was a specific pathogen. It was an idea of India and of India's equivocal place in the colonial world, as both victim and source, as both danger (to itself and to the West) and opportunity (with respect to medical science and sanitary policy). Cholera, wrote Haffkine in 1895, reprising a familiar trope, was 'a disease having its origin in the East.' It followed, then, that 'the efforts which have for their object its stamping out or mitigation, or the prevention of its spread' were necessarily concentrated on 'those localities in which the disease has a permanent abode, and from which it starts periodically in epidemic form to invade other countries.'[103] India was the cause, the target, and, just possibly, the solution.

3

A MODERN PLAGUE

Flushed with the success of his recent military campaigns in northern Italy, on 19 May 1798 Napoleon Bonaparte embarked at Toulon with a large French invasion force, bound for the eastern Mediterranean. His intention was to conquer Egypt and Syria and so open up a new front in the escalating war with Britain, and then, in alliance with Tipu Sultan, ruler of Mysore, to use this as a base to attack British India. The destruction of the French fleet by the British Navy under Horatio Nelson at Aboukir Bay in August 1798 checked French ambitions, but Bonaparte remained in Egypt for a further year, battling Ottoman armies and besieging several cities, including Jaffa.

In a famous painting by Antoine-Jean Gros, completed in 1804 and now on display in the Louvre (see fig. 1), Napoleon, resplendent in his military uniform, was portrayed visiting a lazaretto or pesthouse in Jaffa and touching (or gesturing toward) the bubo, the glandular underarm swelling, of a plague victim. It was as if plague, too, were his to command and to conquer, a military idiom often employed in the literature of disease in general and plague in particular. Was Napoleon (or his artist) recalling the 'king's touch' by which medieval French and English kings supposedly cured their subjects of scrofula?[1] Possibly his gesture was intended to show to the French soldiers who had fallen victim to plague that this was not a disease to be feared, or that he at least was superior to its contagion. Was it a gesture of compassion, 'as he willingly exposed himself to the plague in order to bring comfort to his men'?[2] Whatever the Napoleonic gesture was meant to signify, the painting itself was a representative piece of nineteenth-century Orientalist art, situating plague as an affliction of a threatening, if geographically indeterminate, East, with Napoleon the defiant or compassionate hero, for whom the battle against disease was only another kind of conquest. Here, in pictorial form, was an example of what has aptly been called 'epidemiological Orientalism.'[3]

'Plague,' though, is a slippery term. It is used in English to describe a specific disease (bubonic plague), a zoonosis originating among rodents but spread to humans through rat-fleas and caused by a bacterium now known as *Yersinia pestis*. But we also use 'plague' in a wider sense to describe a pestilence of whatever nature, sometimes alongside or interchangeably with other descriptive tags, like influenza or AIDS. More broadly still, it can refer to the massive or repeated occurrence of anything we consider harmful, threatening, or destructive, like a 'plague of locusts.' The confusion, fear, and repugnance captured by this more general usage inform and energize the specifically medical meaning of the term. Thus, in Albert Camus's 1947 novel *La Peste*, set in colonial Oran, on the fault line between the Orient and the West, bubonic plague becomes a pathogen of a peculiarly threatening, enveloping, and insidious kind, a pestilential metaphor for the human condition.[4]

Gros's *Pesthouse at Jaffa* represents only one of the several ways in which bubonic plague—*pestis orientalis* as it was named by contemporaries—entered imperial history and the pandemic narrative. In January 1801 an expeditionary force of 8,000 soldiers, half of them Indian, was dispatched by sea from Bombay to defeat the remnants of the French Army in Egypt. Here was an early instance of a pattern, repeated many times during the nineteenth and first half of the twentieth centuries, of deploying Indian troops overseas in the service of the British Empire. It was also an illustration, as later with cholera and influenza, of the army as a specific site of medical observation and, conversely, a vehicle for disease dissemination. During the year the troops spent in Egypt plague again made its appearance. Of the 391 Indian soldiers who perished during the campaign, 127 died of plague. To James M'Gregor, the army's chief medical officer in Egypt, plague was one of the diseases 'peculiar to Egypt' (the other being ophthalmia). He attributed it to the climate and soil, the poverty and squalor, in which, he believed, most Egyptians lived. M'Gregor was confident, however, that, with prompt action, plague could be successfully contained and effectively treated.[5]

Without previous personal experience of the disease, M'Gregor trusted to the work of his compatriot Patrick Russell. Before becoming known for his studies of Indian snakes and flora, Dr. Russell had been physician at the British factory at Aleppo in the 1760s. He published a treatise on plague in the city, in which he identified a high fever and the appearance of buboes as indicative signs of the disease. Given Britain's extensive trade with the Levant, Russell's concern was that plague might again afflict Europe, as it had as recently as the Marseilles outbreak of 1720–1.[6] But Russell made no reference to India in his treatise, nor did M'Gregor imagine plague as other than endemic to the Middle East. Indeed, when the army returned to Bombay and Madras, precautionary quarantine measures were adopted in case the 'Egyptian infection' might be inadvertently introduced into India.[7]

Pandemic Preludes

Up to that point, early in the nineteenth century, India had appeared largely innocent of plague. The Black Death, which so devastated and demoralized fourteenth-century Europe, had scant impact on South Asia, if it even penetrated there at all. It is only from the early seventeenth century and the reign of the Mughal emperor Jehangir that incontrovertible accounts of bubonic plague in India exist.[8] Given that this was a period of extensive commercial contact and growing pilgrim traffic between India and the Red Sea, and a time of growing European mercantile activity, it is theoretically possible that plague was only now spreading to India, almost three hundred years after the Black Death, in part through increased contact with the West.[9]

However, as with cholera, the British occupation of India created novel opportunities for observing this disease, and in the decades after the Egyptian campaign several local outbreaks of bubonic plague were reported from Gujarat, Rajasthan, and the sub-Himalayan region of Kumaon and Garhwal.[10] Through historical and geographical accounts of contagious disease like those of J. F. C. Hecker and August Hirsch from the 1830s onward (see Chapters 1 and 2), these local episodes became incorporated into a wider narrative in which India emerged not as a threatened outlier but as one of the principal sites, even perennial reservoirs, of the disease. The geographical locus of 'Oriental plague' lurched eastward from Egypt to India (and beyond to China), just as the history of pandemic plague was being pushed backward to the Black Death and the 'plague of Justinian' centuries before that.[11] The most widely reported of these Indian episodes was the 'Pali plague' of 1836–7. Named after the town in Rajasthan where the epidemic began, the outbreak sparked panic and flight from the worst-affected area. Of Pali's 12,000 inhabitants, 8,000 fled, and 1,200 succumbed to the disease. But, despite reaching the North-Western Provinces, the Pali plague remained relatively localized and disappeared of its own accord.[12] When bubonic plague arrived in Bombay in 1896–7 some observers suggested that it, too, might have originated in Rajasthan and the sub-Himalayan region, or that there were two different strains of the disease—a mild West Asian strain long resident in the Middle East (the plague Napoleon encountered at Jaffa) and a far more virulent 'Indo-Chinese' strain, kept in deadly circulation by the 'teeming millions' of South and East Asia.[13]

Plague was a temporal as well as spatial marker. To Western contemporaries the plague that began in Bombay in 1896 and then spread across northern and central India, reaching its peak of mortality around 1907, threatened nothing less than the return of the Black Death.[14] India's plague was discursively annexed to Europe's greatest demographic and epidemiological disaster, a trauma kept alive for the British by the London plague of 1665–6 and for the French by the Marseilles outbreak of 1720–1. For the West to view plague in Bombay as the return of the Black Death signaled two things. One was the fear that a plague pandemic would become a Frankenstein monster free to terrorize the entire world unless it could somehow be stopped in its tracks. There was concern that, like the fourteenth-century plague and more recent cholera pandemics, the disease would spread rapidly and inexorably from Asia into Europe, causing panic and mortality on a scale matched only by its medieval precursor. The West needed to guard against this 'Oriental' scourge by halting its westward transmission. A second effect of identifying the plague of the 1890s with that of the 1340s was to reawaken the recurrent fear that pandemics reenacted the atavistic horrors of the past, hurling society backward into the dark pit from which it had so laboriously emerged. Cholera might, with qualification, be identified as a new disease, but, for the West, plague was the bearer of deeper historical resonances. It was a medieval contagion unleashed on a modern world. When in 1903 the naturalist Alfred Russel Wallace decried British rule in India for allowing plague and famine to stalk the land, it was partly on the grounds that, even at the height of the modern age of science and innovation, in Bombay and Calcutta 'horribly insanitary conditions' existed that rivaled 'the worst plague-infested cities of Europe in the middle ages.'[15] In the 1930s, Victor Heiser, the globe-trotting representative of the Rockefeller Foundation, expressed a similar fear, describing plague as threatening the return of the Black Death, posing, like cholera before it, a danger to the entire 'civilized world.'[16]

And yet it was in India that by far the greatest number of people died in what is now labeled the third plague pandemic. Of just over 13 million plague deaths recorded worldwide between 1894 and 1938, 12.5 million (close to 90 percent) were in India.[17] China, Manchuria (where plague may have taken pneumonic form), and Java in Southeast Asia also suffered severely, while Australia, Africa, South America, and California were more marginally affected. In this geographical sense, the pandemic was undeniably a global phenomenon. And yet the plague of the 1890s and 1900s did not reach Europe, or rather it was detected in a few cases in European ports without establishing itself. There and in most other parts of the world, it remained confined to a smattering of coastal enclaves or 'plague ports.'[18] Plague proved to be pandemic more in terms of the global anxiety it aroused than with respect to its transcontinental spread and eventual death toll. Millions died of plague in India, at least 7 million by the time W. J. R. Simpson spoke of the disease in London in 1907 (see chapter 1), and 12 million by the time it began to peter out in the 1920s. Plague rumbled on in India; by then, however, the rest of the world ceased to regard it as a pandemic threat.

Even at its height plague seemed highly discriminatory. The great majority of those who died in Hong Kong, India, and Manchuria were not Europeans but 'Asiatics.' In 1900 *The Lancet* noted the comparative immunity of Europeans to plague and the 'comforting though curious impression that plague is a disease of Asiatics'— 'comforting,' that is, for Europeans.[19] Plague continued to present itself to most Western observers as a disease of race, class, and, above all, place—the rat-infested homes and insanitary hovels of the 'Oriental' poor.[20] Plague seemed to endorse the idea that not all races and places were equal.

By being so largely confined to India (and East Asia) while leaving the West essentially unscathed, plague heightened the Occidental perception of India as a still medieval society, one on which modern ideas of health and sanitation had barely impinged, where ignorance, fatalism, and squalor still reigned. Certainly, plague exacted a terrible price from India: the scale of mortality, the extent of human suffering and socio-economic dislocation, were enormous. And yet the paradox was that in many ways India's plague was less the return of an ancient scourge than the making of a modern pandemic, one in which railroads, steamships, newspapers, and factories combined to incubate, disseminate, and spread word of the disease; a pandemic in which, and through which, modern science, modern politics, and modern modes of representation and self-expression struggled to gain ascendancy. The decade of the 1890s is better seen as marking the birth of India's scientific and social modernity than as a precipitous descent into medieval squalor and obscurity.

India put its stamp on the pandemic in several ways. Most of plague's victims were located there, and it was primarily in relation to India that Europe recoiled from this revenant horror. Much of the scientific investigation into the etiology and transmission of plague was conducted there, as were some of the earliest attempts to control the disease through mass vaccination and rat extermination. India's experience in the 1890s and 1900s framed and informed the historical and epidemiological debate about what bubonic plague was and must therefore have been like in earlier times. Because in India plague could be so directly observed and investigated, it provided the template for what has been termed the 'plague concept,' the authoritative model by which to understand and interpret the long-term history and epidemiology of the disease.[21] India in the 1890s and 1900s not only endured bubonic plague; it might almost be said to have invented it.

The Bombay Plague

The experience of plague in India in the 1890s was initially that of Bombay. The city was an epitome of modern connectivity. One of the leading ports and largest urban centers of the entire British Empire, Bombay conducted extensive maritime trade with ports across the Indian Ocean and, especially after the Suez Canal opened in 1869, with Europe. Once the disease struck Bombay it became, according to a former city health officer, Dr. G. J. Blackmore, in 1909, 'the great plague distributing centre of the world.' Bombay bore primary responsibility for 'the present pandemic.'[22] The city looked inward as well as outward, its influence extending far into the interior. When famine struck in 1876–8, thousands of villagers trekked to the city in search of food and shelter: many died there. By the 1890s, as its cotton textile industry flourished, Bombay had become at least a temporary home to more than 800,000 people, many of them, including 80,000 millhands, migrant workers from upcountry Bombay or northern India. As well as its wealthy merchants and industrialists, Bombay had densely populated working-class districts, crowded tenements, and sprawling, insanitary slums. It reeled under recurrent bouts of malaria, smallpox, cholera, and tuberculosis; it had appallingly high levels of maternal and infant mortality. In 1895 the annual death-rate was over 30 per thousand; in 1896 it rose to 41. In the worst plague years the rate shot up still further: 68 per thousand in 1899, and 97 in 1900, before falling back to 77 in 1901.[23] Bombay was a modern city, but its poverty and endemic ill health were as symptomatic of its industrial modernity as they were indicative of years of municipal underfunding and sanitary neglect.

The third plague pandemic probably began in Yunnan in southwestern China in the 1850s. By 1894 it had reached the southern port and British colony of Hong Kong. Despite attempts to suppress it, the disease continued to spread and resulted in an estimated 100,000 deaths on the island before eventually subsiding.[24] Given the extent of shipping between Hong Kong, Bombay, and Calcutta, it was only a matter of time before plague, carried by stowaway rats and their fleas, made landfall in India. The date of the arrival of the disease in Calcutta is unclear—it may have been as early as October 1896—but in Bombay the first cases were reported in July and August 1896 from Mandvi, close to the docks, where dead rats were discovered in grain stores and merchants' houses. However, as with influenza in 1918, there was initially confusion about exactly when the disease had arrived in the city, by what route, and whether it was plague at all. The first authenticated case was reported by a Goan practitioner, Dr. A. G. Viegas, on 23 September 1896, but this was greeted with skepticism by health officials reluctant to face the grim truth. Only in October was his diagnosis confirmed.[25]

A hastily convened Bombay Plague Committee announced a raft of 'remedial measures' to check the progress of the disease. These included confinement of plague patients in hospital, house-to-house visitations to locate additional cases, the isolation of infected households, the destruction of infected bedding and clothing, and the flushing out of drains and sewers with seawater and disinfectant to extirpate what was thought (like cholera) to be an infection caused by 'filth,' poverty, overcrowding, and deficient sanitation.[26] The provincial government went further, assigning municipalities wide-ranging powers to disinfect buildings, destroy property, and isolate or hospitalize plague suspects (see figs. 2 and 3).[27] From 79 plague deaths in the city in September, the figure rose to 313 in October, and over a thousand in December 1896. In April 1897 it was rashly believed that the epidemic might be over (a recurring delusion in the history of Indian epidemics), but it returned with renewed vigor and by the end of that year more than 11,000 plague deaths had been recorded. Officials suspected the actual total was much larger.[28]

To the savagery of the disease was added the violence of a regime in sanitary overdrive. In targeting bodies and dwellings rather than the disease itself (of which little was at first understood), attempts by the state and by municipal authorities to control plague and curb its spread led to an upsurge of protests, demonstrations, and riots. On 10 October 1896, a crowd of angry millworkers besieged Bombay's Arthur Road Infectious Diseases Hospital (perceived as a place where people were sent only to die or be killed) and threatened its staff. On 29 October, nearly a thousand millhands, 'that ever-present source of danger' in the eyes of the authorities, attacked the same hospital after a woman worker had been taken there as a plague suspect.[29] Again, on 9 March 1898, weavers from the Julaha community, migrants from North India, blocked the hospitalization of a twelve-year-old girl from their community who had shown plague symptoms. In the resulting fracas a magistrate was injured and buildings set alight.[30] These episodes captured the intensity of working-class hostility to enforced segregation and compulsory hospitalization. Fueled by rumor, driven by fears for personal safety, provoked by suspicion of the authorities, plague riots became one of the characteristics of the epidemic. They were certainly not the only reaction, for, as historians have shown, there was no single Indian response to plague; and yet such incidents articulated the way in which the disease, and more especially authoritarian attempts to contain it, generated bitter conflict and a deep questioning of state authority.[31]

Plague was on the cusp of becoming a global pandemic, not just an Indian epidemic. The first nine international sanitary conferences had been primarily concerned with cholera; now attention shifted to plague. The tenth conference, which opened in Venice in February 1897, was dominated by alarming reports of plague's arrival in India and delegates sought assurance that the authorities there would impose strict measures to prevent its onward spread.[32] As plague was still thought of as being transmitted through the movement of people and commodities, a convention was agreed requiring immediate action to be taken, principally with respect to India's ports and maritime trade. This was backed up with the threat of an embargo on all goods leaving India by sea. Since the 1860s the Government of India had gradually ratcheted up measures for the control of cholera, smallpox, and other contagious diseases, including legislation to bring India's maritime passenger traffic under closer sanitary surveillance. Pressure from the international conferences in the early 1890s had added weight to this momentum, but in 1897 existing measures no longer appeared sufficient. Rattled, even before the Venice conference met, by the scale of plague deaths, the Indian government responded with a rapidity and forcefulness that were surprising given its previous reluctance to act more vigorously against cholera. That plague had 'taken root in Bombay' and was surfacing elsewhere, in Karachi and Poona, was certainly concerning, but the existential threat to India's overseas trade was even more compelling. The viceroy's council concluded in January 1897 that 'for the safeguarding of our commerce the Government must be prepared to take steps to allay the fears of other nations.'[33]

The upshot—the Epidemic Diseases Act of 4 February 1897—was one of the most draconian pieces of sanitary legislation ever enacted in British India and, in terms of India's public health history, one of the most momentous measures ever adopted.[34] Reintroduced in 2020 to combat Covid-19, it also provides one of the most telling parallels between the government's handling of the plague pandemic of the 1890s and that of the coronavirus of more recent times. The Act's 'wide and summary powers' gave the government authority to override existing laws whenever they were deemed inadequate to prevent an outbreak or the spread of an infectious disease. It authorized the inspection of any ship, leaving or entering an Indian port, and the detention of any of its passengers and crew; the inspection of passengers traveling by rail or any other means; and the 'segregation, in hospital, temporary accommodation or otherwise, of persons suspected by the inspecting officer of being infected with any such disease.' Pilgrimages could be halted, fairs and festivals banned. Disobeying the Act was a criminal offence, but no legal redress could be had against anyone operating under the Act. Although intended to sanction anti-plague measures, the Act did not specify plague alone: it could, in theory, be deployed against any epidemic disease.[35] In this authoritarian Act, with its disregard for individual rights, one can glimpse something deeper—the increasing interventionism of the colonial state, the expansion of its public health ambitions, and a growing predilection for regulatory measures and coercive control.

And yet, despite this drastic step and the blanket measures it enabled, there was much uncertainty not only concerning the nature of plague and the manner of its transmission but also as to who were the main victims of the disease and why. It was evident in Bombay that the more affluent classes suffered least: Europeans, Parsis, and high-caste Hindus were far less likely to catch plague and die from it than the lower castes. Mortality figures revealed the skewed nature of the epidemic, with one in every eight plague deaths among millworkers (even though many had already quit the city). The poorer classes 'suffered most severely,' it was acknowledged, and this race–class–caste distinction was soon broadly replicated across India.[36] Moreover, in many parts of India plague rode on the back of dearth and the violent inroads of hunger. The early plague years saw some of the deadliest famine mortality in colonial India's entire history: the time of plague was a time of famine.[37] In Bombay city in 1896–7 plague operations and famine relief measures overlapped, with almost 52,000 people, mostly from the poorest Hindu and Muslim communities, on relief between August and November 1897.[38] During the first year of the epidemic, between October 1896 and September 1897, on average 2 million people a day across India were on relief works, rising at times to 4 million. In 1899 the monsoons again failed, and in that and the following year as many as 4 million people died from hunger-related causes in British India and the princely states.[39] Pandemic plague had recruited a deadly local ally.

It was, though, not the poor alone who sickened and died. Bombay was India's richest city and yet it suffered proportionately more than any other urban center, more even than Calcutta, a city of comparable size and equally insanitary conditions. For some officials, plague was also a disease of the itinerant grain and cloth traders whose merchandise helped spread the disease or who lived in hazardous proximity to infected grain stores and cloth depots. These were among plague's earliest victims, at Mandvi, close to the Bombay docks, in 1896–7.[40] And were women more at risk than men? Some administrators certainly thought so. As the census commissioner for

Bihar and Orissa later remarked: 'The habits of women expose them much more to the attacks of the rat flea than do those of the men; they live less in the open air, they go barefooted, they sweep the floors and handle the grain, they nurse the sick and assemble round the corpses for the purposes of mourning just at the time when there is the greatest risk of infection.' He concluded, 'Wherever ... there is plague there is likely to be heavy female mortality.'[41] In terms of race, class, and gender, plague appeared highly discriminatory. If this was a pandemic, it was far from treating everyone alike. And yet, in theory, the Epidemic Diseases Act was applicable to everyone.

On the Move

Plague was on the move, setting both people and pathogens in motion. From its epicenter in Bombay city, the disease swept rapidly outward, along the lines of road and rail and through the panicked flight of urban populations. By the end of 1896 there had been 2,086 deaths from plague across the Bombay Presidency: this figure rose sharply to 46,944 in 1897, and 86,191 in 1898. In 1899 there were 15,874 plague deaths in Bombay city, but 96,596 across the whole province.[42] Moreover, plague was beginning to settle into a recurring temporal pattern, dying away one year only to resume a year or two later during what was coming to be recognized, with some resignation, as 'the plague season.' The contagion was becoming entrenched not just in towns and cities but increasingly in the countryside. Intended to contain the epidemic and allay mounting public disquiet, the measures taken in Bombay had the opposite effect. As fear of the disease, and still more of the state's sanitary and medical measures, took hold, Bombay citizens took to flight (see fig. 4). In what the colonial authorities dubbed a 'wild unreasoning panic,' a huge exodus occurred: thousands quit the city in October and November 1896 to return to their home villages or seek safety upcountry. By late January 1897, an estimated 378,900 people had quit Bombay, more than a third of the population. Karachi witnessed a similar exodus: almost a quarter of its 105,000 inhabitants had fled by late January 1897.[43] The city didn't seem safe. It was better to be elsewhere.

In scenes again familiar during India's national lockdown in March 2020, Bombay's railroad stations in late 1896 thronged with people who were desperate to escape the pestilence, or evade sanitary measures, or who, because of the loss of their employment, were left without money, work, or any means of subsistence. As one official put it:

> While the panic was at its height and the exodus in full flow, the scenes at the railway stations were striking—a motley crowd of natives of every caste and creed pressing and shouting for tickets, and then, as the train steamed in[,] a hurrying anxious throng, old and young alike tottering under enormous bundles of household goods. As special after special left the station, the relics of the disappointed crowd sooner than miss the next opportunity would settle down to sleep on the platforms. The busy scenes at the station stood out in marked contrast to the quietness of Bombay; whole streets of shops were closed, business was paralysed and the desolate emptiness of thoroughfares ordinarily teeming with life was most remarkable.[44]

In many instances, however, the plague refugees simply carried the disease with them. Railroad passengers (or their clothes and chattels) bore the disease north into Gujarat and Rajasthan, east into Central India, the North-Western Provinces, and Bengal; plague pushed south to Poona, Hyderabad, and the southern Deccan, infecting princely states as well as British provinces. The disease first erupted in Mysore in August 1898: by mid-January 1899, there had been 10,000 plague deaths in the state, 6,000 of them in Bangalore.[45]

The spread of plague not only transports us from the cities to village India; it also gives us insights into how the disease arrived and became lodged in a given locality. In late November 1899 a Julaha weaver named Khizir, having been discharged from the mills in Bombay, traveled by train to Allahabad and then on to his home village, Mau Aima, twenty miles away. He was accompanied by his son Faizu and daughter Sungri. The village had a population of 6,000: many Indian villages were similarly large and with closely packed houses, conditions in which rats, fleas, and the plague they transmitted could thrive as easily as in any city slum or tenement.

Unfortunately, Khizir and his family, who appeared healthy on their arrival, brought plague with them to Mau Aima and the telltale buboes began to appear. Faizu died on 4 December, several other deaths quickly followed, and soon the whole village and its outlying hamlets were infected. Some residents had already fled. But it was only at the very end of December that the deteriorating situation attracted the attention of Allahabad's civil surgeon, who then ordered the removal of the sick to a makeshift hospital, the isolation of contacts, and the disinfection or destruction of infected houses. Three weeks later the entire settlement was evacuated. No further cases were reported after mid-May 1900, and villagers were allowed to return home. In this instance, villagers and landowners appear to have fully cooperated with the health authorities, perhaps because they could see for themselves the inroads the disease was making. But in all, of the 156 plague cases reported in Mau Aima only 35 recovered; 121 died.[46]

Infection, flight, evacuation, death: these were scenes repeated across much of India during the early plague years, and they unleashed an extraordinary experiment in sanitary surveillance and state control. In Punjab, for instance, the epidemic began in August 1897, when a Brahmin returning from Hardwar brought plague to the village of Khatkar Kalan. First, members of the Brahmin community sickened and died; then the disease spread to other castes and nearby villages. Plague was officially confirmed in October 1897 and by the end of that month there had already been 72 cases and 39 deaths. The authorities began an unprecedented inspection of homes and villages, seeking out plague suspects and victims, ordering the evacuation of infected villages or *mohallas* (sections of towns), removing entire populations to specially constructed plague camps, establishing police cordons, and setting up makeshift hospitals. In some instances, officials encountered resistance. At Garhshankar in April 1898 the police opened fire on protesters opposed to evacuation: 9 villagers were killed and 35 wounded. According to Punjab's deputy sanitary commissioner, 'the incident, regrettable though it was, had a marvellous salutary effect.' The 'affray' became a 'turning point in the plague operations,' and the authorities consoled themselves with the thought that the deaths from the police firing were 'small compared to what the mortality from plague would have been had those severe measures not been taken.'[47]

Plague was undoubtedly a story of colonialism as state violence, incorporating and extending existing administrative practices of coercion and confinement.[48] But it was also a story of Indian agency, a narrative of Indian, rather than colonial, life and death. The investigation into plague cases and routes of infection wove a rich tapestry of human life and local incident—who visited which relative when and why, who worked for whom and in what capacity, who traveled to which market or shrine, who received the dead person's clothes, who evaded the police cordon by bribing guards, who snitched on their neighbor for concealing corpses or sheltering the sick. Europeans dictated policy and assumed overall charge, but it was Indian assistant surgeons and hospital attendants who routinely carried out plague operations on the ground, negotiated with villagers, tended the sick and dying, doled out medicines, compiled statistics, drew maps of villages and *mohallas*, and helped author the official narratives in which their names were barely even mentioned (fig. 5). Then, too, there were the village Chamars, the 'untouchables' who performed the dangerous work of disinfection and corpse removal and who, not infrequently, paid for it with their own lives.[49]

The modern modes of transport—the steamships and railroads—that facilitated the spread of disease were also enlisted as instruments of surveillance and control. Passengers on steamers departing from Bombay, Karachi, Calcutta, and other ports were systematically stopped and searched—whether they were pilgrims bound for Jeddah or coolies embarking for Burma. In February 1897, the Government of India suspended the *hajj* from Indian ports.[50] In Bombay in 1899, 65,822 vessels were checked, and 1.2 million passengers and crew examined.[51] The Venice convention required that medical checks on ships should include the physical examination of every traveler immediately prior to departure. Passengers were made to stand in line at the dockside to be individually checked for plague symptoms—a high temperature and lymph node swellings. 'They open their body clothing,' it was reported, 'and a Medical Officer feels each man's chest with both hands, which enables him to detect any increase of temperature. The superficial glands in the neck, armpits, and groins are then examined. The tongue and eyes are looked at.' If any suspicious signs were detected, the passenger was detained and subjected to a more thorough examination.[52]

A particular fear was that rail passengers leaving Bombay would transport the disease across the subcontinent to Calcutta (where it was finally confirmed as having arrived in April 1898). At inspection stations along the main routes thousands of travelers were stopped and examined (fig. 6). At Kalyan on the Great Indian Peninsula Railway 3,320 people were scrutinized on trains leaving Bombay, though of these only 234 were found to have plague. As the disease seeped into eastern India, inspection stations were established on the East Indian Railway, the largest at Khanna on the Delhi–Howrah line. The scale of these inspections is staggering, especially given the poverty of their achievement. By September 1898, nearly 1.2 million passengers had been examined at inspection stations in Bengal. Of the 17,994 detained, only 7 died—none from plague.[53]

This was intervention on a massive, if remarkably unproductive, scale. Rather than imposing order, it encouraged extortion and nurtured resentment. There was a class as well as racial dimension to these inspections. Unless visibly ill, first-class passengers were spared; second-class passengers were examined in their carriages; but third-class passengers were hauled out and examined on the platforms—men and women, in full public view. Officially, at Khanna it had

at no time been the practice to detain all passengers coming from infected areas. Detention under observation has been confined to persons who are regarded as suspicious by reason of their appearance, or symptoms, or the dirty condition of their clothes or effects. It has extended occasionally to persons who could not be easily traced and could not be relied upon to give notice of the occurrence of plague among them, and to emigrants and persons of the coolie class travelling in large bodies.[54]

But, even though 'respectable' Indians were meant to be excluded from this ordeal, many, to their fury, were treated as if they were common coolies, or asked to pay bribes to escape more humiliating treatment. Because so many middle-class lives were affected, personal testimony surfaces through plague to a degree seldom evident with cholera; plague, moreover, occurred at a time of growing nationalist assertion and hardening resentment of colonial rule. Later one of India's foremost revolutionaries, Shyamji Krishnavarma, an Oxford-educated MA, gave a scathing account of his abusive treatment while journeying by train in March 1897, soon after the new sanitary regulations came into force. At Ratlam a European officer, seeing Krishnavarma and his fellow Indians passengers, commanded them

> in a very insulting and imperious tone as if he was ordering a menial servant or a slave 'Come out, come out, I cannot wait for you', although we had not the least idea that it was necessary for us to alight from the carriage for the purpose of medical examination. His dictatorial manner of procedure so much provoked us that we were naturally impelled to ask him 'Is that the way to address a gentleman?'

Krishnavarma reluctantly stepped down from the carriage only to notice that an Englishman, traveling second-class, was examined in his own compartment 'and treated with every consideration,' while he, a first-class passenger, was 'summarily ordered to leave the carriage and roughly handled.' He 'resented this invidious distinction and openly declared that it was a most flagrant case of partiality.' At this, the officer 'became extremely violent and shouted out in a rage that he would have us arrested at once.' Krishnavarma was charged with assaulting a public servant in the execution of his duty, but, as he was not without influence of his own, the charges against him were dropped. Even so, he was left with an abiding sense of grievance.[55] Typically, it was the state's antiplague measures, rather than plague itself, that sparked such intense anger and acute sense of colonial injustice.

Turbulence and Trust

In Hong Kong in 1894, Kitasato Shibasaburo and Alexandre Yersin had identified the plague bacillus, later named *Yersinia pestis* in Yersin's honor. But, as with cholera, miasmatic, environmental, and social interpretations of disease etiology remained influential in India, and the association of plague with Indian bodies and Indian homes largely determined the sites of state intervention and the people and places targeted. A notice issued by the Punjab government in 1898 epitomized this:

> The germ to which plague is due has been described by doctors as a ground germ. It clings to particular buildings and localities, unless it is conveyed at a more rapid rate from place to place in the human body, or in clothing, bedding, rags, hides or skins or other material which fosters it. It is this characteristic of the disease which explains the measures which Government has adopted to stamp it out. The danger lies in infected houses and localities, and in infected clothing, bedding and other articles. It is necessary therefore to separate the sick from the healthy, to exclude all alike from infected houses and localities till complete and scientific disinfection has been carried out, and to disinfect property before access is allowed to it.[56]

A Bengal government resolution issued a month later carried a similar message, contrasting plague with cholera and smallpox as a far more infectious disease. 'Not only was the plague more dangerous than either of those diseases, but its mode of infection was ... more subtle. The dust of floors, the plaster of the walls, every garment of the patients, became a source of plague.'[57] Thus, while at one level bubonic plague had all the weight of a pandemic that could erupt wherever the bacillus happened to be present, in its immediate manifestations it was understood to be profoundly local—residing in rags and old clothing, in walls and floors, in the bodies (alive or dead) of the infected. In Bombay and Karachi the doorposts of houses harboring plague were marked with a cross inside a circle (see fig. 3)—overtones of the London plague of 1665–6 when infected buildings were similarly daubed with a cross. Houses designated 'unfit for human habitation' were demolished, their floors dug up, their contents burned (fig. 3). As these measures intensified, the Indian press began to seethe with reports of homes violated by search parties, property wantonly destroyed, women molested. Even the dead were not immune. As mortality mounted, long delays occurred at cremation grounds and graveyards, with bodies denied burial or the funeral pyre until a doctor had certified the cause of death. Whatever dangers the disease itself might bring, colonial authoritarianism created the greatest sense of grievance and hardship. In that sense, to recall Shklar's distinction between misfortune and injustice, the British were held far more culpable than any disease-causing deity or demon.

Nowhere was hostility more evident than in Poona. Plague had reached this city of 120,000 from Bombay in October 1896, and within weeks large numbers of plague cases, then deaths, were occurring. A medical inspector was appointed to keep watch on passengers arriving from Bombay, but little was at first done to prevent infection. That changed in February 1897. The assistant collector, W. C. Rand of the Indian Civil Service, was appointed to oversee plague operations; his assistant was an army medical officer, W. W. O. Beveridge, previously on plague duty in Hong Kong. Empowered by the Epidemic Diseases Act and believing that, as in Hong Kong, British troops were essential for the enforcement of 'stringent' antiplague measures, Rand brought martial vigor to Poona's plague. Although Indians offered to help, as far as Rand was concerned no 'native agency' was available for this work 'or could be relied on if it were.' Instead, British troops searched Indian homes, looking for suspected plague cases and for corpses hidden to evade burial restrictions. Soldiers enforced the disinfection of buildings and the removal of plague contacts and their families to segregation camps outside the city. In barely two months, between 13 March and 19 May 1897, 218,124 homes were searched, 338 plague cases identified, and 64 corpses removed. Houses in the city center were searched on average eleven times; 2,000 houses were fumigated and 3,000 whitewashed.[58]

Poona was a proud city, once the capital of the Maratha Empire and a center of vocal opposition to colonial rule. Its inhabitants were not disposed to accept such coercive and intrusive measures without demur. Poona was home to Bal Gangadhar Tilak, a prominent Hindu nationalist, whose English and Marathi newspapers published a torrent of complaints about the conduct of British troops, including the violation of prayer rooms and kitchens and the rough treatment meted out to residents, especially women: women entered the plague narrative as much as victims of colonial aggression as of the disease itself. Rand brushed aside such protests, declaring it 'a matter of great satisfaction to the members of the Plague Committee that no credible complaint that the modesty of a woman had been intentionally insulted was ever made either to themselves or to the officers under whom the troops worked.'[59] He further claimed to have made use of 'native gentlemen' to explain 'to the public the objects of the search, to act as interpreters between the soldiers and the public and to point out to the soldiers the portions of houses which custom forbade them to enter.'[60] But that was not how most Indians saw the situation: high-caste Hindus, Brahmins like Tilak, felt insulted and humiliated, their role as leaders contemptuously snubbed. Inspired by Tilak's polemics and convinced that high-caste homes and bodies had been violated, on 22 June 1897 the brothers Damodar and Balkrishna Chapekar shot Rand and his escort.[61] Rand died ten days later. His assassination and its political reverberations became a crucial point of departure for militant nationalism in India. Equally, the slaying of one of its senior officials sent shock waves through the colonial administration. The immediate response was to seek punishment and revenge. The Chapekar brothers were put on trial and executed; Tilak, accused of complicity in their act, was sentenced to eighteen months' imprisonment. But even this momentous episode did not, in the short term, check a regime determined to extirpate this modern plague.

By 1899–1900, however, the government was beginning to waver, fearing that as plague penetrated further into Punjab and the North-Western Provinces such extreme sanitary interventionism was administratively and financially unsustainable and, by inciting unrest, could only prove politically and sanitarily counterproductive. There were plentiful signs of resistance. At Cawnpore on 11 April 1900 an attack on a segregation camp by leatherworkers, millhands, and butchers was provoked by reports of women being detained involuntarily. In sentiments that echoed the Rebellion of 1857–8, rumors, placards, and press reports warned of a violent uprising if the state persisted in its draconian measures.[62] What the British increasingly confronted was a coalition of classes—from the new middle class and the 'martial races' of the north and northwest to Muslim pilgrims denied travel to Mecca and Hindus to their festivals, as well as millworkers, municipal scavengers, and low-status communities like the Chamars and Julahas. Fearing a still-greater political backlash, the British saw no alternative but to retreat from the most provocative antiplague measures and to divide the 'respectable' middle classes from 'turbulent' and 'unruly' lower-caste, working-class communities.

An essential strand in this revised strategy was to grant the middle classes and urban elites privileged status. While coolies continued to be examined and slum dwellings searched and demolished, the homes of the upper castes and well-to-do were spared, their bodies (mostly) exempt from examination at rail inspection points; where their dwelling places were spacious enough, they were permitted to nurse the sick in their own homes and gardens. In fact, even before this, many Indian communities had already shown their capacity for self-reliance and determination to pursue their own antiplague initiatives. Among these responses was the opening of caste or community hospitals, where the 'many intricate questions relating to caste habits, food, religious scruples and other similar difficulties' could be accommodated.[63] While government hospitals filled with millworkers, laborers, and domestic servants, private hospitals, some with less than a dozen beds, catered for the needs of individual communities. Bombay had more than thirty of these, for Parsis, Jews, and Jains, for various Muslim groups, and for higher-caste Hindus, such as Brahmins, Marathas, and Pathare Prabhus.[64] Poona had separate plague hospitals for Muslims, Parsis, and Hindus, the last-mentioned managed by a committee of Brahmins and open to all except low-caste Hindus.[65]

Health officials and colonial administrators now actively sought the cooperation of the Indian elites, the 'native gentlemen' whose help and mediation they had previously spurned. 'It is impossible,' declared W. B. Bannerman, director of Bombay's Plague Research Laboratory in 1904, 'for Government or its officers to influence people to any great extent without their help.'[66] Although this accommodative strategy was primarily intended to give momentum to Western medical and sanitary measures—such as the segregation of the sick and vaccination against plague—it also created space for practitioners of Indian medicine—the *vaids* and *hakims*—to treat plague victims or report cases to the medical authorities. To this equivocal relationship between colonial medicine and the indigenous therapeutic systems there was a long and complex history.[67] Since the early cholera years, Indian physicians had proffered their own medical remedies and treatments, only to be largely dismissed and derided by their British counterparts, who remained confident of the superiority of their own techniques. The plague crisis created an opportunity for *vaids* and *hakims* to gain official recognition, to assert their therapeutic credentials, and highlight the failure of Western medicine to deliver effective treatments.[68] In this more conciliatory spirit the 'local indigenous medical man' was hailed by the Punjab government in 1909 as 'a highly respected individual,' one with 'great local influence with the people, who look to him for guidance in the presence of disease.' Rather than being shunned as ignorant quacks, such people might now 'be employed and entertained by local bodies as plague missionaries with great benefit to the cause.'[69]

By the early 1900s plague policy had moved away from state authoritarianism toward public participation and Indian ownership. Official pronouncements emphasized the primary need for public cooperation, even if this meant that the more 'heroic' forms of sanitary intervention had to be withdrawn and plague might, in consequence, spread further and faster. Here was a very modern public health dilemma. In an epidemic (and potentially pandemic) crisis of this kind, was it better to be *dirigiste* and, for the sake of speed and efficiency, use the full powers of the state to 'get things done'? Or was it ultimately wiser, and more effective, to enlist public participation, even if this was slower to have an impact on the disease and, in the short term, less medically productive? The relaxation of the earlier interventionist policy has been seen as permitting a lapse into administrative apathy and imperial complacency once it was clear that Europe was not threatened by an imminent return of the Black Death.[70] It has been interpreted as paving 'the way for a remarkably laissez-faire attitude to plague over the next two decades, even as it ravaged the Indian countryside killing hundreds of thousands a year.'[71] By contrast, Punjab's *Plague Manual* stated categorically that 'the cardinal principle of all plague administration must be that no pressure or compulsion, in any shape or form, is to be brought to bear on the people.' 'Encouragement, persuasion and the provision of facilities for carrying out the measures advanced' were 'the only legitimate means of influencing and guiding public opinion in the direction desired.' Every effort must be made to win the cooperation of the people, 'to enlist their sympathies and bring home to them through their natural leaders and in any other way that may be practicable, that it rests mainly with themselves to bring about, by their own action, the cessation of plague.'[72] Was this the state shirking its responsibilities or adopting a more sensible and socially inclusive strategy? Certainly, the move to a more community-oriented stance was one that critics of state policy during the Covid pandemic of 2020–1 looked back on with favor and saw as one of the 'lessons' to be learned from the colonial past.

Plague as Experience

According to the medical historian Charles Rosenberg, discussing how historians 'frame' disease, 'We need to know more about the individual experience of disease in time and place, the influence of culture on definitions of disease and of disease in the creation of culture, and the role of the state in defining and responding to disease.'[73] The last of these, for India, is much the most accessible: indeed, the colonial narrative of epidemic and pandemic diseases is so dominant that it often leaves the historian scrambling to find any alternative voice or reliant on scraps of information and opinion that, when read 'against the grain' of the colonial archive, provide an alternative worldview or insight into individual experience.

One of the ways in which the colonial authorities most commonly recorded and represented plague was through statistics. By the late nineteenth century, the regime had become a statistical Raj where the sheer volume of morbidity and mortality data, rather than illuminating suffering and loss, threatened to eclipse the lived experience of epidemics. Statistics created an illusion of orderly, effective rule, smoothing over the jagged confusion and hectic uncertainty that the fear of disease, or alarm over state intrusion, actually created. Statistics constitute their own kind of myth. As Jacqueline Rose remarked with respect to Covid: 'Counting is at once a scientific endeavour and a form of magical thinking. It can be a way of bracing ourselves for and confronting an onslaught, and at the same time a doomed attempt at omnipotence, a system for classifying the horror and bundling it away.'[74]

The volume of data compiled on India's plague exceeded that for any pandemic before it or possibly since. The government published reams of statistics on plague cases and mortality; for over a decade, between 1897 and 1910, each major province maintained its own extensive plague proceedings. Bombay and Calcutta municipalities between them produced eleven reports on plague. What the outside world saw of India's plague was a statistical blizzard—a plethora of detail about how many people died and where, of what caste, age, occupation, and gender; how many were sent to hospitals, confined in segregation camps, inoculated; even how many thousands of potentially plague-carrying rodents were trapped, examined, and incinerated.[75] This data storm communicated to the outside world something of the scale of plague's hold over India and articulated, in numerical terms, one understanding of what a modern pandemic signified. It reassured the authorities in India and international observers that the colonial state was not idle, and that plague was, however slowly, coming under control. But the statistical record was actually far from reassuring. Between 1896 and 1900 plague seeped inexorably eastward into northern and central India. In many of these new locations, in Punjab and Bihar, or the interior districts of the Madras Presidency, it became endemic, erupting epidemically every couple of years.[76] What began as a tidal wave of contagion dissipated into small pools of residual infection, the collection and publication of plague statistics a measure of how a once-feared pandemic had become normalized into bureaucratic routine.

Statistics and the growing volume of medical reports represent only one way of understanding plague and its human impact. There was—by contrast with cholera and later influenza—an unprecedented articulateness about Indians' plague experience. Indians did more than merely cope with plague: in one form or another, they took ownership of it, whether through their active engagement in measures to defeat the contagion or in their hostile response to the shock of state intervention and mismanagement. The advent of plague coincided with an upsurge in nationalist sentiment, which episodes like Rand's assassination further intensified, and the rise of a highly vocal and assertive 'native' press. Newspapers in English and the vernaculars scrutinized official reports and statistics; they hoovered up complaints and recycled rumors; they challenged government policy and pointed the finger of blame at officials. While claiming (if only for fear of censorship) to take a detached view, they eagerly seized upon tales of fear and oppression, weaving them into a dark narrative of discontent. We may now see India's plague years as demonstrating the value of a (relatively) free and outspoken press. But in the colonial view India's 'native press' was inherently irresponsible, guilty of peddling what we might now call 'misinformation' or 'fake news.' 'They habitually fail,' one critic maintained, 'to distinguish between fact and mere rumours, are prone to accept as authentic, and to publish without enquiry, any wild tale, or, as it is termed in India, any piece of "gup" that seems likely to interest their readers and increase their circulation.'[77] But never before had the press shown such an ardent interest in epidemics; never before, except in the growing disquiet over famine, had the government been so consistently held responsible for abusing its subjects and bringing suffering to the people over whom it ruled.[78] Through the press plague was transformed from a calamity—an act of god, perhaps, or a 'natural disaster'—into a cause of hardship and oppression for which the colonial government could be directly blamed. The sense of injustice Judith Shklar described had started to kick in.

Personal testimony, to a degree unmatched in previous epidemics, also played its part. Shyamji Krishnavarma's indignation at his experience on the platform at Ratlam was matched by the fury of the social reformer and educationist Pandita Ramabai, who decried the treatment of women patients in government hospitals. No female nurses attended them, she protested in 1897, and so 'poor Purdah women who would never think of uncovering even their faces before strangers, had to submit to the most repulsive and humiliating treatment by male doctors, and ... be exposed to public gaze.'[79] Plague entered the everyday lives of Indians; for some, for weeks, months, even years, it was their lives, the proximate cause of hardship, the imminent manifestation of encroaching death. But what is also most striking is how many women, like Ramabai, added their voices to the collective disquiet. This, in part, was a reflection of the extent to which women, especially from the middle classes, felt the impact of state intervention—the house searches, the station inspections, the forced hospitalizations that brought the state to their door and into their homes. But this female engagement was also indicative of a new articulateness among women themselves, as they entered higher education, joined the educational and medical professions, organized themselves into committees and societies, or otherwise found a public voice.[80]

Even among women, though, there was no single experience or uniform response. At one extreme stood Sister Nivedita, born Margaret Noble, who shortly before the outbreak of plague had left London to join her spiritual mentor, Swami Vivekananda, in Calcutta. When the contagion struck the city in 1898, Vivekananda issued a 'plague manifesto,' calling on Indians to fight the disease. Through the work of the Ramakrishna Mission he set up in March 1899, and through her own speeches and activism, Nivedita made this cause her own, nursing the sick, and appealing to Indian students to join in combating plague. The epidemic gave Nivedita a novice's insight into Indian suffering and impelled her toward an increasingly critical view of British indifference and colonial neglect.[81]

By contrast, in her Marathi autobiography Lakshmibai Tilak wrote extensively about plague's impact on herself and her family. At first for her, a young Brahmin wife, the disease was only a shadowy presence. She heard of it through family visits to Nashik, where it was spoken of as a 'new disease.' 'The victim would get a couple of lumps in his armpits,' Lakshmibai explained, 'and before you know what was happening he was dead.' Villagers 'panicked when they heard this story.'[82] Soon after, in an incident that echoed Krishnavarma's experience, she was traveling by train with her son Dattu who was suffering a mild fever and she grew anxious at having to leave the carriage at Daund junction to be inspected, fearing he might be suspected of having plague. 'As we got off the train we were cordoned off,' she wrote. 'All the compartments were instantly locked. Before each compartment stood doctors, sepoys and police who created a cordon to hem people in like cattle in a pen. The doctor would examine every passenger and only those who passed were allowed to go ahead.' She was 'very scared,' but, having taken the precaution of cooling Dattu's hands and feet with water beforehand, he passed unhindered. For the moment, they were safe.[83]

Then rats began to appear in her house in Ahmednagar: two rodents nibbled food put out as a ritual offering, then suddenly they spun round and fell dead. 'I had heard a lot about rats dying in this fashion,' Lakshmibai recalled, 'but this was the first time I had seen it.' Her husband immediately pronounced that they were 'plague-carrying rats.' A few months later, after time spent in quarantine, the family returned to Ahmednagar: so too did plague, and again rats began to die. By now plague was on everyone's lips. Dattu was sent to relatives for his protection. But when Lakshmibai's daughter Tara was diagnosed with plague, the Tilaks moved to a segregation camp, where they remained for eighteen harrowing days and nights. Plague raged all around them. It was mid-winter and bitterly cold. 'We were surrounded by the sick,' who in their agony screamed at night and pounded on the walls of the huts. Food and sleep were hard to come by, and of the sick only one in ten survived. 'I thought,' Lakshmibai recalled, 'if Yama [the Hindu god of death] had a kingdom anywhere it had to be here. The place was terrifying, the night was terrifying, the surroundings were terrifying, and the state of my heart was terrifying.'[84]

Tara's death seemed imminent. But Lakshmibai, who had become interested in 'home remedies' and 'native medications,' didn't give up. She put poultices on Tara's fever-racked body and fed her castor oil mixed with sugar and milk. She wrapped her in a blanket with her feet next to the stove. Having done all she could, she told Tara, 'Now you are free to die. I didn't want to feel I had left anything undone.' She was distraught and fully expected her daughter to die, but Tara recovered, and the family was free to leave the camp. But, educated by her plague experiences, Lakshmibai had moved a long way from her Brahmin orthodoxy and high-caste scruples and now felt a duty to serve others. She returned to the camp to help relieve patients' suffering and see that they were properly fed and cared for.[85] Only gradually did the trauma of plague fade from the Tilaks' lives.

Lakshmibai's memoir testifies to how plague burrowed, rat-like, into individual experiences and personal memories. It demonstrates the multiple sites at which plague and antiplague measures were encountered—in the home, at railroad junctions, in hospitals, in segregation camps. Unlike Krishnavarma's, it is not a narrative overtly critical of the colonial regime; rather, it shows one woman's determination to fight the disease through self-help and service to others.

Plague lodged in pictures as well as words. As a means of observing disease and recording its impact and treatment, photography flourished during India's plague years as never before. It was part of what made plague visually modern. Although present in India since the 1830s, photography had rarely been used in relation to disease. But in the 1890s and 1900s the camera was pressed into service to record plague—not only to show the disease's outward physical manifestations, but, more especially, to document the measures taken to contain the contagion and minister to the sick. Suddenly, there was an abundance of photographs showing graveyards and burning-grounds stacked with corpses; the interior of plague hospitals and segregation camps; plague committees touring streets and inspecting homes; Indians being inoculated against plague (see figs. 7 and 8). Photography archived the experience of plague, but, even though Indian as well as European professional photographers were employed to capture plague scenes (like Karachi's R. Jhalbhoy), it did so largely from a Western perspective.[86] Photographs helped fix plague in the public memory; because they are easily accessed and for the dramatic scenes they represent, the images were widely reproduced in the Indian media during the Covid pandemic of 2020–1. They illustrated, though, not so much the horror of plague (fig. 9) as the rigor of colonial medical and sanitary intervention; more than the suffering of victims, they showed European doctors and nurses ministering to the Indian sick (figs. 10, 11, and 12).[87] If reminiscences and memoirs shed light on Indian agency and anger, photographs, by contrast, reinforced an idea of Indians' dependence on state aid and Christian succor. This was not quite the 'king's touch' or the iconography of Napoleon in the pesthouse at Jaffa, but there was a family resemblance. Further, photographs (along with postcards and sketches of plague scenes published in illustrated newspapers) gave India's stricken plight and remedial measures an international presence. Here was an important ingredient in modern pandemicity—the ability to document pictorially disease and disease control almost as it happened and thousands of miles away. For as long as international fear persisted, India's plague made global photographic fare.

The Vaccine Controversy

As with cholera, one of the elements common to all four of the diseases discussed in this book is inoculation—the hunt for an effective vaccine and the claims made for its efficacy and ownership. To vaccine strategy in India there were three broad considerations. Could a suitable vaccine be made, would it work, and could it be produced on a sufficiently large scale? Would it be acceptable to the Indian population? And what part should the state play in developing, delivering, and taking responsibility for a vaccine?

Early on in the plague epidemic, in October 1896, the Government of India sent for Waldemar Haffkine, who had already demonstrated the effectiveness of his anticholera prophylactic. He set up a small laboratory in Bombay and began experimenting with a vaccine made from heat-treated plague bacilli. The results were encouraging: Haffkine tested the vaccine on himself in January 1897 and then trialed it on volunteers, including prisoners in Bombay's Byculla jail. Haffkine was convinced that mass inoculation against plague was 'the only measure known to science' for effectively combating the disease and asserted that its value had been shown by 'accurate observations and measured in an unmistakable manner.'[88] But, as with his anticholera vaccine, senior figures in the Indian Medical Service (IMS) remained unconvinced. The director-general of the service, Robert Harvey, insisted that the method Haffkine employed was only 'hypothetical,' its effectiveness unproved. For the present, 'the process is too crude and imperfect to justify any [use of] compulsion on the part of Government.' The operation was admittedly painless but could cause a high temperature and local irritation. 'This,' Harvey concluded, 'makes people shy of undergoing inoculation unless they have something to gain by it, and the fear of plague is in many instances insufficient to overcome these objections.' In his judgment, the sanitary measures already adopted were a better option.[89] A few months later, in July 1898, Harvey, now the Government of India's sanitary commissioner, repeated his skepticism. The question was 'not one of theory, but of practical administrative experience,' he declared, and experience had already shown that fear of inoculation could 'drive the people to frenzy.' Unless 'universally accepted,' inoculation could have little value in controlling plague: it was 'idle to dream of an alien government successfully imposing universal inoculation on the people of India.'[90]

Popular resistance seemed to endorse Harvey's doubts. In Calcutta in May 1898 rumor was rife that inoculation was going to be made compulsory; there were attacks on supposed inoculators, at least one of them fatal.[91] Inoculation was rumored to cause 'instantaneous death,' impotence, or sterility. Tales circulated in Punjab that 'the needle was a yard long; you died immediately after the operation; you survived the operation six months and then collapsed; men lost their virility and women became sterile; the Deputy Commissioner himself underwent the operation and expired half an hour afterwards in great agony.'[92] That such rumors were incorporated into official reports can be taken as evidence less of the extent of popular opposition than of administrators' readiness to believe in Indians' irrational beliefs and superstitious nature, and yet they resonate with opposition to inoculation in the subcontinent to this day and, indeed, among anti-vaxxers around the world. A century on, it might seem, not much has changed.

However, there were indications that the prophylactic was not only effective but acceptable to most Indians. Whatever India's sanitary commissioner might think, provincial governments turned to inoculation as one of the few effective tools at their disposal. In Punjab the lieutenant-governor authorized a program to immunize two-thirds of the population within six months: this required Haffkine's vaccine to be manufactured on a scale unprecedented at the time, 70,000 doses a day. The campaign began well, with 232,000 individuals inoculated between May and the end of September 1900 and half a million by the close of the 1903 vaccination season.[93] Then disaster struck. On 30 October 1902, in the village of Mulkowal a botched inoculation resulted in the death from tetanus of nineteen people. This 'mishap' was probably due to the carelessness of the European inoculator, Dr. Elliot, in using contaminated forceps to open a vaccine vial, but the immediate blame fell on Haffkine for failing to ensure the safety of vaccine production in his Bombay laboratory. The Mulkowal incident gave fresh fuel to critics of the vaccine and those who harbored a personal animus against Haffkine as a Russian Jew and an outsider to India's medical establishment. It was years before he could clear his name.[94] Haffkine has been hailed as the 'forgotten pioneer' of vaccine technology in India, but his achievement came at great personal cost.[95]

Inoculation has served—in the colonial past as in recent historiography—as an index of what India could achieve in terms of mass prophylaxis and as evidence for the rationality (or otherwise) of a population confronted with a deadly disease. How great a setback then were the deaths in Punjab? Pratik Chakrabarti observed that 'the negative impact of the Mulkowal incident featured much more strongly in colonial official minds than it did among the villagers of the Punjab.' Strikingly, there continued to be a strong demand for inoculation in Punjab when, after a brief suspension, it resumed in January 1903.[96] That said, though, one of the reasons for the formation of a Sanitary Association in Bombay in 1904 was to persuade middle-class Indians that plague inoculation was safe despite the 'Mulkowal disaster.'[97] Even in Punjab, the provincial plague manual listed several measures—quarantine, evacuation, disinfection, rat destruction—ahead of Haffkine's prophylactic and stressed that inoculation was only effective for six months.[98]

W. B. Bannerman, who succeeded Haffkine as director of the Bombay plague laboratory, declared in 1905 that inoculation was 'the most efficient, the cheapest, and most practical measure that can be adopted.' And yet, he added, it was 'essentially a state measure.'[99] Haffkine's vaccines against cholera and plague enabled the Government of India to show that it was meeting its international commitment to combat diseases that loomed large in the global pandemic imagination. However, while inoculation offered a short-term fix, it did not prevent plague, like cholera, from remaining endemic in India, nor did it resolve the problems—poverty, malnutrition, overcrowding, deficient sanitation—that underlay its continuing presence. When plague began to fade out in India in the 1920s it is unlikely that inoculation was solely, perhaps even primarily, responsible. The absence of famine was one factor; improving health education and facilities another. Fabian Hirst's perhaps overly negative conclusion was that the long-term decline of plague was probably due not to inoculation but to a decline in the 'aggressive power' of the pathogen and the rise of herd immunity among rodents.[100]

The Plague Effect

Plague gave a much-needed boost to medical science and scientific research in India. For years, the colonial medical establishment had proved itself cautious and conservative, out of touch with, even openly hostile to, modern medical advances. The opening phases of the plague pandemic seemed to reinforce this position: there was reluctance from many in the IMS to embrace the new science of bacteriology or see the value of Haffkine's prophylactic. The habitual emphasis on Indian exceptionalism persisted as medical and sanitary officers blamed India and Indians for harboring yet another 'filth' disease. The 'unreasoning panic' of the early plague years was replaced by what colonial observers identified as Indians' 'resignation' or 'fatalism.'[101] However, the combination of international pressure and local crisis obliged the colonial authorities to shed their inertia and embrace modern medical science. International concern did not end with the Venice convention of 1897. Several countries sent their own investigative commissions to Bombay; India, the main or at least most immediate source of plague infection, was also the principal site for its scientific investigation. Britain's own plague commission, which reported in 1901, examined the cause and nature of plague outbreaks, the manner of the disease's transmission, possible measures for its containment, and the effectiveness of prophylactics. The commission confirmed bubonic plague as a bacillary infection and its origin as a rat epizootic transmitted to humans by fleas, a connection previously demonstrated by the French Pasteurian Jean-Louis Simond in India in 1898.[102]

The rat-flea theory was at first contested. In 1898 an official publication stated that the role of rats was unclear 'but it is certainly not so common a cause of infection as the sick person and his [sic] surroundings.' That position had so far changed ten years later that it was emphatically stated that plague epidemics among humans were 'solely attributable' to rat epizootics.[103] In 1905 the Government of India set up a specialist bacteriology unit which rapidly morphed into a separate research department. Along with other breakthroughs, such as Ronald Ross's discovery in 1897 of the role of anopheles mosquitoes in human malaria, plague stimulated fresh interest in laboratory science, in medical entomology, and in immunology. From a place of relative obscurity and riding the international wave of investment in tropical medicine, India's medical establishment gained world renown and became a dynamic center for innovative research.[104] This was a remarkable turnaround. Before the 1890s laboratory science had received scant professional support or state funding. Plague helped change that. And even though in the racial hierarchy of colonial science, senior research posts were reserved for Europeans, Indians working on plague, as well as on cholera and other infectious diseases, firmly established their own scientific credentials. Among them, S. S. Sokhey at the Haffkine Institute in Bombay, C. G. Pandit at the King Institute in Madras, and S. C. Seal at Calcutta's All-India Institute of Hygiene and Public Health played a crucial role in investigating the etiology and ecology of plague. Here was another kind of ownership, one whose legacy extended into Indian public health administration long after independence.

* * *

Epidemics, Adam Kucharski has argued, have four stages: a spark, a period of rapid growth, a peak, and a slow decline.[105] Plague had an abrupt beginning in Bombay in 1896: this was the spark. From there the contagion penetrated to other towns and cities in western India and then spread further into northern and central India: 1897–1900 was a period of persistent growth. The third stage, the

India-wide peak, came between 1901 and 1907. This was the time when plague seemed most threatening—to India and to the world. Thereafter, plague's decline was stubbornly slow. Once established in town and country, plague showed a frustrating tendency to remain and resurface; it did not pass with the lightning rapidity of influenza in 1918–19. Only in the 1940s and 1950s, with DDT to kill fleas and antibiotics to treat patients, was plague finally forced into retreat.[106] Moreover, the distribution of plague deaths across India was very uneven. Of 12 million fatalities between 1896 and 1930, three-quarters occurred in just three provinces—Bombay (2.4 million), the United Provinces (2.9 million), and Punjab (3.5 million). The Madras Presidency, by contrast, escaped relatively lightly, though still suffered a quarter of a million deaths between 1901 and 1942.[107]

Why did India have so many deaths? Why did it suffer so disproportionately to other parts of the world that over 90 percent of all deaths during the third pandemic happened in this one country? There are no easy answers, but there are clues. Like cholera before it, the dissemination and survival of plague in India were favored by patterns of human activity—by densely populated cities, towns, even villages, where a large number of susceptible humans were repeatedly exposed to infection; by the constant movement of people, accentuated by flight; by the storage and transportation of cotton, cloth, and grain, which provided conducive media for rats and their fleas; and by homes and workplaces where rats lived, largely unhindered, alongside people. Socio-economic conditions assisted the spread and recurrence of the disease: poor sanitation in the slums and tenements of Bombay; the drought and famine that lethally coexisted with plague in the 1890s and 1900s. And, finally, though the colonial administration eventually developed reasonably effective tools to combat plague and the science to support them, the initial impact of British measures was highly counterproductive— flushing out drains and demolishing houses, for example, simply encouraged infected rats to migrate further afield. Wholesale coercion prompted flight from the cities; it made the population, even when not actively hostile, reluctant to comply with sanitary measures. At times the colonial authorities appeared more anxious to assuage international alarm and to uphold their own authority than to grapple with seemingly intractable domestic health issues.

Research in India also showed that the ecology of plague was extremely complex. It was affected by a wide range of variables—by season and climate, temperature, rainfall, and humidity, by the storage and movement of the grain on which rats fed, by the proximity to human habitation of specific kinds of rodents (principally black rats) and their fleas. In western and northern India the 'Oriental rat flea,' *Xenopsylla cheopis*, proved a highly effective vector for the transmission of the plague bacillus from rodents to humans. However, *X. cheopis* was not widely found in southern and eastern India, which helps to explain why those areas were far less affected by plague.[108] Moreover, this species of flea was not native to India. It may have arrived in India from Egypt only in the second half of the nineteenth century, with the opening of the Suez Canal, possibly with imported cargoes of raw cotton; once again, India's links with the Middle East, rather than with East Asia, suggest a possible plague connection. Where the history of cholera encourages us to look at one set of environmental relationships, a triangulation between bacillus, water, and the human uses of water, plague invites us to consider another kind of three-sided history—one where extended contact between humans, rodents, and insects resulted in species-crossing epidemics. In this we can discern echoes of an ancient relationship between animal or insect diseases and settled human populations, a story as old perhaps as the Neolithic revolution, crop farming, and the domestication of animals. But in the modern world, in the age of globalization, that animal–insect–human nexus has intensified and spawned not just local contagions but also the threat, if not always the reality, of a worldwide pandemic.

4

WAR FEVER

In the age of Covid-19 there appeared—to the historically minded—
much that was 'eerily and unpleasantly familiar' from the Spanish
Flu pandemic of 1918–19.[1] The terrifyingly rapid and seemingly
unstoppable spread of viral infection; the scenes of profound
distress, engulfing grief, and mass mortality; the despairing search
for remedies, for medicines, vaccines, and hospital beds; the
struggle of overstretched and exhausted doctors and nurses to
cope with escalating numbers of seriously ill patients; the desperate
pleas and panicked responses of governments; the fear, anger, and
bewilderment of entire populations—all these seemed closely to
mirror, if not exactly to replicate, the devastating influenza pandemic
that swept the globe almost exactly a century earlier. In the time of
the coronavirus, the history of past pandemics, and the specter of
1918–19 in particular, returned to haunt and horrify the present.

Once overlooked, 'lost,' or 'forgotten,' the Spanish Flu has now
come to occupy a prominent place in the annals of pandemicity.[2] No
modern pandemic has given rise to so many 'worst-case scenarios,'
alarming prophecies, and worrying analogies. Like its epidemiological
avatar Covid-19, this, too, was a deadly viral infection; like Covid,
this, too, ravaged the world and left millions dead or bereaved. But
recognition of the exceptional potency of influenza—its lethality,

its transmissibility, its global propensities—did not begin in 1918. It came much earlier. In his *Handbook of Geographical and Historical Pathology* in the 1880s, August Hirsch singled out the disease as having all the characteristics of 'a true pandemic.' Influenza, he observed, occupied 'an exceptional place' among all known contagious diseases: 'no other of them has ever shown so pronounced a pandemic character as influenza.' And, to support his claim, he listed fifteen pandemics between 1510 and 1875, including some which had brought destruction to the Americas as well as wreaking havoc in the Old World. Here, almost uniquely in his view, was a disease capable of traversing 'the whole inhabited globe.'[3]

Russian Flu

As if in fulfillment of Hirsch's dire prognostications, in 1889–92 influenza swept the globe in a manner that, with hindsight, can be seen as a pathogenic dress rehearsal for the far more devasting pandemic of 1918–19. Although it was dubbed the 'Russian Flu,' it was clear to medical experts at the time that Russia was not the most likely source of this pandemic, which may have had its origins in China or the Mongolian steppes. The contagion was, however, first identified as it rampaged across the Russian Empire—much as the 'Spanish Flu' of 1918 was so named only because it was first reported in neutral Spain (at a time of censorship among the warring great powers) and not because it originated there. The need to ground pandemics in a particular place and time, and so to shift blame onto others, has been a recurring theme of their globality, often distracting from the more immediate reasons why, whatever a contagion's origins, some societies have proved far more susceptible than others.

In the late 1880s and early 1890s it was possible by means of postal communications and telegraph services, through newspaper columns and official reports, to plot with some precision the course of the disease as it moved across Russian Siberia into eastern Europe, then on to London, Paris, and New York. More than any disease before it, even cholera, this was recognized by contemporaries, even as it happened, as a pandemic.[4] Influenza may not have been a new disease, as Hirsch had reminded his readers, but, even in an age of rapid advances in medical science, it proved impossible to check. Quarantine measures were of little avail, and as many as one million people died worldwide. Gradually, of its own accord, as the pool of susceptible hosts shrank, or possibly as the virus mutated into a less infective form, the pandemic faded away. Like Alexander the Great, it had no more worlds to conquer.

British India was not immune to the 'mysterious Russian disease,' but it arrived there relatively late, in January 1890, and attracted little attention at the time. This after all, unlike still-rampant cholera, was a contagion for which India could not be blamed. The disease appears, though, to have been fairly widespread: like the Spanish Flu in 1918, it almost certainly entered India through the port of Bombay, with the disembarkation of British troops, who then passed it on to upcountry military stations. Influenza sped across northern India, infecting Delhi and Lucknow and penetrating as far as Calcutta. In Bombay business activity was temporarily suspended; apart from soldiers, factory hands, office workers, schoolchildren and prisoners were struck down but remarkably few deaths were recorded.[5] Only a handful of accounts of the Russian Flu in India were published. It generated little statistical data and, once the pandemic peak had passed, influenza largely disappeared from the medical literature. In the 1890s, and especially with the advent of plague only a few years later, India had many more deadly and persistent diseases to ponder. If there were lessons to be learned, nobody learned them. It was only with the hindsight of 1918 that commentators scrolled back to the earlier influenza episode and recognized in it something 'strikingly similar' to the Spanish Flu.[6]

The Measure of Mortality

By contrast with Russian Flu, the impact of the 1918–19 influenza epidemic on India was utterly devastating. Upwards of 12 million people, possibly as many as 18 or 20 million, died from influenza or from associated pneumonia and respiratory complications. A conspicuous trait of this runaway pandemic was its exceptionally high mortality rate, ranging five to twenty times higher than during a normal influenza season. As with the coronavirus pandemic of 2020–1, virtually no country was left unscathed by the Spanish Flu, but India, along with other colonial or semi-colonial territories, bore the brunt of the disease. Its death-toll was much the highest for any single country, some recent surveys suggesting that as much as 45 percent of the entire global mortality (now thought to be in excess of 40 million people) occurred in India. This mortality was equivalent to between 4 and 6 percent of the entire population of around 320 million, a much higher figure than in Europe and North America where it was generally less than 1.5 percent.[7] In some parts of India—Bombay, the Central Provinces, the United Provinces, and Punjab—mortality edged close to 10 percent. Influenza was no more 'democratic' than the preceding pandemics. As many people (915,000) died in India's Central Provinces as in Britain and the United States combined (approximately 228,000 and 650,000 respectively). By some accounts, though there are no reliable data to confirm this, more than half of all Indians were infected with the virus. Moreover, the impact of the disease was fierce, immediate, and unavoidable. Seldom in the history of Indian epidemics before Covid-19 was eyewitness testimony so eloquent about the pervasiveness of a disease and the suffering it caused.

In India, where the great majority of people still lived in villages, this was a largely rural affliction. One observer, reporting from coastal Maharashtra in early October 1918 at the height of the pandemic, wrote: 'Every village I came in contact with or had reason to hear of had its same story of a large proportion of its inhabitants sick—commonly I should think the greater proportion and often two-thirds, and each village had its considerable toll of deaths.' He (or she) continued: 'What strikes one about it is its sudden—almost instantaneous—universality over whole tracts of country at once. One cannot remember any epidemic where effects were so simultaneous in all places at once—it penetrating into even every small village seemingly.'[8] Cities were not spared, however. In Delhi, since 1912 the capital of British India, three-quarters of the population were affected. 'Delhi [is] in the throes of a horrible attack of influenza,' the chief commissioner wrote to the viceroy on 19 October 1918. '[It is] very fatal when neglected. Yesterday's deaths amounted to 264. Nearly everyone is down with it.'[9] Calcutta, too, was 'like a city of the dead.'[10]

Globally, the pandemic caused by the H1N1 virus is thought of having occurred in three waves: the first roughly from March to August 1918, the second from late August to December, and the third from early 1919 until about May that year. But, like the history of cholera pandemics, this chronology does not map precisely onto the South Asian experience and the subcontinent's wide regional variations: the first (or, as some epidemiologists would now term it, 'herald') wave did not commence until mid-June in Bombay, reaching Calcutta and Madras in late July; the second started in Bombay in mid-September, reaching its climax in Calcutta in late November; and the weaker third wave shattered into a series of local outbreaks that lasted, with diminishing effect, into 1920.[11] Globally, influenza traveled mainly by sea. The Indian epidemic began with the arrival of infected troopships at Bombay and Karachi in May–June 1918, with early cases in Bombay reported, as with plague in 1896, close to the docks. In this first wave older people proved especially vulnerable to infection, but mortality rates remained low. In Bombay in early July it was reported that the 'Spanish Sickness' was 'not ordinarily dangerous to life,' even if it was a 'sharp tax upon the aged and the very young.' Later that month it was predicted that the epidemic was nearly over.[12] The mildness of this initial phase and the low fatality rate fed the hubristic assumption that there was little to be feared from the disease (as with the Russian Flu thirty years earlier), leaving both the public and the medical profession unprepared for the devastation that followed.

From October to early December 1918, as the virus morphed into a more deadly and contagious form, India was struck by a second, far more lethal wave of the disease.[13] Such was its virulence that victims died within days of developing symptoms. The total mortality in India in October 1918, the peak of fatality, was said by one Indian Medical Service (IMS) officer to be 'without parallel in the history of disease.' It is a measure of the greater virulence of the second wave that in Bombay, with a population of just over one million, there were 1,640 deaths in the first phase and nine times as many, 14,678, in the second. In a single day, 6 October 1918, 768 deaths from influenza were recorded in the city, greatly exceeding the highest daily total from plague in the 1890s and 1900s.[14] Across the Bombay Presidency more than a million deaths occurred during October and November 1918, roughly two-thirds (675,222) in October alone.[15] Nasarwanji Hormusji Choksy, medical superintendent at Bombay's Arthur Road hospital, remarked that 'in its rapidity of spread, the enormous number of its victims and its total fatality …, influenza reached a virulence before which even plague with all its horrors fades into insignificance.'[16]

Like plague before it, but with far greater rapidity, influenza radiated outward from Bombay into northern and central India, where some of the heaviest mortality occurred. In this second phase, and in common with mortality profiles around the world, individuals between the ages of fifteen and forty proved exceptionally vulnerable. Neither the earlier wave of the disease nor the Russian Flu of thirty years previously had conferred much, if any, immunity. In Western countries the death-rate among women was generally equal to or lower than among men; but this was not the case in India.[17] There, more women died than men. Because of the gender bias in family care, women, who may have been less nourished in the first place, neglected their own health for the sake of their husbands and children; when they too fell ill, no one remained alive or able to feed them and nurse them back to health. Pregnant women were particularly at risk. Children under ten suffered less, as did older adults. And, as ever in India, there were wide regional variations. Like plague before it, influenza had markedly less impact on eastern and southern India, though even in the Madras Presidency 650,000 people had perished from the disease by the end of 1918.[18] In Calcutta, where the first wave struck in July and the second between September and December 1918, mortality jumped by 50 percent over the previous year, from 21,360 to 31,371, with most of the additional 10,000 deaths due to influenza and related respiratory conditions.[19] The city's health officer, H. M. Crake, was stunned by the 'lightning like rapidity' of the second deadly wave. 'I have never seen any epidemic,' he wrote, 'of such a truly explosive character. It is no exaggeration to say that all classes of the community in all parts of the city were attacked.'[20]

Speed and destruction defined the epidemic. In the Central Provinces, where an estimated 6 to 7 percent of the population died, the epidemic spread 'with great rapidity, paralysing towns and decimating villages.'[21] In what was described by the provincial sanitary commissioner as 'incomparably the most violent outbreak of disease of which we have any knowledge,' hundreds died within days. 'The ravages of the disease were seen at their worst,' he reported, 'in the villages, where the complete helplessness of the people combined with scarcity of food and clothing produced a calamity which baffles description.'[22] In Punjab, where close to a million influenza deaths were recorded between early October and the end of December 1918, its sanitary commissioner painted an even more apocalyptic picture. At the height of the crisis, the scenes were

> such as to render adequate description impossible. The hospitals were choked so that it was impossible to remove the dead quickly enough to make room for the dying: the streets and lanes of the cities were littered with dead and dying people: the postal and telegraph services were completely disorganised; the train service continued, but at all the principal stations dead and dying were being removed from the trains; the burning ghats and burial grounds were literally swamped with corpses, whilst an even greater number awaited removal; the depleted medical service, itself sorely stricken by the epidemic, was incapable of dealing with more than a minute fraction of the sickness requiring attention; nearly every household was lamenting a death, and everywhere terror and confusion reigned.[23]

As in the plague epidemic twenty years earlier, one response was flight. Migrant millworkers and laborers quit Bombay, Calcutta, and other industrial cities to return to their towns and villages, some saying that 'they preferred to die at home.'[24] But many perished or fell ill even before they could flee. Three textile mills in Cawnpore, together employing 7,000 workers, reported over 5,000 absentees during the height of the epidemic and 170 deaths.[25] But, as with plague, flight had dire consequences. 'During the panic caused by the epidemic,' wrote India's sanitary commissioner, F. Norman White, 'the trains were filled with immigrants from infected centres, many of them being ill.'[26] Railroad stations and junctions then became nodes for the onward spread of the contagion, pushing it further on into the small towns and villages. The influenza epidemic may have taken its greatest toll in some of India's most backward regions, but, like plague before it, it was still a modern disease, exploiting so much that made India modern. White stressed that influenza was *not* a new disease—there had, he noted, been previous pandemics—and yet the disease clearly arrived on the back of half a century of innovation and change.[27] India's economic, social, and technological modernity—its roads, railroads, tramlines, and steamer services, its factories, mills, mines, and plantations, its newspapers, telegraphs, and postal service, even its dance halls and cinemas—either fueled the epidemic or spread news of its inexorable advance.[28]

Influenza's Impact

Unlike cholera's long reign, influenza was a Hobbesian nightmare—nasty, brutish, but mercifully short. Given the sudden onset of the pandemic and its short time span, coupled with the absence of any provocative government intervention, India's rumor mills were not as active as during the opening phase of the plague epidemic. Even so, there was some speculation about the causes of the epidemic and colonial responsibility for its spread. In mid-1918 there was a widely circulating (and not unfounded) report that British troopships had been responsible for bringing the disease to Bombay, an allegation the government struggled to deny or dismiss.[29] It was rumored in October 1918 that either Lord Willingdon, the governor of Bombay, or his wife had caught influenza. But, if so, he or she soon recovered, prompting one Indian newspaper to ask what Willingdon's 'fat-salaried departmental lieutenants [were] doing to alleviate the suffering of the afflicted.'[30]

The anti-British tenor of these reports was matched by a more general association of influenza with the Great War. Still ongoing for most of the pandemic, through recruitment drives, troop movements, and daily newspaper reports the war in Europe and the Middle East was clearly familiar to a large portion of the Indian population. To many Indians the mysterious epidemic was not influenza but a 'war

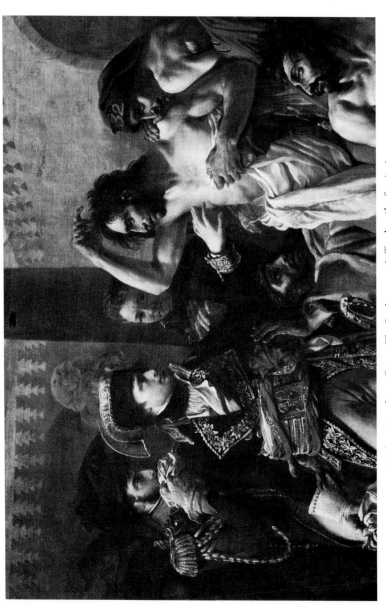

1. Antoine-Jean Gros, *The Pesthouse at Jaffa*, detail of painting.

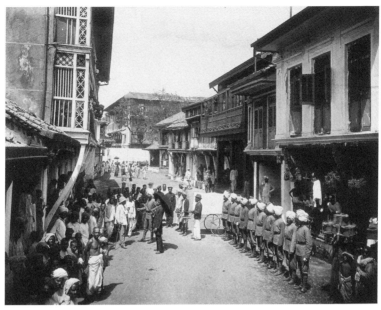

2. A Group of Officials Making a Visit to a House in Bombay Suspected of Holding People with Plague, 1896.

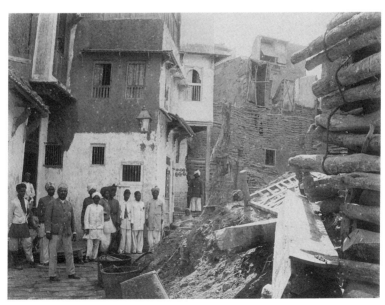

3. Plague-Infected House which Has Been Demolished, Karachi, 1897.

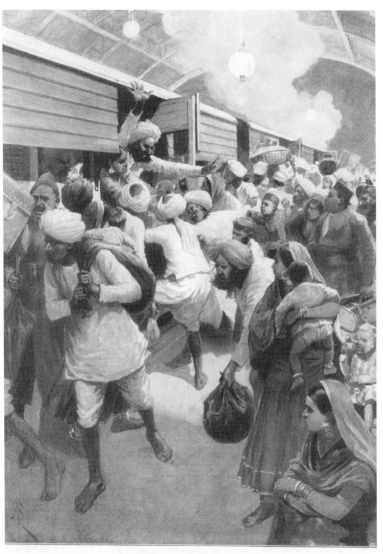

THE PLAGUE IN INDIA: THE EXODUS FROM BOMBAY.
By A. Forestier.

4. The Plague Exodus from Bombay, 1896.

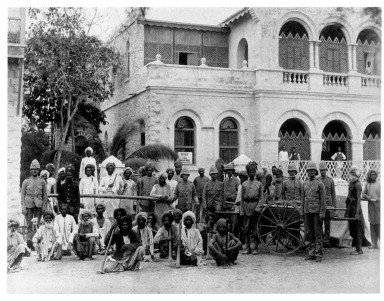

5. Staff from the Rambagh Section of the Karachi Plague Committee, Karachi, 1897, outside Plague Office.

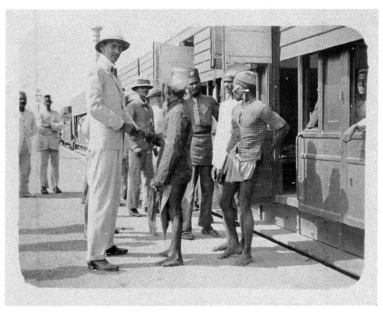

6. Medical Officers Watching the Arrival of a Train at Sion Railway Station, during the Epidemic of Plague in Bombay, 1897.

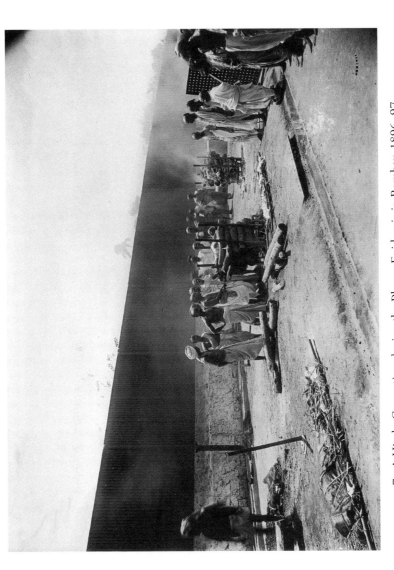

7. A Hindu Cremation during the Plague Epidemic in Bombay, 1896—97.

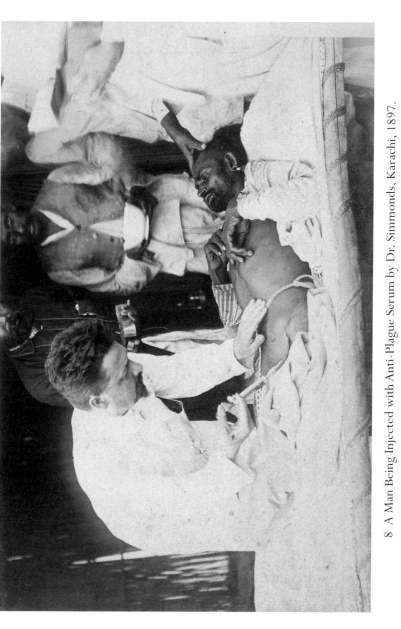

8 A Man Being Injected with Anti-Plague Serum by Dr. Simmonds, Karachi, 1897.

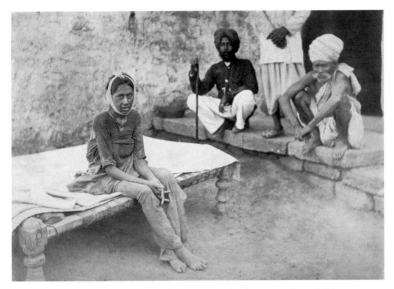

9. Female Patient with Bubonic Plague, Karachi, 1897.

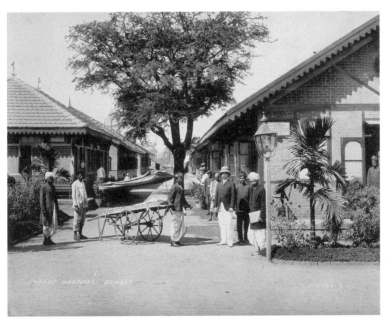

10. Bombay Plague Epidemic, 1896–7: Plague Hospital, with Stretcher Carriers and Staff Standing Outside the Building.

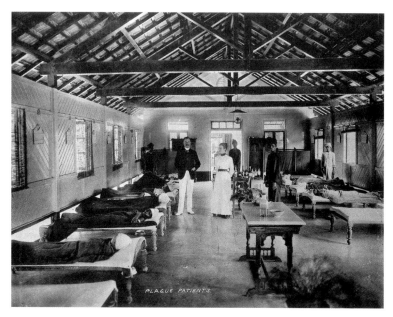

11. Bombay Plague Epidemic, 1896–7: Interior of a Plague Hospital.

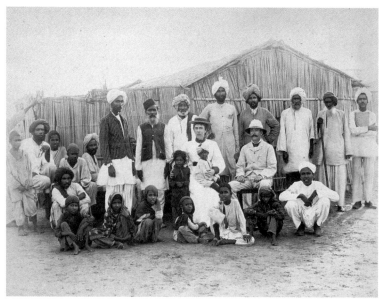

12. Hospital Staff during the Outbreak of Bubonic Plague, Karachi, 1897.

disease.'[31] In Punjab, where 'fantastic' rumors 'sprang up and died down like weeds,' one local paper claimed in July 1918 that the 'war fever' had originated in Berlin and that 'the tyrannical Germans have transmitted it to India by some special means.'[32] In September an individual identified only as 'B' wrote to the newspapers from Poona claiming that the pandemic had been unleashed by 'vapour from the gas bombs' in France and was now 'spreading all over the globe.'[33] This assertion may not have originated with 'B' or even in India: similar rumors of poison gas and biological warfare were circulating elsewhere in the war-troubled world.[34] Here was a potent myth for a world thrown out of kilter by war. Despite attempts to dismiss it as absurd and unscientific, the gas story persisted and worried officials who feared that it might inflame antiwar and anticolonial sentiment. India's sanitary commissioner insisted that whatever 'wild rumours as to the nature and causation of the disease' might suggest, influenza was categorically not a 'war disease.' 'Such wild unfounded rumours,' White wrote, 'as those which attributed the pandemic to the extensive use of poison gas on the Western Front, or to the evil machinations of our unscrupulous enemy [Germany], would scarcely have deserved mention, had they not been so current in India during the months of October and November [1918].'[35] To a degree unmatched by previous pandemics, and not repeated until Covid, influenza established a synchronicity and connectivity between India and concurrent events around the globe. A few years after influenza had subsided, the United Provinces' census superintendent wrote: 'To enlarge on this calamity is unnecessary. Everyone witnessed it in some part of the world or another.' He linked the global disaster to the scenes he had personally witnessed of 'villages that had in a month lost more than half their inhabitants, and great rivers choked with corpses, which could not be disposed of in the ordinary way.'[36]

In the official reckoning, a more educated public and greater access or recourse to medical aid explained why the urban middle classes suffered much less than the rural poor. In Punjab, for instance, case mortality among Europeans was less than 5 percent and little higher among town-dwelling Indians, at about 6 percent. But the rate was over 50 percent among rural inhabitants 'who had no knowledge of the treatment to be adopted and could not obtain medical aid.'[37] Likewise, of the United Provinces it was said, 'According to medical opinion the only treatment for influenza is absolute rest and good nursing.' This was 'more or less possible for town dwellers in the autumn of 1918, but for the cultivators it was not.'[38] In upcountry Madras, reported the provincial sanitary commissioner, the 'scientific' treatment of the disease was impossible, as 'the general ignorance of the masses combined with the absence of suitable medical organizations contributed greatly to the abnormal death-rates.' Some people even resisted medical treatment 'under a superstitious belief that the epidemic was a visitation of the Goddess or Amman and that any treatment by drugs would be offensive to her.'[39] The colonial citation of Indian belief in disease deities as a negative, even obstructive, trope had not disappeared, nor had blaming the poor for their own affliction.

Yet after December 1918, following this maelstrom of mortality, the epidemic rapidly lost momentum; within a few years influenza had sunk to statistical insignificance. There was no clearly defined third wave, though localized outbreaks persisted into 1920–1. In Calcutta in 1922 only 927 deaths from influenza were recorded out of a total mortality of 30,395. The city's health officer, while duly noting continuing deaths from influenza, was far more perturbed by a 'terrible epidemic' of smallpox in 1920 which cost 3,000 lives.[40] In Bombay, where nearly 4,000 deaths from influenza had been recorded in 1918, the number in the city dropped to 1,605 in 1920 and 1,389 in 1921, then fell to 528 in 1922, 250 in 1923, and 118 in 1924. However, perhaps as an after-effect of the pandemic, the number of deaths attributed to respiratory diseases (bronchitis and pneumonia) remained much higher: 18,737 in 1920; 21,982 in 1921; 13,614 in 1922.[41] But by the mid-1920s pre-existing infections—smallpox, cholera, malaria, tuberculosis—again grabbed the medical headlines.

Influenza was the greatest epidemic disaster India ever experienced, at least within the annals of recorded history. Quite how many people died will always be a matter of dispute, with estimates ranging between 12 and 20 million.[42] Since a census had not been taken since 1911 it was unclear what the population of India actually was in early 1918 and so the true scale of the mortality could never be calculated with any precision. India's death registration system was crude, reliant in the countryside on the reports of illiterate and medically untrained village watchmen. The cause of death given was notional at the best of times. Requests for district-by-district influenza mortality returns were rebuffed by colonial officials in Bengal on the grounds that 'the agency employed for the reporting of vital occurrences' was 'unable to diagnose properly the different causes of mortality.'[43] In such a monumental catastrophe the dead were too many to be counted and watchmen themselves lay among the sick and dying.[44] Flight from cities, towns, and villages further complicated the record. Since there was no category for influenza in the mortality returns—it was not even a certifiable disease— fatalities were entered under the all-purpose heading of 'fever,' resulting in uncertainty as to how many of these deaths were in fact due to influenza or to concurrent malaria, or they were attributed to 'respiratory disease' when influenza may have been the primary cause. The disposal of the dead added a further strand of unreliability. Around the world, the 'piling up of bodies' and the 'ominous accumulation of the unburied dead' contributed enormously to the pandemic horror.[45] But nowhere was this confusion of the dead more evident than in India where many of the deceased were placed unceremoniously and unburied on wasteland or in jungles, their bodies devoured by animals and birds, or their rotting corpses were committed, uncremated and unregistered, to rivers and streams.

The death of so many people in such a short space of time was exceptional even in India's woeful history of disease, even in relation to the famines and catastrophes of the nineteenth century. How do we begin to explain, still more understand, such colossal, almost incomprehensible levels of sickness and death? What made India so vulnerable to the ravages of the influenza virus even in a pandemic which caused at least 40 million deaths—probably more—worldwide? And what does influenza in its size and scale contribute to our broader understanding of pandemics and of India's relationship to them? More than any other pandemic, the influenza of 1918–19 was cited in connection with Covid in 2020–1. But was this analogy really warranted?

India at War

In 1973 the historian Ira Klein published an influential article in which he surveyed the period 1871–1921 in India and documented the extraordinarily high rates of mortality resulting from famine and recurrent bouts of cholera, smallpox, and plague (among other epidemics) and reaching a 'woeful crescendo of death' with the 1918–19 pandemic.[46] Beyond its global impact, for Klein the significance of the influenza episode lay in accentuating and driving to new heights an escalating trend in disease and death that dated back to the 1870s. He argued that British attempts to modernize India were themselves partly to blame for this 'woeful' trajectory: by disrupting natural lines of drainage and creating swamps where none had existed before, irrigation canals and railroad embankments facilitated the spread of malaria; new steamship routes, the opening of the Suez Canal in 1869, and the extensive rail network created from the 1850s onward, all exposed India to outside epidemics in a manner not previously possible. At the same time, the glaring deficiencies of colonial rule, its laggardly response to famine, and the wholly inadequate public health system it instituted failed to check or reverse this fatal spiral.[47]

There is much to be said in favor of this broad argument. However, nowhere in the article did Klein single out for consideration the specific factors that lay behind the catastrophic impact of influenza on India or do more than suggest that an accumulation of pre-existing health issues and an ongoing history of colonial neglect were responsible for this cataclysmic episode. Yet, contrary to Klein's claim about an ever-increasing tide of death and disease, there was a growing conviction among officials that the battle for India's public health *was* being won—against plague, smallpox, cholera, typhoid, and all the other diseases to which India had been prone. And even if famine had not been entirely extirpated, it seemed, since 1907, to have been in abeyance and that the provisions of the Famine Code, dating from the 1880s, were helping to check its recurrence. Many issues— malnutrition, infant mortality, maternal health, tuberculosis, and, above all, malaria—remained, but, at least in the cities, it was as if a corner had been turned. At the close of 1917 Calcutta's health officer announced that the past year had been the healthiest the city had ever known. Deaths from cholera and smallpox, which had been falling for years, had touched 'phenomenally low' levels. Plague deaths, at their lowest since the onslaught of 1898, had shrunk consistently since 1905. Indeed, plague had 'almost vanished' from the city's vital statistics.[48] India's eastern metropolis could, it seemed, now bask in a new age of public health.

Such optimism proved unfounded. In 1918, the ink barely dry on the health officer's report, Calcutta was savaged by one of the deadliest epidemics it had ever known, and mortality soared to unprecedented heights. At 35 deaths per thousand of the population, the city's death-rate was suddenly the highest figure recorded since 1907. No one had expected that. As the health officer put it, 'the setback in the progressive decline in mortality which had been a characteristic of the returns since 1913 is to be regretted.'[49] In Bombay, too, the sudden virulence of influenza was unanticipated. In 1915 the annual death-rate was lower than in any year since before the famine of 1876–8.[50] To add to the confusion, not only was the first onset of the disease relatively mild in nature, but in the opinion of some medical experts the disease was not even influenza but perhaps dengue or sand-fly fever, imported from the war zone in Mesopotamia (Iraq). India's sanitary commissioner was alarmed at the possibility it might be yellow fever rather than the influenza already rampant in Europe.[51]

Crucially, influenza struck India—and the world—in a time of war.[52] The Great War of 1914–18 had a massive impact on India and undoubtedly facilitated the epidemic that hastened in its wake.[53] India's involvement in the war began with soldiers sent to the Western Front in September 1914, before being relocated a year later to other battlefields, mostly in the Middle East. By the time the war ended in November 1918, 588,717 Indian soldiers had fought in the long and arduous Mesopotamia campaign. In all, close to a million soldiers from British and princely India served in the war, almost half of them from Punjab. Of the total number of soldiers enlisted, 53,486 were killed and 64,350 wounded. This was an undoubtedly heavy and grievous loss but one that can be seen, in retrospect, as being of slight demographic significance compared with the prodigious death-toll from influenza.[54] In one Punjab district, 694 serving soldiers died: in the same district by the end of November 1918, 30,000 individuals had perished as a result of influenza.[55] That India could mobilize a million men, supply vast quantities of arms, clothing, and military materiel, fund hospitals and troopships, and put the increasingly industrial economy on a war footing said much about the capabilities of the modern colonial state in a time of emergency. But evident, too, was the enormous strain this placed on the Indian economy, the creaking administrative infrastructure, and the fragile, indeed skeletal, system of public health. As Norman White later conceded, these were 'years of great stress and anxiety. The, at best, meagre health and medical services had been depleted by the war effort and were just sufficient for routine work, if all went well.' But, he grimly added, 'Things went persistently badly.'[56]

Globally, the mobilization of millions of soldiers was critical in enabling the growth and spread of the pandemic, starting, in all probability, in crowded army recruitment camps in the United States.[57] The role of the war in India's influenza epidemic followed similar lines. Like the troopships that brought influenza into western Europe from American ports, ships carrying returning or invalided troops from Port Said in Egypt and Basra in Iraq almost certainly introduced influenza to Bombay and Karachi in May–June 1918.[58] But many other factors also connected influenza with the war. Intensive recruitment for the Indian Army was still ongoing in the middle months of 1918 when influenza first struck, and the disease quickly impacted on the number of able-bodied men available or willing to present themselves for enlistment (there was no conscription in India). Once the disease had arrived, troop movements and army cantonments became central mechanisms in the India-wide dissemination of the virus (post office employees were another, if smaller, category of mobile individuals who helped spread the disease).[59]

It was later claimed that the army had benefited India by providing troops in cantonments with prompt and effective medical attention and so saved many lives, and that, through the payments made to serving and pensioned soldiers, Punjab in particular was 'greatly enriched by the War.'[60] In reality, both British and Indian soldiers recorded a large number of influenza cases and deaths, with Indian troops further suffering from pneumonia and the respiratory complications that caused so many additional fatalities. Of the 18,757 British soldiers stationed in India, 770 had died of influenza by the end of November 1918, and a further 56 from pneumonia. Among the 45,310 Indian troops there were 5,082 deaths from influenza but 2,064 from pneumonia. During the epidemic the death-rate for British soldiers was just over 8.9 per thousand from influenza and 0.7 from pneumonia, while among Indian soldiers the rates were substantially higher, 15.2 and 6.2 per thousand respectively.[61] The death-rate in the Indian Army was several times higher in 1918–19 than it had been before the war, an adverse trend for which influenza was primarily responsible. In the columns of army statistics for 1918 influenza towered over insect-borne and waterborne infections.[62]

Indian soldiers' greater susceptibility than European troops to pneumonia and other airborne diseases had been a feature of the army returns for many years, possibly due to their inferior accommodation in army lines or insufficient medical attention. India's sanitary commissioner put it in explicitly racial terms, stating that pneumonia was 'very much more toxic for Indians that it [was] for Europeans … the toxaemia is more profound.'[63] In this respect, as in many others, race loomed large in analysis of the pandemic, though whether this was the 'innate racial susceptibility' of non-white populations or a consequence of 'conditions of life that favor the transmission of influenza infection' remained unclear.[64]

By its destructive inroads, influenza, like cholera before it, underscored the centrality of the army to British rule and the reliance on Indian manpower to maintain the imperial war effort. But that dependence came at a heavy cost. The intensity of military recruitment in some areas of India stripped the agrarian economy of many of its most able-bodied workers, leaving only those less fit to sow and harvest. In Punjab, the Raj's principal recruiting ground but also one of its most agriculturally productive provinces, nearly one in eight of all males of military age were enlisted: in some districts— Rawalpindi and Jhelum—it was close to one in three.[65] Punjab was also a major food producer and exporter, and the absence of adult males left rural households more vulnerable than ever to the effects

119

of poor harvests and epidemic disease: the second wave of influenza struck many areas of India as autumn harvesting was about to begin or as the land was being prepared for new crops. In Punjab whole villages were wiped out by the disease, with adult males proving particularly vulnerable. The death-rate for 1918 (81 per thousand) was more than twice that for the previous year (38 per thousand). With self-interested hindsight officials in Punjab expressed their relief that the epidemic had not struck sooner: if it had, it would have robbed the army of much-needed recruits.[66]

Famine and Fever

In 1918–19 India experienced 'famine' on several fronts. There was, first of all, a severe 'fodder famine' due to widespread drought greatly exacerbated by the vast quantities of grass and straw extracted to feed army animals in India and Iraq. This in turn impacted on the volume of milk available for human consumption, with knock-on effects for the health of Indian consumers. It also led to the death of the cattle needed for ploughing and other agricultural tasks. As the governor of Bombay reported in January 1919 to the secretary of state for India: 'Cattle are beginning to die in considerable quantities in the Deccan and we can't get fodder enough to alleviate the trouble. Large quantities of valuable fodder are being exported from here to Mesopotamia by the Army.'[67] As the epidemic struck, there was a chronic shortage of firewood for domestic fuel, accentuated by the huge number of cremation pyres blazing across Hindu India. Imported kerosene, used for lighting and cooking, was costly and in short supply.[68] Then there was a 'famine of tonnage.' Severe shortages and distribution delays, linked to the war itself, restricted imports by sea and the capacity to move goods overland by rail: this began to impact on prices, which by late 1918 reached record levels for food grains, kerosene, cloth, and other essential commodities.[69] Hoarding and profiteering stoked popular anger in ways not seen since the early plague years. In the Madras Presidency in September 1918, grain riots and looting rippled through tense bazaars, sparking several days of unrest. Crime statistics scaled new heights.[70]

Most narratives of famine in colonial India concur in ending in 1907 before jumping more than thirty years to mass starvation in wartime Bengal in 1943.[71] Yet in 1918–20, famine, brought on by drought, poor harvests, and food shortages, stalked several provinces. After 1877 and 1899, themselves peak famine years, 1918 saw the worst drought in modern Indian history. Not surprisingly, therefore, in that year famine and influenza became 'a set of mutually exacerbating catastrophes.'[72] As Chinmay Tumbe has argued, drought, rising food prices, and undernutrition explain 'both India's uniqueness, compared to other parts of the world, as well as the variation of influenza-related mortality *within* the country.'[73] A recent survey similarly concluded that, at a time when therapeutic intervention had little impact, intercountry differences in the influenza death-toll of 1918–19 were 'strongly mediated by the state of economic advancement, with poverty and deprivation and associated comorbidity playing a vital role over and above the virulence of the virus.'[74]

Although it is often asserted that the influenza pandemic was so destructive globally because it attacked some of the healthiest members of the population, individuals whose immune systems went into fatal overdrive (the 'cytokine storm' effect), this does not adequately explain the Indian situation. Certainly, in the deadly second wave of the epidemic adults were most affected, but the Indian reports strongly suggest a close correlation between poverty, food deprivation, and general debility on the one hand and influenza and pneumonia on the other. Almost from the outset, influenza was described by Indians and Europeans alike as 'really a disease of hunger and exhaustion.'[75] 'The people who suffer most,' confessed Punjab's sanitary commissioner, 'are the poor and the rural classes, whose housing conditions, medical attendance, food and clothing are in defect.'[76] Underlying malnutrition and the concurrence of other infections such as malaria, cholera, and tuberculosis undoubtedly increased susceptibility to influenza. In Punjab, which had experienced a series of deadly and debilitating plague and malaria epidemics over the previous decade, heavy rains in 1917 created ideal conditions for the resurgence of malaria, though exactly how many of the deaths registered in 1918 were due to malaria rather than influenza was impossible to determine: pandemics tend to sweep up and devour a great deal of mortality that has other, more immediate, causes.[77] Indeed, it is one of the tragedies of our pandemic understanding that while influenza was seen globally as the great killer, in India malaria, with an estimated one million fatalities a year, was a more persistent cause of death.

British officialdom was in two minds about recognizing a relationship between the influenza epidemic and the prevalence of poverty, food shortages, and hunger, fearing how this might be used to attack British rule and undermine colonial authority. Famine was a word the state elected not to utter. In 1918–20 the Government of India chose to speak only of 'distress' and to insist (ironically in its own 'Famine Proceedings') that levels of mortality and hardship were nothing like what they had been in the dark days of 1899–1900: there were now, the viceroy stressed in an urgent telegram to London, no starvation deaths and in April 1919 only 337,000 individuals on relief works compared to 5.25 million in 1899.[78] But this was not the common view. Since the 1890s famine had become a highly political issue, particularly following the Poona Sarvajanik Sabha's investigations in the Deccan in 1897, Dadabhai Naoroji's denunciation of *Poverty and Un-British Rule* in 1901, and R. C. Dutt's searing exposé of British economic policy in 1904. The fact of famine, or the fear of famine, added to the growing swell of nationalist indignation, seeming to offer incontrovertible evidence of sustained economic exploitation and the callous indifference of the colonial power. When in September 1918 B. D. Shukul, a member of the Indian Legislative Council in Simla, called for an investigation into agricultural conditions in India and began to cite the nationalist case for famine as a direct consequence of British rule, the government was quick to shut down the debate.[79]

But famine became a nationalist cause to a degree that epidemics did not (the early plague years apart), and in 1918–19 officials were keen to skirt the issue by stressing the international nature of the pandemic, a term now seized upon in some administrative quarters as a convenient explanation for India's vulnerability. White, India's sanitary commissioner, stated that the country's great mortality was *not* caused by malnutrition: influenza was a pandemic, a global and not uniquely subcontinental phenomenon, and even prosperous, well-fed countries like the United States had suffered from it. And yet, elsewhere in his report, he quietly conceded that, while malnutrition was not a direct cause, 'the insufficiently nourished members of the community offered a very feeble resistance to the disease' and this contributed to the 'fatal issue.' He further noted that Kidderpore, close to the docks in Calcutta, with 'its large poverty-stricken coolie population living under the most insanitary conditions, suffered much more than the other wards of the city.'[80]

Officials in the districts and the provinces tended to be more forthright. Eyewitnesses themselves, many were affected by the scale of suffering and the massive loss of life they saw around them, and perhaps felt a pang of conscience that such appalling scenes were happening on their watch. Bombay's governor, Lord Willingdon, wrote to the viceroy in October 1918 in some despair: 'We are on the verge of serious famine conditions,' and noted how hardship had been exacerbated by influenza.[81] A month later, Delhi's chief commissioner remarked: 'There is no doubt that many deaths have been caused by malnutrition, and those who have carried out house to house visits in distributing medical aid report numerous cases of great distress.'[82] In the United Provinces the sanitary commissioner remarked that if influenza was more fatal in India than elsewhere, it was 'not due to the fact that sanitary conditions are worse in India, but to the fact that economic conditions are worse. The people of India are worse housed, worse clothed and worse fed and can consequently offer less resistance to disease than those in England and America.'[83] In Bengal, Charles Bentley concurred, pointing to the 'almost prohibitive' cost of cloth, rice, ghee, oil, and sugar in 1918, which had 'greatly aggravated the distress among the poorer classes.' The 'result of inadequate nourishment and clothing' was that 'the vitality of the population generally was lowered and this contributed to the large death-rate from fever (including influenza).'[84]

As the first impact of the epidemic receded, the evidence for incipient or actual famine proved impossible to ignore. In southern Bihar, for instance, when relief works opened they attracted 3,000 people; a further 74,000 were put on gratuitous relief.[85] Similar test works were opened in selected districts of Punjab and the Madras

Presidency.[86] In the Central Provinces, where influenza raged with exceptional severity and the death-rate leapt from 36 per thousand in 1917 to a colossal 103 per thousand in 1918, official responses to the epidemic were delayed because 'district officials were much preoccupied by the prospect of impending famine'—a calamity for which, unlike influenza, they had long been prepared and for which the provincial Famine Code gave step-by-step directions.[87]

But even within specific regions and provinces it is possible to observe what Nancy Bristow has, in a different context, called 'the inequitable distribution of suffering.'[88] As already noted, the countryside was particularly hard hit by the epidemic, but even there certain communities—particularly 'untouchables' (Dalits) and *adivasis* (tribals)—proved exceptionally vulnerable.[89] As David Hardiman showed, the Bhils in the forested Dangs of eastern Gujarat were severely affected in 1918 or thereabouts by a disease described by them as *manmodi* or the 'break-neck disease.'[90] This curious vernacular term occurs elsewhere in the literature on western India, for instance, in the autobiography of Lakshmibai Tilak, who was living at the time in the Deccan. She described *manmodi* as 'almost worse than plague.' However, she made no mention of any deaths, and while she wrote knowledgeably about plague, she did not identify this as influenza: might it have been an outbreak of another disease— dengue, for example?[91] Other tribal communities beside the Bhils also suffered, like the Santhals in western Bengal and Bihar, among whom influenza, accentuated by drought and hunger, 'wrought great havoc.' Officials, though, were quick to blame the victims, claiming that tribals lacked basic medical knowledge, took to drink, or exposed themselves to heat and cold in ways that hastened the fatal onset of influenza and pneumonia.[92]

Whereas with cholera and plague, the physical manifestations of the disease were closely observed and widely described, and added to the perceived horror of the disease, relatively few accounts exist for India describing what influenza looked or felt like. The rapid physical collapse, the nasal hemorrhaging, the cyanosis as the victim's skin turned purple or blue, and the delirium, frequently described in the American influenza narrative, were seldom recorded in India, perhaps because death came so quickly and entire communities were rapidly overwhelmed. The descriptions we have are largely confined to medical texts, K. C. Bose, for example, noting in his medical report on influenza in Calcutta that 'cyanosis was often seen and generally was the herald of death.'[93] Perhaps to most lay observers influenza appeared less like a new disease than an extreme version of the malarial fever with which it was so often confused and conflated.

Public Health Responses

The colonial medical and sanitary regime was not entirely unresponsive to the influenza epidemic, but, in contrast to its abrupt and heavy-handed intervention in the early plague years, it did, or felt able to do, relatively little. In Bombay, the government issued leaflets in English, Gujarati, and Marathi, telling people how to stay safe, and, in the 1918 equivalent of 'social distancing' in 2020, advised them to remain at home, to rest in bed if they felt feverish, and to avoid stations, cinemas, dance halls, and other crowded places.[94] The impracticality of much of this advice, especially in relation to the poor ('do not travel in over-crowded tram-cars'; 'avoid unnecessary exposure and fatigue'), was as apparent to many observers in 1918 as it was to Covid commentators on similarly impractical pronouncements in 2020.[95]

If epidemics were, as Charles Rosenberg suggested, a drama, then at times the influenza pandemic resembled a theatre of the absurd. Among other places the government encouraged people to avoid were skating rinks. Skating rinks in India? In fact, ice- and roller-skating rinks had enjoyed something of a craze in India since the mid-1870s—in places as far removed as Quetta, Simla, Calcutta, and Bombay (the Elysium on Fort Street).[96] But these were almost entirely frequented by Europeans (and perhaps Eurasians), mostly during the Christmas festivities, and the advice anyway simply replicated recommendations made to the public in the United States and Britain. The recycling of such advice is indicative of how India, at least official India, struggled to take ownership of the deadliest pandemic in modern history. Skating rinks were hardly a venue frequented by India's urban poor or rural masses, those among whom influenza was most likely to cause sickness, debility, and death.

For want of central direction from the Government of India or from the provincial authorities, much responsibility fell on the municipalities. Temporary dispensaries were set up to supply milk and medicines; blankets and 'pneumonia jackets' were issued. People were urged to keep warm, take aspirin or quinine, and eat nourishing food.[97] Facemasks (shades of Covid-19) were recommended, following a pattern adopted from the United States, and especially encouraged for health workers, but in practice in India they were rarely worn.[98] Elsewhere government or municipal dispensaries provided medical relief: the United Provinces mobilized its fleet of more than a hundred traveling dispensaries. But there were few clinics or dispensaries operating in the villages, where they were most needed; many were closed because of staff sickness or because they had rapidly run out of medicines.[99]

In Bengal the government authorized district boards to employ an additional sixty-six sub-assistant surgeons. It warned of the 'intense infectivity' of influenza and advised the public to avoid coughing and sneezing in confined spaces, eat nourishing food, and guard against chills. But in some districts, like Nadia, doctors did no more than distribute 'flu pills.' 'No wonder,' complained Calcutta's *Amrit Bazar Patrika* in February 1919, 'that people ... died like flies, unmedicated and untreated. Men, women and children are still dying by thousands, but who cares?'[100] In 1918–19 there were no state-directed lockdowns as during the Covid pandemic of 2020, but many industries, business houses, and administrative agencies temporarily ceased to function simply because of the widespread sickness and death of their employees. Unlike in 2020, cinemas and theaters in Bombay (though not, it seems, Calcutta) remained open and appear to have faced no restrictions. Not everyone was happy about this. In his account of influenza in Bombay, E. S. Phipson, a former city health officer, singled out cinemas as a particular danger to public health. In Bombay, he wrote, they had become very numerous, and, while they gave cheap and popular entertainment to the masses, they also created 'the almost perfect medium for the interchange of microbic infections.' They were 'dark, inadequately ventilated and the atmosphere is invariably warm and humid.' They had 'several performances every evening with no intervals for the cleansing and perflation [airing] of the building.' Only certain vested interests, he complained, stood in the way of their closure.[101]

Without antiviral drugs, without basic medical supplies or a clear understanding of how the disease might best be treated, some officials had recourse to eclectic remedies of their own. One European in Orissa, with no medical training, resorted to handing out 'such things as chlorodyne, camphor, essence of ginger, essence of peppermint, and anything I thought would do good.'[102] Bengal's sanitary commissioner observed that 'the lack of knowledge and of any real specific against the disease rendered efficient general treatment impossible.' A great many different remedies had been recommended, he noted, the sheer number and variety of which suggested that 'the majority of them are of little real use.'[103]

The Epidemic Diseases Act was not invoked (though in some provinces, like Bombay, its implementation was briefly considered); there were no house searches or physical examinations at railroad stations; no segregation camps; no compulsory hospitalization. There was no coordinated response by the health services, no agreed policy as to how to deal with the unfolding catastrophe. The Government of India almost made a virtue of its own inertia, arguing that 'during epidemic times' depression became 'widespread ... in the minds of the general population.' It was best, therefore, not to add to the gloom by unnecessarily closing theaters and other 'resorts of amusement,' as the effect on public morale might be 'worse than if nothing was done at all.'[104]

As during the coronavirus of 2020–1, great importance was attached to finding a vaccine. By 1918 India was accustomed to the idea of prophylactic inoculations and was well equipped for their manufacture. Since the early nineteenth century vaccination against smallpox had steadily gained ground, despite the suspicions it had initially aroused and opposition from minority sections of both Hindu and Muslim communities. As seen in chapter 3, further to his cholera work, in the 1890s Waldemar Haffkine rapidly devised a vaccine for use against plague and this was ultimately credited with helping to contain the disease. Influenza invited a similar response. In 1919 quantities of an anti-influenza vaccine were prepared in Indian laboratories and issued for use, especially to the military.

Some medical officers spoke highly of the results, perhaps because influenza was already on the wane, making the outcome appear favorable, but no data were collected to assess its efficacy and some physicians were certainly agnostic as to its value.[105] Since influenza was widely thought at the time to be caused by a bacillus, discovered by the German bacteriologist Richard Pfeiffer in 1892, and not, as later research showed, a virus, the vaccine distributed in India cannot have been effective against influenza.[106] In reality, neither in India nor anywhere else did medical intervention bring the pandemic to a close. The disease disappeared when it had run its natural course.

Apart from deficient knowledge of the causative microorganism, many other difficulties presented themselves in trying to tackle influenza in 1918. One acute problem was that many officers of the IMS, numbering barely 700 even in peacetime, had been drafted into war service in Europe, across the Middle East, and especially in Iraq. The principal rationale for the IMS was as a state-run medical service for the Indian Army, and in an emergency like the Great War military health took precedence over public need.[107] Some members of the service had died by 1918 and not been replaced; others had yet to revert to civilian posts. The war further exposed the underlying fragility and skewed priorities of colonial India's health administration. The epidemic struck India 'at a time when she was least prepared to cope with a calamity of such magnitude,' wrote S. P. James. 'War demands had depleted the personnel, and many of the staff available were incapacitated by the disease.'[108] Doctors had to be seconded from the Royal Army Medical Corps (RAMC), whose normal remit was the care of British troops in India, even for routine hospital work, despite their lack of local expertise.

The obstacles faced by medical staff in 1918 are evident from the experience of a Scottish doctor, Thomas Herriot. Having qualified in Edinburgh in 1912, Herriot was drafted into the British Army in February 1915. He served in France and was made a temporary captain in the RAMC a year later. Sent to India in 1918, he was put in charge of the military hospital at Jullundur in Punjab. The first he knew of 'Spanish influenza' was from reading a newspaper article about it, but this meant little to him until the disease arrived in the province.[109] He had scant expertise to guide him.

As Punjab's sanitary commissioner later explained, 'Prior to the present epidemic influenza was regarded with apathy and scepticism by the vast majority of the [medical] profession' in India.[110] The first wave of the disease entered Punjab only in August 1918: it caused, according to the official narrative, 'inconvenience but no alarm,' and the death-rate remained reassuringly low. The second wave, arriving in September, was much more virulent. In October mortality for Punjab shot up to 13.9 per thousand (the 'normal' average was 2.2); in November it reached a 'staggering' 34.2 per thousand.[111] With other medical personnel off sick with influenza, Herriot was burdened with the duties of his colleagues as well as his own and had no time to carry out the diagnostic tests he wanted to conduct. (This was not untypical. Calcutta's health officer had a similar experience, noting, 'Unfortunately with half my staff down with influenza, very few precise observations were made in the early stages of the epidemic.')[112] The first cases Herriot encountered were among Indian soldiers. From them influenza spread to the bazaar, to laborers, and domestic servants, and hence Europeans. Malnutrition and comorbidity were undoubtedly factors in the high levels of mortality in Punjab. In this time of pandemic confusion, it was at first assumed that the disease must be malaria, which had been rampant in the province for years, but laboratory tests failed to reveal either malaria parasites or plague bacilli. If, Herriot wrote, the disease was in fact influenza, 'no information had been received, either from other stations [in India], or from England which would help in diagnosing the disease.'[113] He was on his own.

Before the epidemic was over there had been a million deaths from influenza in Punjab: one in twenty of the entire population perished. Like Bombay, Punjab had been one of the provinces worst affected by recent famines, by plague and malaria, again suggesting that influenza was at its most destructive among populations already ground down by disease and hunger.[114] Conditions in 1918 were exacerbated by the failure of the monsoon and the poor outturn of crops, including the fodder needed for cows and buffaloes to produce the milk that was central to the Punjabi diet and that physicians recommended as an aid to recovery. Since the nights were bitterly cold, many Indians slept indoors to keep warm, Herriot noted, 'in the little mud huts where there was overcrowding and no ventilation,' an environment in which influenza and pneumonia thrived.[115] Patients in the Jullundur hospital were racked with pain; some, delirious with fever, proved hard to medicate and control. Their temperature soared to 102 or 103 degrees; they were exhausted yet unable to sleep. As their health deteriorated and pneumonia set in, cyanosis caused patients' faces to turn 'a peculiar violet lavender hue.' This 'grave sign' gave little hope of recovery. For those who did survive, convalescence was painfully slow. Herriot, though, drew some consolation from the fact that of the 214 cases he treated, only 21 died, a ratio roughly in line with Indian Army case fatalities generally in 1918–19.[116] Given the bewildering array of symptoms patients presented and the continuing medical uncertainty as to the nature of the disease and how to treat it, Herriot would have liked to use his Edinburgh training to examine blood and urine samples, but he lacked the time and the apparatus to do so. His Indian assistant, who normally helped with laboratory work, was laid up with influenza. The only authoritative source Herriot could turn to was out-of-date articles in *The Lancet*. He struggled to keep track of his patients' rapidly changing or fast-deteriorating condition, to record their alarming symptoms, and to apply what seemed the appropriate treatment.[117] He could only muddle through: even before the epidemic was fully over, he was invalided out of India and returned, broken in health, to Edinburgh. He died, aged 62, at Berwick-upon-Tweed, in 1949.

Self-reliance

Colonial medical activity, or the lack of it, was only part of the equation. In the early plague years of the 1890s and 1900s, the popular and middle-class reaction had been against draconian state intervention. In 1918, by contrast, the complaint was that the government was far too inactive.[118] Having little to offer of their own, medical and sanitary officers were reduced to blaming the impact of the epidemic on the sudden and global eruption of a crisis that was beyond the capacity of *any* medical service to control or, still more, on public ignorance and the 'absolute helplessness' of the people.[119] But the inactivity of the state, its general disavowal of ownership and responsibility, made it the more likely—and necessary—that Indians, especially urban, middle-class Indians, would come forward with their own measures of self-reliance—organizing relief parties, visiting the sick, distributing food and medicine, and overseeing the disposal of the dead.[120]

Here was one strand in a decolonizing agenda as Indian activism supplanted state lethargy and apparent unconcern. In an urban context at least, colonial claims about the 'helplessness' of the people look absurd when measured against the remarkable upsurge in civil action, self-help, and philanthropy. Nowhere was this more evident than in Bombay. In September 1918 the municipal corporation set up a Medical Relief Committee: all but one of its five members were Indian. The committee promised to take whatever steps were necessary to combat the epidemic and to recruit as many doctors, hospital assistants, and medical students as possible 'to undertake a systematic house to house visitation at regular intervals to render medical aid and advice to the patients suffering from the disease and to distribute suitable medicines free of charge to such patients as may be willing to take them.'[121] Three weeks later, the *Times of India* published a lengthy account of all that was going on in Bombay—the work of Christian missionaries, college professors and their students, and boys from the American mission high school. Volunteers corps had been formed: one, organized by Dr. L. L. Joshi of the Bombay Indian Christian Association, was supported by funds and medical supplies donated by Parsi, Hindu, and Muslim philanthropists. A dispensary had been opened in Girgaum to distribute for free medicines supplied by the municipality, while volunteers were touring city precincts and slums to provide patients with 'medicines [and] nourishment.'[122]

Drawing on indigenous philanthropic practices but further impelled by rivalry with Christian missionaries and aware of the inadequacy of state measures, religious bodies and secular welfare associations, ranging from the Arya Samaj and Ramakrishna Mission to the Seva Samiti and Bombay's Social Service League, had since the 1890s gained extensive practical experience of relief work in times of famine, earthquake, pestilence, and flood. Now that expertise was mobilized to help individuals and communities struck down with influenza.[123] Nor was this philanthropy confined to the big cities. Parsis in Surat, for example, organized a relief committee that distributed medicine and other supplies to nearby villages.[124] In Bengal, Bhagyadhar Mullick, a professor at the Scottish Churches College, set up an influenza dispensary at his home in Baghbazar in Calcutta before returning to his natal village in Howrah district to continue his charitable work. He caught influenza—that 'dreadful malady'—and died a 'martyr's death.'[125] Influenza had its heroes. In Punjab, 'the epidemic called forth a great deal of self-sacrifice and social service on the part of the better educated.' Medical students 'scattered over the country to do what they could in the way of relief, and funds were generously provided for the supply of medicine and comforts.'[126] None of this suggests 'helplessness' or fatalism in the face of disaster.

In December 1919 Bombay's Social Service League (which had been established in 1911 and which in 1918 ran its own relief fund) presented silver medals and certificates to students who had enrolled as volunteers during the 'disastrous influenza epidemic.'[127] Speaking in August 1924 at the British Empire Exhibition's India Day in London, Lady Cowasji Jehangir spoke of the contribution that India's women, including Parsis like herself, had made to the nation's well-being over the previous fifty years. She recalled that at the time of the 'dreadful epidemic of influenza which swept through our land, carrying off six million lives, our women worked day and night, going fearlessly from house to house, giving advice, nursing the sick and bringing whatever human courage and help and consolation could be brought to those whom the dreadful scourge had attacked.' This, she added, was evidence that India was 'awakening' and that the glory of India was not 'a tradition of bygone years, but a living reality of today.'[128]

Indians owned the epidemic in other ways, too. The demonstrable inability of Western medicine and state public health to curb the epidemic or provide effective relief for the mass of the population gave added inducement to practitioners of Ayurveda, Unani, and homeopathic medicine to offer their services and encouraged both patients and practitioners to be eclectic in their search for remedies. The Bengali poet Rabindranath Tagore responded to the influenza crisis by preparing his own Ayurvedic medicines. He devised a concoction known as Panchatikta Panchan, a febrifuge consisting of neem leaves and other medicinal herbs, and administered it to pupils in his school at Shantiniketan. By his account students fell sick whenever they went home but were free from the disease when they stayed with him. 'About two hundred people live here,' he wrote to his friend, the scientist Jagadish Chandra Bose, 'yet the local hospital has almost no patient ... I am inclined to believe that this is definitely the miracle of the Panchan.'[129]

Ayurvedic remedies and Shastric cures for influenza—'war fever'—were widely advertised in newspapers at the time. Some heroically claimed to cure influenza in a single day or to have saved thousands of lives.[130] This left IMS officers seething with indignation (much like their successors during Covid-19) at such 'questionable remedies.'[131] But, undaunted, supporters of Unani and Ayurveda declared that their medicines had been highly successful against influenza and used this as grounds for demanding greater state recognition and funding. When the All-India Ayurveda Conference met in Delhi in late January 1919, at a time when influenza still raged, the chairman spoke of Ayurveda as 'the first born truly scientific medicine' in the world and 'a monument of Aryan civilization.'[132] The pandemic gifted proponents of India's non-Western medical systems a new confidence and a new opportunity.

* * *

Uncertainty will always remain as to exactly how many people died in India in the 1918–19 influenza epidemic, but there is no doubting that mortality there was 'by far the highest for any single country.'[133] That between 12 and 20 million people perished represents a catastrophe of almost unimaginable proportions. But what is also important is why so many died in India compared with other regions of the world, how this awful visitation was understood and responded to at the time, and how it has been interpreted in the century since. Influenza in 1918–19 was unquestionably a pandemic: given its unprecedented geographical reach, the speed of its movement, and the phenomenal mortality it caused, it was the most truly global of any pandemic before or since. One response to the enormous death-toll in India was for the colonial medical establishment to give a collective shrug—to argue that influenza was a natural disaster, a cruel force of nature, to which no society, however well equipped with hospitals, doctors, and medicines, was immune, and that no government could possibly have foreseen or prevented. Since it was such a freakish aberration, British rule in India was accordingly (in its own eyes) blameless. With more than 300 million people, India was the world's most populous country and therefore bound to suffer in proportion to its huge numbers and, given its alleged 'helplessness,' probably more. Influenza, in this view, was a Malthusian reckoning. The explanation for India's extraordinary mortality was then seen to lie, in one official version of events, if not exactly with nature's caprice, then with Indians' poverty, physical (and perhaps racial) weakness, their ignorance and lack of medical and sanitary awareness: Indians died, so the argument ran, because they were foolish or vulnerable, not because colonialism had failed them.

The converse of this self-exculpatory reasoning was that India's extreme susceptibility to influenza owed much to two specific factors, neither entirely unique to India, but which pressed with exceptional severity on the people of India in 1918–19. One of these was deeply entrenched poverty and malnutrition, actual or incipient famine, and the conjuncture of influenza with other infectious diseases. Together these sapped the vitality of the people and left large numbers exposed to influenza or incapable of resisting its inroads. These background conditions had (as Klein demonstrated in his 1973 article) long prevailed in India, but they were greatly exacerbated by drought, failed harvests, and high prices in 1918–19. To this lethal concoction was added a second deadly ingredient—the war. While some individuals profited from the increased demand for Indian goods and services, overall the Great War imposed enormous hardship on India. The recruitment of so many men to fight for the empire and the Allied cause deprived India of many of its most productive workers; it left regions like Punjab, which had already suffered a spate of life-sapping epidemics, extremely vulnerable to hunger and disease. The war created shortages, high prices, and scarcities—in food, cloth, oil, fodder for livestock—intensifying the hardship Indians already felt. The war weakened the already fragile public health system, diverted medical personnel elsewhere, and distracted administrative attention from the engulfing pandemic. The movement of military personnel, with troops returning from overseas or moving between cantonments, was a significant factor both in the inception of the disease and in its subsequent dissemination. War and famine together account for a large part of India's exceptional vulnerability in 1918–19. And yet, paradoxically, given their greater visibility and political prominence, war and famine also obscured or helped explain away the extent and awfulness of the suffering and loss wrought by influenza. It is to this erasure, this orphaning of influenza from India's history, that we turn next.

5

ORPHANS OF THE STORM

In December 1923 Bombay's Excelsior Cinema screened D. W. Griffith's silent movie *Orphans of the Storm*. Starring the Gish sisters, Lillian and Dorothy, and using innovative cinematic techniques, this historical melodrama retold the story of the French Revolution of 1789 from the perspective of two poor, orphaned girls and a scheming, dissipated noble. 'The guillotine is seen at its deadly work,' gushed the advertising blurb, 'and there are tremendous crowds of frantic men and women fighting wildly against the aristocrat in the hope of freedom.'[1] Such was the popularity of the two-and-a-half-hour epic—Griffith's 'best and biggest picture' and 'a film every person in Bombay must see'—that it returned to the Empire Theatre in October 1926 for a second run.[2] With hindsight one can see a bitter irony in this. In 1923 India had only just emerged from the most destructive 'storm' in its history—the influenza epidemic of 1918–19—and only months before the film's first screening in Bombay, India's census commissioner had revealed that at least 12.5 million people had died in this pathogenic deluge. The 'frantic' scenes of men and women struggling to evade the epidemic and escape its clutches seemed now, barely four years on, to be ignored or forgotten. And the real 'orphans' of that 'storm' and of the famine that accompanied it—the thousands of children made parentless, the widows left husbandless—had, it seemed, slipped out of common recall and, for decades to come, into historical obscurity.

Calculating Loss

Only gradually did the enormous scale of the calamity of 1918–19 become apparent, and that slow-motion revelation may be one reason why India's devastating experience of Spanish Flu was not fully recognized at the time and has, until recently, been ignored or downplayed. India's sanitary commissioner, Norman White, produced an interim statement in early 1919 in which he estimated 6 million influenza deaths up to the end of November 1918, with 5 million dead in British India and a further 1 million in the princely states.[3] For many years thereafter 5 or 6 million was the death-toll widely cited: remarkably, this redundant figure is one some historians still quote.[4] White's 'preliminary' report was never followed by a more systematic investigation, though as early as November 1918 a member of Bombay's legislative council, Ebrahim Haroon Jaffer, called for a committee of experts to investigate this 'mystery disease,' which, he said, had left physicians 'groping in the dark.'[5] White himself left India and the IMS soon after, as if turning his back on the calamity.

The worst of the epidemic was over by the time India's decennial census was held in March 1921, and it took a further two years for the results of that exercise to be collated and published. By that time (early 1923), the estimated mortality, calculated in terms of excess deaths and the fall in the population since 1911, was put at 12.5 million for British India and the princely states combined.[6] As noted in the previous chapter, the tendency in recent years has been to revise the number of deaths in the pandemic substantially upward, globally to 40 million or more and for India to as many as 20 million. This latter figure represents more than 6 percent of India's population at the time.

There is a revealing episode in the contemporary assessment of the impact of influenza (and concurrent famine) on India. On 20 January 1919 the Welsh-born, American-raised missionary and agricultural expert Sam Higginbottom wrote to a friend in North America, a

Mrs. Gibbud, about the devastation he was witnessing in Allahabad, where he was principal of the agricultural college, and especially in the state of Gwalior, where he was an agricultural adviser. 'Influenza has been fearful,' he wrote in anguish. 'Hundreds of bodies daily floating in the river.' Higginbottom reckoned from what he had seen in the villages in October and November 1918 that Gwalior had, at a conservative estimate, lost at least 10 percent of its population to influenza and, assuming that India as a whole had suffered equally, the death-toll among India's 320 million people would therefore amount to 32 million. High death-rates among prisoners further suggested to him that the mortality had been far greater than government sources indicated.[7] The story was rapidly passed on by Higginbottom's correspondent to the Canadian press. Sensational headlines appeared in the *Toronto Star* claiming 'the greatest tragedy' to have 'visited the world in years' was unfolding in India; famine (influenza was barely mentioned except as 'the plague') was causing millions of deaths and funds were urgently needed for India. 'Words fail to portray the ghastliness of this stupendous tragedy,' the paper declared, 'and photographs taken in different parts of the country depict scenes too gruesome for publication.'[8] A Famine Relief Fund was established and by July 1919 had collected more than $40,000. Higginbottom's missionary contacts were instrumental here, providing the organization for fundraising and seeing in India's abject misery an opportunity for Christian conversions. As Higginbottom wrote from Allahabad: 'medical missions have a great field here ... now is the time for the presentation of Him who came that they might have a more abundant life.'[9]

The Government of India was outraged by the Canadian press coverage, fearing at a time of great political uncertainty the immense damage such stories could do to the reputation of British rule in India and abroad. In a stern rebuke to Higginbottom in August 1919, the secretary of the Government of India's Revenue and Agriculture Department rejected the American's claims as a series of gross exaggerations and serious 'mis-statements' —today they would be labelled 'misinformation'—and reasserted the official line that the death-toll from influenza was unlikely to exceed 6.5 million and that the 'distress,' never amounting to famine, had been handled effectively and without significant loss of life.[10] Higginbottom was by this time embarrassed that his private correspondence had been made public and recognized that he might have miscalculated the extent of mortality across India. He asked the government to help him out (especially in the light of an impending tour of the United States and Canada in which he feared awkward questions would be asked of him), but it sternly refused to do so and declined to accept the funds that had been raised for a famine which, it believed, had never even existed.[11]

Two aspects of this episode are particularly striking. One was the way in which famine rather than influenza became the headline story, not only for the Canadian press and missionary fundraisers but also for the Government of India in its testy defense of its crisis management. The second is that while Higginbottom's calculation of 32 million deaths was misjudged in extrapolating data from one badly hit rural area (Gwalior) to the whole of British and princely India with its wide regional variations in infection and mortality, his figure does not appear so wildly out of line with more recent recalculations of influenza deaths (up to 20 million), especially if famine mortality and the deleterious effects on health of widespread hunger are also factored in. Higginbottom may have been wrong, or at least rash, in his arithmetic but right in attempting to open up an alternative narrative, one that was radically at variance with official propaganda and the colonial determination to minimize the demographic impact of the influenza–famine catastrophe of 1918–19.

On any graph of Indian mortality for the late nineteenth and early twentieth centuries, 1918 stands out as a solitary peak, towering high above the returns for any other year. And yet in the report of the Government of India's census commissioner, J. T. Marten, published in 1923, and in the various provincial censuses, the magnitude of the influenza epidemic was played down. It became subsumed within a narrative stretching back over the whole decade and studded with recurrent epidemics of plague, cholera, malaria, and kala-azar, a tale of good harvests and plentiful rains punctuated by occasional poor seasons and then crippled by wartime scarcities and rising prices. The 1918–19 agricultural season was, Marten conceded, 'disastrous,' but famine relief measures were 'so highly perfected' that scarcity was now 'not necessarily accompanied by high mortality.' Regrettably, though, India could not escape the influenza pandemic which

> visited almost every portion of the country and wiped out in a few months practically the whole natural increase in the population for the previous seven years. Emergency measures were taken. Transport, the export of foodstuffs and the distribution of the necessities of life were all placed under Government control, and it was only the wonderful resisting power of the people acquired from years of steady economic improvement that enabled the country to tide without absolute disaster over a year of unprecedented difficulty and strain.[12]

The words 'difficulty' and 'strain' did scant justice to the utter calamity of influenza and famine, and one might reasonably wonder, if the death of millions of people did not constitute an 'absolute disaster,' then what did? Rather than admit any direct liability for the scale of India's mortality, colonial accounts focused instead on what the government *did* do or had already put in place, mostly with respect to famine rather than the epidemic, and the underlying trend of 'steady economic improvement' (for which the government claimed responsibility) which made possible the (less than evident) 'wonderful resisting power of the people.'

The provincial reports on the 1921 census assigned varying degrees of prominence to the epidemic. Many stressed the host of economic and social factors that had affected the population over the decade since the previous census, setting the massive mortality and disruption caused by influenza alongside other epidemics or balancing the many years of prosperity against the few seasons of hunger. Enormous though the mortality of 1918–19 was acknowledged to have been, the epidemic was slotted in alongside other 'natural' disasters—cyclones, floods, droughts, earthquakes— for which, in the official view, there could likewise be no human culpability, but which were part of the inherent vulnerability of Indians and the precarious physical environment in which they lived. In such narratives influenza almost became normalized, a moment of extreme 'stress' perhaps, but one that did not radically affect the overall picture. India, it was repeatedly stated, had been 'exceedingly prosperous' until 1918.[13] Even in Punjab, where a million people died of influenza, 1918 was seen as no more than a temporary aberration in an otherwise healthy decade.[14] The rapidity with which influenza melted away after early 1919 made this rosy outlook on India's economic prospects and social well-being the more plausible; so did the evidence of a birth-rate rapidly rebounding from the sharp demographic downturn of 1918–19.[15] If not entirely complacent, these contextualizing accounts of India's influenza were oddly reassuring.

Orphans and Opportunities

Pandemic histories are primarily concerned with causation, with the arrival and spread of a disease, the nature of state responses and societal reactions, and the tally of lives lost (case numbers or morbidity being historically far more difficult to quantify). Little time is usually spent in considering how such monumental losses impacted on those who survived, the orphans, in a literal or metaphorical sense, of the pandemic storm.[16] Determining with any precision how many people died in India's influenza epidemic was—and still is—extremely difficult. Trying to calculate how many orphans and widows influenza left in its wake is even more problematic. Historians have noted that the population of India recovered relatively quickly after 1919, buoyed up by high levels of fertility. But the 1921 census reports made no explicit mention of how many widows and orphans remained, and, like almost all aspects of the epidemic, the impact of influenza was complicated— and in part overshadowed—by concurrent famine.

Since influenza killed a significant proportion of young to middle-aged adults, it must have robbed many a family of parents and breadwinners. Orphans, deprived of family support and debilitated by hunger and disease, must have died in large numbers even before they could be counted among the inmates of orphanages and rescue homes. One orphans' home at Pandharpur in the Bombay Presidency, set up in the wake of an earlier calamity, the famine of 1876–8, admitted 41 orphans in 1918–19, 8 of whom then died from influenza.[17] The government was not unaware of the orphan issue.

As early as November 1918 the Bombay administration registered concern at the number of infants orphaned by the epidemic, especially in and around Poona, and noted that missions and other charitable organizations lacked adequate funds and personnel to look after them. It entrusted to district officials responsibility for the orphans' care and proposed the setting up of crèches to accommodate them until they could be reclaimed by relatives or handed over to orphanages and educational institutions.[18] In January 1919 the Bombay government again noted that many orphans and 'helpless old people' had been left on its hands, especially in the southern (Deccan) districts.[19] Likewise in its 1919–20 administration report the government of Bihar and Orissa acknowledged that influenza had caused 600,000 deaths and that the situation had been exacerbated by 'a year of famine.' It had accordingly become necessary to provide gratuitous relief for individuals unable to work or support themselves, their numbers 'swollen by the orphans left by the ravages of influenza.'[20] But this report, like many similar sources, gave no further details as to their numbers or subsequent fate.

As the Sam Higginbottom case has shown, missionaries, too, became actively involved. In making an urgent appeal for funds, the National Missionary Council meeting at Lahore in December 1919 cited the 'terrible ravages' caused by influenza which had left thousands of destitute and orphan children, a 'calamity' made worse by 'the high prices prevailing throughout the world owing to the great war.' One missionary reported being besieged by a thousand orphans, 'the heritage of India's influenza and famine troubles.'[21] Because of the concern missionaries showed for the sick and bereaved, and the material support they provided, in some parts of India famine and epidemics had contributed since the 1870s to a significant increase in evangelization and the growth of the Indian Christian community.[22] The influenza and famine of 1918–19 accelerated this trend, at the same time provoking criticism from Hindus who felt that their religion was being undermined.

The number and destiny of widows are even more uncertain than those of 'influenza orphans.'[23] Wifeless men were likely to remarry, but that was far less probable with Hindu widows, at least for those of the higher castes among whom widow remarriage was rare, if not expressly prohibited. New charitable homes were opened for them, as they were for orphans: some, according to their age, were sent to schools and other educational institutions. Philanthropy was spurred in part by fear that women without husbands, left homeless and destitute, would sink into a still worse state of beggary and prostitution (much as uncared-for orphan children might be trafficked).[24] In Benares a home for 'distressed women' saw its numbers substantially increased by the epidemic: here they were taught needlework and sewing, educated in Hindi, and required to attend daily readings from the Ramayana.[25] In Poona the Seva Sadan, or Social Service Society, headed by Ramabai Ranade, herself a widow, not only cared for those widowed by influenza but also relied on a number of widows to carry out house visits and nurse the sick. The society further provided women with 'facilities for becoming teachers, nurses, and seamstresses' and 'other means of being independent of relations and charity.'[26] There is evidence, too, that in districts hard hit by influenza female participation in the workforce (including that of widows) grew after the epidemic owing to labor shortages, though this shift had been reversed by 1931.[27]

India's economy, already skewed by the effects of the war, was put under further strain by influenza, though, as with the demographic recovery, the process of readjustment seemed relatively swift if hardly, from a human perspective, painless. It was not only towns and villages that were ravaged by the disease. So, too, were mining and plantation communities. For instance, the workforce in the Kolar goldfield in the princely state of Mysore had previously been hard hit by plague in 1898 with more than 700 deaths. Now in 1918–19 it suffered 13,600 cases of influenza (roughly half of all its Indian employees) and recorded 960 deaths.[28] Influenza also resulted in a very high death-rate among workers on the coalfields of eastern Bihar, 'into which masses of enfeebled persons had crowded for work.'[29] Across India thousands of workers and their dependants died; many more fell sick and, being unable to work, lost their livelihood. Conversely, the ravages of influenza created an intense labor scarcity: in Sind, for example, landowners were desperate in early 1919 for laborers to pick cotton and harvest rice.[30] But labor shortages also prompted a significant (if short-term) hike in wages, and impelled a new tide of migration from drought-prone, impoverished areas of rural India like Bihar and Orissa to the mines and plantations. In the United Provinces, where prices had soared and the scarcity of basic commodities was acute, the great mortality of 1918–19, with an estimated 2 million dead from influenza alone, caused a severe dearth of labor and wages 'rose abruptly.'[31]

Flight had throughout been one of the basic responses in India to the threat or onset of epidemic disease, the intense desire to escape the sickness and seek somewhere safer. This response was evident, too, during the influenza epidemic: in industrial cities like Ahmedabad the workforce was depleted as much by flight as by the 'Spanish sickness.'[32] But, as the immediate threat passed or as famine further undermined rural subsistence, epidemics also impelled new cohorts of workers to seek employment in factories, plantations, and mines. In 1917–18, 11,000 workers and their dependants had left southern Bihar for the tea districts of Assam; in 1918–19, the year of influenza, the number shot up to over 196,000. Emigration 'swelled to a flood.'[33] From the employers' perspective this was the tea estates offering a 'haven from starvation ... to these poor people,' but it was also a commercial prospect not to be missed.[34] The Jorehaut Tea Company in Assam reported that 'a severe outbreak of influenza' among the labor force in 1918 was followed by a 'quite abnormal' influx of coolies, with 3,500 new workers enrolled. According to the report presented to the company's annual general meeting in June 1919: 'It was essential that every advantage should be taken of this opportunity of replenishing our labour force,' especially as 'such an opportunity' might not 'occur again for some years.'[35] Not for everyone was influenza an unmitigated disaster.

Stimulated by rising commodity prices, the removal of wartime restrictions, and an improving supply situation, many of the European-owned sectors of the economy experienced high levels of profitability and growth that seemed, in a matter of months, to swallow up the losses caused by the epidemic and famine crisis. The Singlo Tea Company of Assam, which reported record profits in 1920, took on an additional 751 laborers. Influenza was acknowledged to have resulted in a heavy death-toll in the Assam tea gardens, 'but otherwise the health of the coolies' showed 'a remarkable improvement.' Singlo's estate doctor went so far as to observe with some complacency that 'had it not been for the influenza epidemics [in 1918–20] the death rate in the Assam gardens ... would have been no greater than London.' This, from a company perspective, was 'a very satisfactory state of affairs.'[36]

In response to plague in the late 1890s and early 1900s, the colonial medical establishment had, belatedly, taken the opportunity to intensify research into the epidemiology of the disease and to absorb the discoveries, techniques, and benefits of the bacteriological revolution. No such transformation occurred during or in the aftermath of the influenza epidemic, a salutary reminder of the dangers of assuming a Whiggish view of medical history and the inexorable rise of modern medicine. India's new-found bacteriological expertise and pioneering investigations of water- and insect-borne diseases did not translate into a pioneering virology, if only because in India, as elsewhere, there was a continuing belief that the causative agent was Pfeiffer's bacillus rather than the virus that research in the 1930s later revealed it to be. R. H. Malone, of the IMS, was appointed to conduct an inquiry on behalf of the Indian Research Fund Association (created by the government in 1911 and the forerunner of India's post-independence Council of Medical Research) into the bacteriology of influenza and the preparation of a vaccine.[37] A clutch of articles appeared in India's medical press, including a substantial report by E. S. Phipson on the epidemic in Bombay, and by a number of Indian authors like Calcutta's highly respected K. C. Bose.[38] But otherwise, as influenza waned, medical attention shifted back to the diseases that had long preoccupied India's medical researchers and public health experts—malaria, cholera, smallpox, plague, kala-azar, and tuberculosis. Of the scores of medical articles and monographs on influenza produced globally in the decade after 1918, less than a dozen were written in, or related to, India.[39]

In J. A. Turner's authoritative account of *Sanitation in India*, published in an updated edition in 1922, twice as much space was given to yellow fever, a disease that had never established itself in India, as to the influenza epidemic in which millions of Indians had died.[40] In 1924 the editor of the *Indian Medical Gazette* profiled the 'seven scourges' of India, but influenza was not among them.[41] When the prestigious Far Eastern Association of Tropical Medicine met in Calcutta in 1927, the government issued a handbook celebrating its medical and sanitary services. The work of various research institutes was described; plague, malaria, cholera, smallpox, and kala-azar featured prominently. Influenza received a single brief mention (and that only in relation to vaccine production).[42] In India there were no innovations, no vaccine discoveries, no lasting achievements, to present to the world as evidence of the medical gains and material benefits of colonial rule. The influenza epidemic was not an episode of which medical science and public health officers in India could feel proud, or over which they could claim scientific ownership. As Mike Davis put it, 'science does not celebrate defeat', and the failure of medicine, in India and around the world, in 1918–19 'was quickly repressed in popular memory.'[43] Influenza became subject to a kind of amnesia. Consoling though it is to believe that events of such magnitude and destructive power yield compensatory achievements and leave behind some positive legacy, for India that was almost entirely not the case.

The Politics of Colonial Memorialization

An editorial in the *Indian Medical Gazette* in July 1921 observed wearily: 'Most of us have already almost forgotten the great influenza epidemic of 1918–1919.' Only when there was some local recrudescence or some new report was published was there any reminder 'of the dark days through which we passed.'[44] And yet the experience of influenza could not so easily be 'lost' or 'forgotten.' In an autobiographical chapter of a book published in 1935, James Best recounted his experiences as an officer of the Indian Forest Service during the First World War. Having had his request to serve in the armed forces rejected, he was stationed instead in Hoshangabad district in the Central Provinces, where his wartime duties included supplying timber and fodder for the army. Only toward the end of this chapter did Best refer to 'the influenza plague' in the autumn of 1918 and the 'terrible death-toll' resulting from it. Entire forest settlements were deserted, he recalled, as the inhabitants fled in terror; in some villages half the population perished. Such was the devastation caused by the epidemic that it was remembered locally as *garbar*, 'the confusion.' 'One did what one could for them,' Best wrote, referring to his attempt to provide medical aid for stricken villagers, 'and some of the sights are difficult to forget.' In the winter of 1918 when he and a companion went snipe-shooting in the dried-up bed of the Narbudda (Narmada) River, it was hard to avoid 'stepping on the thousands of rotted corpses which lay about everywhere ... Some still had rags of clothing on them, others lay broken up by the crocodiles and Narbudda turtles.'[45]

That is the point at which Best's chapter ends, but his brief narrative of the epidemic is both significant in itself and representative of many other reminiscences written from a European perspective about India in 1918–19. His account supplements and confirms, on the basis of personal observation and experience, what can be gleaned from official commentaries and statistics. Rural India, especially remote areas like Hoshangabad, and tribal communities in particular, suffered, as previously noted, exceptionally high rates of sickness and mortality. Forestry officers, salt officials, and other state agents who worked in such out-of-the-way locations were well placed to observe and record the epidemic's impact, and felt impelled to do so if only because it so drastically affected the health and available labor of their Indian workers and subordinates.[46] Even the phrase Best culls from local memory—that this was a time of 'confusion'— echoes evidence for popular recollection of the event from other sources and the connection made in both public discourse and the official perception between the ravages of disease and a more general sense of crisis and dislocation caused by the war: this was influenza as 'war fever.'[47] As late as the 1950s, villagers in Mysore still referred to the calamitous events of 1918–19 as 'the plague coming out of black gunpowder,' suggesting a continuing association with the war.[48] Nor was it uncommon, as in Best's account, for Europeans to recall mass influenza mortality through the abandonment of human corpses— too many to burn, too numerous to bury—in rivers and jungles or on waste ground, where they were consumed by birds, fish, and reptiles. The devouring of human flesh by wild animals added immeasurably to the horror with which the epidemic was remembered.[49]

But there is more to be garnered from Best's description. He described his efforts, along with those of others (whom we assume to be Europeans), to collect large quantities of the herb *chiretta* and to boil it up as a medicine for distribution to the sick: this, he averred, was a 'great success' and had a very beneficial effect on those he treated.[50] This incident is remarkable because *chiretta* was a medicinal herb widely used as a tonic and stimulant in indigenous medical practice but it was not a conventional ingredient in the Western pharmacopoeia. It silently attests to the fact, for which there is other evidence, that Western medicine had little of value to offer in this epidemic and that many Indians (and Europeans) looked to indigenous or folk remedies instead, both in the cities and in remote rural areas where the reach of Western medicine was anyway limited. Like many other European accounts of the epidemic, Best stressed the apparent 'helplessness' of the local population and the humanitarian aid that even he, a forestry officer devoid of medical training, was able to provide for the stricken population.[51] Moreover, he noted, his was not the only assistance given. He also recorded the 'splendid' efforts made by Quaker missionaries and their converts ('mission boys') in caring for the sick.[52]

Best makes no mention of falling ill himself (death-rates among Europeans were low), but what he remembered was boiling up and distributing *chiretta* and the ghastly sights to which he and his snipe-shooting companion were exposed. It was not uncommon for the Indian experience of catastrophe and the personal and collective trauma that resulted from famine, flood, and epidemic to be represented in this way as a demonstration of European philanthropy and benevolence or as an affront to European feelings and sensibilities, and often as both together. In the process such first-hand accounts neglected or subsumed within their autobiographical narration the prodigious suffering of Indians themselves, as if such pain lay beyond their imagination and emotional reach.[53] It was in similar vein that India's sanitary commissioner, Norman White, long after recalled: 'No one who took an active part in our impotent efforts to control the disease … is likely to have forgotten his experiences.'[54] What were his 'experiences,' arduous though they may have been, compared with millions of Indians' suffering and grief?

For Best the influenza epidemic formed only one episode within a larger story—his personal experiences as a colonial forestry officer and, more especially, the war years and their impact on India. Indeed, he introduced the subject of the epidemic by remarking that influenza and the disruption it caused were a source of 'added anxiety' to his already demanding and stressful life in Hoshangabad. Apart from the snipe-shooting incident, he concluded his account of the war years by observing that on arrival at Taku railway station in November 1918 he first learned that the Armistice had been declared.[55] An epidemic in which between 12 and 20 million people died in India is thus sandwiched within a narrative of the Great War, a war in which Best was unable to fight, and yet of which he was acutely aware even at such a great distance from the fighting.

War, Memory, Nationhood

The time in which the influenza epidemic fell was a period of intense memorialization for India. The Great War was preeminent in this. Close to a million Indian soldiers fought in major theaters of the war and of these nearly one in eight died or was seriously wounded.[56] The British authorities were fully aware of the importance of India's military contribution to the imperial war effort and were reminded of their debt by nationalist politicians in India, by the princes who supplied soldiers, ambulances, and hospital ships, and by administrators themselves who realized the highly detrimental impact that failing to honor the war dead would have on the morale of serving soldiers, on future recruitment, and an already wavering British prestige in India.[57] A series of 'victory durbars' were held in Punjab in the months following the Armistice at which the lieutenant-governor profusely thanked the districts that had contributed most men to the Indian Army.[58] Commemorative monuments were erected to India's war dead—at Neuve Chapelle on the Western Front, at Basra in Iraq, at New Delhi's India Gate, and at Patcham Down in Sussex, where Sikhs and Hindus from the Brighton military hospital had been cremated.[59]

There was no such memorialization for the far larger number of Indians who died from influenza. The 53,486 Indian soldiers and non-combatants killed in the war were greatly outnumbered by the 675,222 Indians—men, women, and children—of Bombay Presidency who in this one province alone died in October 1918 or the further 247,348 who perished in the following month.[60] But sheer numbers were not—are not—the sole basis on which the dead are remembered or on which they enter the public record and collective memory. Soldiers and non-combatants died for a discernible cause—the defense of an empire or the expectation that India would be rewarded for its wartime sacrifices by a postwar settlement that would progress the cause of Indian home rule. Influenza had, in a political sense, no meaning, no remembrance-worthy rationale. Indeed, it was a sorry paradox, and one officials were keen to play down, that it was British troopships from Basra and other Middle Eastern ports that were the means by which the pandemic first entered India in 1918, just as troop movements and cantonments were a significant factor in its onward dissemination within India. Commemorating the war dead obscured a greater, still deadlier tragedy—the millions who died from influenza.

Apart from the war, memorialization had an additional presence in this period. From the time of the partition of Bengal in 1905 onward, Indian patriots who were executed for their political 'crimes' or who died from other causes were celebrated as heroes and martyrs. Their garlanded, flower-strewn bodies were taken in procession through crowded city streets, watched by thousands of mourners, then honored at the cremation ground with prayers, songs, funeral orations, and displays of anticolonial fervor. Memorial statues and *samadhis* (shrines) were erected at the site of their burning.[61] Their contribution to the nationalist cause was repeatedly impressed on the public memory, their lives invoked as exemplars of patriotic service, suffering, and self-sacrifice. But this powerful political narrative, too, swallowed up the alternative story of influenza's inglorious dead.

Despite the assertions of some historians, influenza connected only tangentially with India's emerging political crisis. The impasse had begun in the middle years of the war as nationalist politicians strove to capitalize on Britain's military weakness and India's contribution to the war effort to win concessions that would advance India on the path to home rule or a still greater measure of *swaraj* (self-rule). In

1918-20, even as some leading dissidents, like Bal Gangadhar Tilak and Annie Besant, became less strident in their demands than they had been at the height of the Home Rule movement in 1917, a new agitational force emerged in the form of Mohandas Gandhi, who in a matter of months switched from recruiting soldiers for the Raj to riding a rising tide of anticolonial discontent. In mid-July 1918, when the first wave of 'Bombay fever' reached Ahmedabad, Gandhi was still helping to recruit for the Indian Army.[62] By the time the more lethal second wave of Spanish Flu struck in September, Gandhi was suffering a severe and debilitating illness of his own. This was dysentery brought on by stress (not least his work as a recruiting agent), by physical exhaustion, and by a frugal diet. Erik Erikson called it a 'nervous breakdown.'[63] There is no evidence to indicate that Gandhi was suffering from influenza as some historians have claimed in trying to posit a connection between pandemic loss and nationalist resolution.[64]

Gandhi was no stranger to contagious disease. In the course of his career in South Africa and latterly in India, he had frequent cause to reflect on the nature and meaning of disease. When he returned to Durban in Natal from Bombay in December 1896, the ship in which he was traveling was suspected of carrying plague and protesters prevented the disembarkation of passengers for several days. In the following years, Gandhi helped to nurse the plague-sick. On his return to India in 1915, his attempt to establish an ashram at Kochrab in Gujarat was thwarted by a plague outbreak and he was forced to relocate to Sabarmati on the outskirts of Ahmedabad. From the time of his manifesto *Hind Swaraj* in 1909, Gandhi attached great moral significance to disease, seeing it as a consequence either of the ills of modern civilization or of an individual's indulgences and excesses. Given that Gujarat was one of the areas of India worst hit by influenza in 1918 and that the epidemic stimulated a sustained philanthropic response from the Indian middle classes, one might have expected Gandhi to be in the forefront of efforts to care for influenza victims. Certainly, some of his followers at Sabarmati helped distribute medicine to nearby villages, even as Gandhi lay ill. But Gandhi himself appeared rather indifferent to the epidemic, perhaps preoccupied with his own illness.[65] In a letter to his son Harilal in

November 1918, Gandhi noted that the family had been badly hit by influenza: Harilal's wife had been one of its casualties. Gandhi added, more in resignation than alarm, 'But such news is pouring in from everywhere so that now the mind is hardly affected.'[66] In January 1919 Gandhi wrote to his friend C. F. Andrews, 'So you have been suffering from influenza,' but made no further comment on the disease.[67] In February that year, Gandhi told another acquaintance: 'There is hardly a family left in India that has not lost some dear ones. One's feelings almost become blunt when the same news comes from anywhere with merciless regularity.'[68]

While Gandhi's illness provides the most obvious explanation for his apparent personal lack of concern, the absence of any mention of the epidemic in political narratives of the period is striking, especially in view of the criticisms made in the Indian press at the time about the government's laggardly response. Influenza was absent, for instance, from the political memoirs of M. R. Jayakar, a moderate nationalist who supported social welfare schemes in Bombay, and from the autobiography of Jawaharlal Nehru, who recalled Gandhi's 'serious illness' but made no reference to the epidemic then raging around him.[69] Conceivably, influenza had, in their view, no place in political memoirs; perhaps it simply had no great or lasting impact on their own middle-class lives. One has the impression from such reminiscences, as from most historical narratives of the period, that even in the critical months of 1918–19 political life continued uninterrupted: conferences were held, speeches made, resolutions passed.[70] Perhaps, too, there was a collective shrug of resignation. However singular and bitter the experience of influenza, it fitted into an existing pattern—of epidemic disease and administrative inaction. In asking in February 1919 how the government had dealt with the influenza epidemic, Calcutta's *Amrit Bazar Patrika* observed that malaria, kala-azar, and other diseases 'have already converted most of our villages into deserts. The legacy of the great war, we mean influenza, has added further horror to the already horrid situation.'[71]

By the time Gandhi had recovered from his illness, other, arguably more momentous matters were foremost in his mind. The British had reneged on their wartime promises, especially the declaration made by Edwin Montagu, secretary of state for India, in November 1917 that India would be granted a substantial degree of self-government after the war. Instead, the Government of India imposed the Rowlatt Act, which extended wartime restrictions on rights of assembly and further curbed political protest. Gandhi now summoned up all his energy to direct a nationwide campaign of non-violent resistance against the Act. The Rowlatt Satyagraha has been extensively discussed and yet influenza rates barely a mention in historical accounts of this seminal episode.[72]

Agitational politics helped drive influenza from the front pages of Indian newspapers.[73] Instead of the 12 to 20 million influenza deaths in late 1918 and early 1919, what most came to be remembered and memorialized was the Amritsar massacre of 13 April 1919, when (by official reckoning) 379 people were shot dead and a further 1,200 wounded by troops under the command of General Reginald Dyer at Jallianwala Bagh.[74] This was a pivotal moment in the Indian nationalist movement, and widespread horror at the shooting of unarmed civilians created an upsurge of anger and disillusionment with phony promises of self-rule. As in Ireland, influenza in India was subsumed within a more compelling story of patriotic suffering and aspiring nationhood.[75] By the time the full demographic toll from the epidemic became apparent in 1923, India had moved on to non-cooperation, civil disobedience, and a political upheaval that threatened the very survival of the Raj. And by the time *that* crisis was over, India had a new, if inadequate, constitution; Gandhi was in jail and influenza had sunk to insignificant levels. Plague, malaria, tuberculosis, and other diseases entered India's political discourse as analogous to, or indicative of, the affliction of colonial rule, and an article in Gandhi's *Young India* written in the wake of Jallianwala Bagh asked whether a regime that had callously allowed 6 million Indians to perish from influenza 'like rats without succour' could possibly care whether a few dozen people died as a result of Dyer's massacre.[76] But otherwise influenza hardly entered India's vocabulary of outrage and resistance. It was undoubtedly a catastrophe, but it did not describe a wider cause or ignite a greater political imaginary.

Private Tragedy

The study of modern South Asia has turned increasingly to emotion and affect.[77] There is every reason why India's epidemic and pandemic experience should be included in that pursuit. Emotion was unquestionably one of the hallmarks of the Covid-19 pandemic, as television, newspapers, and social media coverage made painfully clear, for India as elsewhere. Equally, it could be argued that one way of decolonizing contagion is to access the private emotions of those who suffered and endured the disease rather than those who, as officials and epidemiologists, pronounced, often loftily, upon its causes and effects. And yet historically, for India, the evidence for personal affect is difficult to uncover. Perhaps, in any fine-grained analysis, we can read it even into medical texts and administrative reports, through the emotionally charged language that is used or by the empathetic manner in which the fear and anguish of the sick, dying, and bereaved are registered even in the most austere officialese or intricate medical jargon. Clearly, influenza in 1918–19 was personal and intimate, but the private grief which the epidemic occasioned is hard to locate. As will be seen in chapter 7, there were ways in which the 'lessons' of 1918–19 were recalled, for instance, at the time of the 1957 influenza pandemic, not least by those individuals personally concerned with public health. From letters sent from the Western Front in 1914–15, we known a great deal about what Indian soldiers thought of the war in which they were fighting, about the fear, anger, and bewilderment they experienced.[78] But, for the present, we have few Indian voices and only scant first-hand testimony for and about those who fought, or fell victim to, influenza. Perhaps this lacuna will change as more research is undertaken on the 1918–19 epidemic, especially in the light of Covid-19. As official narratives and statistics indicate, the epidemic impacted massively on individuals, families, and entire communities across the subcontinent, and yet the evidence for this is, as yet, only fragmentary.

Some evidence does, though, survive from contemporary sources, if only fragmentary and second-hand. For example, in one of many obituary notices that appeared in the Indian press from mid-

July 1918 onward we learn of the 'untimely' death from influenza of eighteen-year-old Syed Edroos, 'a young man of fine disposition and much promise.' He was the only son of a leading Muslim politician and long-serving member of the Bombay legislature, and his death 'caused profound regret and sincere sorrow among all sections of the community.' The funeral procession to the main mosque in Surat on 13 July was reportedly 'one of the largest ever seen in this city' and was accompanied by local dignitaries and a police guard of honor.[79] Few other deaths from influenza over the following months attracted even that much media attention, perhaps because few Indians of prominence and stature died from the disease or because death was felt to be a matter for private grief rather than public commemoration.

While for India's plague years we have a wealth of photographic material, for influenza (so far as I am aware) we have none. In 2020–1 it was possible to memorialize the Covid dead through photographs and online family tributes.[80] But before the 1920s newspapers rarely published obituaries for any but the most eminent of Indians, and the practice of accompanying death notices with a photograph of the deceased only later came into fashion. In 1918–19 deaths were mostly reported arithmetically, as weekly or monthly totals, not by individual names. When particular cases did appear in print, it was often only because they represented the more tragic or sensational end of the Indian spectrum of death and mourning. Thus, in a village in the United Provinces the fate of a young widow whose husband and father had both died from influenza was remarked upon because she committed sati on her husband's funeral pyre.[81] In his memoirs, the Hindi poet Suryakant Tripathi, writing under the pen name Nirala, recalled how he was summoned home by telegram when his wife fell ill with influenza. By the time he arrived at her village she had already died and the Ganges was swollen with the bodies of the dead. 'This was the strangest time in my life,' he wrote, 'my family disappeared in the blink of an eye.'[82] But traumatic though the episode undoubtedly was, it played no further part in Nirala's autobiography.

In the absence of other sources, we might seek surrogates in fiction. Cholera and plague are not infrequently described as the cause of sickness and death of characters in many Indian novels and short stories. In Lal Behari Dey's *Bengal Peasant Life* (first published in 1874), one of the principal characters dies of cholera while on pilgrimage to Puri. In Rabindranath Tagore's short novel *Chaturanga* ('The Quartet,' 1916), Jagmohan dies of plague while trying to help sufferers during the epidemic in Calcutta; and deaths from plague and cholera appear in several of Munshi Premchand's Hindi short stories (such as 'Idgah' in 1938). In the second part of Sarat Chandra Chatterjee's semi-autobiographical novel *Srikanta* (1918), there is a striking description of the brusque medical inspection of coolies embarking for Rangoon. As with many other writers of Indian fiction, the experience of disease was very real and intimate for Chatterjee: both his wife and infant son died of plague in 1908.[83] But, in one of its many apparent absences, influenza had only a slight or fleeting literary presence: we learn little from Indian literature about what Elizabeth Outka aptly termed 'the vertigo of loss.'[84]

One place where influenza was directly cited was in Ahmed Ali's *Twilight in Delhi*, first published in 1940 but presumably based on the author's childhood impressions (he would have been about eight at the time of the epidemic) or on family reminiscences. In this story of a high-status Muslim family in old Delhi, influenza captures a mood of both personal tragedy and communal disintegration. Bilqeece, a sickly wife, dies in the epidemic, but the private grief her loss occasions simply adds to the growing despair within an elite community that already feels its old way of life is in terminal decline. Here influenza is more metaphor than pathogen. Although the British are ultimately held responsible for destroying the proud remnants of Mughal culture, 'fate,' 'destiny,' and 'Nature' play no less a part. Employing the same idiom of natural disaster as the British, in 1918 Ali writes, 'Nature herself was rebellious and seemed angry with the people of Hindustan.' Not content with the thousands of India's war dead, Nature chooses to demonstrate its 'callousness and might' by turning Delhi into 'a city of the dead.' Houses all around the Muslim *mohalla* resound to 'heart-rending cries of lamentation and weeping.' 'There was hardly any house where a death did not take place.' Muslims and Hindus struggle to bury or burn their dead, and yet the Angel of Death is unremitting. 'From house to house he rushed, from door to door, snatching the souls away from human beings burning with fever yet hungry after life, wanting to live on in a world which did not care about them at all.'[85]

Among works of non-fiction, there are other insights to be gleaned. It was not death alone that scarred and traumatized the living but also their own struggle to survive and recover. Some victims of the disease experienced lasting debility and depression, the equivalent of what in 2020–1 came to be described as 'long Covid.' In his memoir, Prakash Tandon recounted how his father Ram Das, a canal engineer in Punjab then in his forties, was struck down by influenza in 1918. 'Postcards with edges torn [to indicate a death] began to arrive almost every week,' Tandon recalled. 'Father went down also and lay hovering between life and death for days … Two of his nephews and both his sisters died within a week.' The family wondered what exactly this 'plague' was, having heard the rumor that it came from the battlefields of Europe. Ram Das made a slow and painful recovery and, once he had sufficiently recuperated, his wife organized a *havan* ceremony 'to cleanse the house of the illness. She distributed sweets and hoped that this foreign affliction would not come our way again. Yam-doot, the messenger of the god of death, had visited our family too often in the past year.'[86] Ram Das, ever the rational engineer, sought his own secular restorative by buying a Singer sewing machine. It is not clear from Tandon's memoir who used the machine and for what, but Ram Das shared the maker's claim that a Singer could actually sing, its mechanical hum for the invalid a cheerful, uplifting sound.[87]

Ram Das and his son survived; many sons did not. In June 1918 the *Times of India* apologized to readers for not being able to publish a lecture given in London by Dinshaw Edulji Wacha, a prominent Parsi businessman and nationalist politician, on the cotton industry in Bombay. This failure was due to the 'confounded influenza epidemic,' then still in its first phase, and the resulting incapacity of the paper's staff.[88] Five months later, on 19 November 1918, at the height of the second wave, Wacha's only son, K. D. Wacha, died from influenza, compounded by pneumonia. The son was 48, the father 74.[89] As a mark of respect, Bombay Corporation adjourned its scheduled meeting and sent condolences to the bereaved father 'who had sustained a heavy blow in his old age.'[90] Despite this personal disaster, Wacha continued with his political work (now for the liberal wing of the nationalist movement) and lived on until 1936. But in 1920 when he published his long-planned memoir of Bombay, he dedicated it 'with tears' to his son who, a little before his death and 'with loving hands and filial devotion,' had helped revise the proofs.[91] In similar vein, the historian Jadunath Sarkar recalled meeting Kashinath Narayan Sane, an eminent Marathi scholar, a few years before the latter's death in 1927 at the age of 83. 'His grown up and distinguished son,' Sarkar noted, 'died of the terrible influenza epidemic which swept all over the world just after the First World War. Sane's heart was made desolate' by this death, 'but his back was unbent. He kept up his regular habit of taking daily exercise by a morning walk.'[92]

These examples imply parental stoicism in the face of immense grief. Perhaps, to return to Judith Shklar's distinction between misfortune and injustice, they suggest that the influenza pandemic was viewed by many of those affected less as a case of injustice (one for which returning soldiers, an imperial war, or colonial negligence might be blamed), but more in terms of a personal misfortune that somehow had to be borne. This was not a political injustice (like Jallianwala Bagh) to be met with public outrage and patriotic anger.

* * *

It is a pandemic paradox that in many ways (and not just in India) the Spanish Flu of 1918–19, and the extraordinary mortality that accompanied it almost everywhere around the globe, were, in its aftermath, largely forgotten. India's experience was doubly elided. The country's massive and unparalleled death-toll was afforded scant recognition compared even with the historical and epidemiological attention given to the same disease in the West, where it caused many fewer deaths and killed a much smaller share of the population. It was largely absent, too, from the dominant narrative history of late colonialism and the Indian freedom struggle, which seldom allowed it more than a line or two, tucked into the brief hiatus between the end of the Great War and Gandhi's first nationwide civil disobedience campaign. The traumatic events of the Second World War, the Bengal famine of 1943, the massacres and mass migrations of Partition in

1947, further obscured the subcontinental experience. It was only in historical demography—notably Kingsley Davis's *Population of India and Pakistan* in 1951 and, more than thirty years later, in 1986, I. D. Mills's essay on 'the Indian experience' of influenza—that concern with India's worst pandemic ordeal was kept alive and updated.[93]

Revival of interest in the Spanish Flu of 1918–20 was a long time coming. Only since the 1980s has the global impact of the 1918–19 virus been extensively revisited, and in this overdue revisionism India, despite having been the world's greatest sufferer, has until recently occupied a fairly minor place. However, since the eruption of SARS, Swine Flu, and more especially Covid, the 'forgotten' pandemic has gained fresh prominence and is orphan no longer, especially in relation to India and the Global South.[94] Given high levels of poverty and undernutrition, the inadequacy of its health infrastructure, and the chronic imbalance between rich and poor, India was deemed particularly at risk from a new influenza pandemic, and the extent of its suffering in 1918–19 was repurposed to illustrate and exemplify the danger posed by a new pandemic threat. India was now viewed, at least by epidemiologists, as the exemplary case to be studied.

This was disease not as metaphor but as an incipient reality. Reviewing the evidence in 2006, Neil Ferguson of Imperial College, London, observed that 'poor populations always endure a disproportionate burden of disease and death from infectious diseases.' Of course, there would never be a 'precise rerun' of the 1918–19 pandemic. But 'health inequality is scarcely less now than in 1918,' Ferguson wrote, 'and the medical advances of the past 90 years are unlikely to benefit much of the developing world in any future pandemic.'[95] India, among those poor and developing nations, was in the firing line. A decade after Ferguson, in a series of articles Siddharth Chandra and his associates urged the global health community to prepare for a new influenza pandemic. This was likely to be a 'truly global phenomenon' and a major 'security issue.' Citing the case of India in particular, they argued the need for in-depth historical studies to give a 'thorough picture' of the 1918–19 pandemic in order to anticipate 'the possible character of any future infections.'[96] History, as the demography and epidemiology of 1918–19 India, was back in fashion. In an article published in 2018, two

Indian researchers, Lalit Kant and Randeep Guleria, reiterated the risks to India of a pandemic on the scale of the Spanish Flu, adding: 'Imagine the devastation a 1918-like pandemic would cause today in India when we are more interconnected. The cities are denser. The speed of travel has increased. Conditions that favoured the spread of influenza in 1918 are still prevalent ... India would not be spared.'[97] By this bleak scenario, millions would die—an unimaginable 62 million by one calculation, an apocalyptic 150 million by another, of which the combined share of India, Pakistan, and Bangladesh would be around 60 million.[98] Sam Higginbottom's estimate of 32 million deaths in 1918–19 appeared modest by comparison.

6

IN THE TIME OF THE NATION

Modern pandemics are semantic events as well as epidemiological phenomena. As in a time of war, old idioms dissolve or acquire fresh meaning; there is a sudden effusion of buzzwords and slang. A new vocabulary of technical jargon is put in circulation by medical authorities and public health experts, enters the language of media and state, and begins to find popular traction. Where previous pandemics spoke of natural disasters—floods, avalanches, storms, and lightning—or, more martially, of invasions and conquests, during the Covid-19 pandemic of 2020–1, while many of these older metaphors were retrieved and refurbished, a more eclectic language emerged. Phrases such as 'case fatality rate,' 'herd immunity,' and 'the R-number' (for the reproduction rate) and acronyms like PPE (personal protective equipment) seeped from scientific discourse into official pronouncements and everyday speech. Terms suggestive of social control gained currency—pandemic 'waves' and 'surges' were to be countered with 'social distancing' or 'lockdowns' (an expression once reserved for the repression of prison riots). After the Boxing Day disaster of December 2004 in which 230,000 people died, Covid became—or threatened to be—'a tsunami.' 'Pandemic' itself, a term so long latent in public discourse, gained through Covid unprecedented use and a nightmarish familiarity. If Raymond

Williams were writing his celebrated *Keywords* today, 'pandemic' would surely be included among the entries.[1]

Many of these English-language expressions and neologisms quickly found their way into Indian public health discourse, into official pronouncements and media coverage of the Covid pandemic. India, too, in this new globe-speak, had its 'lockdowns,' its coronavirus 'surges,' its 'vaccine rollout.' But one other word, not obviously plucked from the medical thesaurus, also gained a new popularity and resonance—'tryst.' On 14 August 1947, in what is widely regarded as one of the great speeches of the twentieth century, prime minister Jawaharlal Nehru spoke eloquently of India's 'tryst with destiny.' 'Long years ago,' he declared to India's Constituent Assembly, 'we made a tryst with destiny … At the stroke of the midnight hour, when the world sleeps, India will awake to life and freedom.' 'A moment comes,' he continued, 'which comes but rarely in history, when we step out from the old to the new, when an age ends, and when the soul of a nation, long suppressed, finds utterance.' But, Nehru added, 'freedom and power bring responsibility.'[2] 'Tryst' was a curious word for Nehru to have used; it suggested a secret assignation, between 'star-crossed lovers,' rather than the open and oft-stated goal of independence for which India had so long and so resolutely striven. But the term struck a chord in India's literary and political culture, if only because it captured the magnitude of India's freedom after centuries of colonial rule and the sense that independence was both a compelling force of destiny and an occasion for the responsible exercise of power.

Over time the term became hackneyed through overuse, but in Covid it found fresh resonance. The pandemic suggested that India's 'tryst' might not after all be with a benign and nurturing destiny but with a malign and deadly disease. 'India's tryst with Covid-19,' ran one journal's headline over a night-time image of migrant workers quitting Delhi in April 2020. The article's author, Vikram Patel of the Harvard Medical School, argued that the recently imposed nationwide lockdown would not in itself eliminate the virus and that fundamental lessons had to be learned from the pandemic about the country's desperate need for adequate healthcare provision. 'India's tryst with Covid-19,' he warned, 'is far from over.'[3] Patel was not alone in redeploying the Nehruvian catchword. 'Delhi's tryst with the third wave of Covid-19 infections,' ran a fairly typical headline in November 2020, while one blogger writing in February 2021 thought fit to give a personal account of his 'tryst with coronavirus and home quarantine.'[4]

'Tryst' might signify little more than a meeting, an encounter, a skirmish. But the word still transported India and Indians back to August 1947, to the heady expectations of freedom, to the fecund promise of independence, and the secular leadership of India's first prime minister. It hinted, more darkly, at the trials and traumas that accompanied independence. Even the photograph of migrant workers that accompanied Vikram Patel's article resembled the familiar images of refugees displaced and dispossessed by Partition. 'Tryst' could be used, if only subliminally, to suggest that India had in some way failed to fulfill its promised destiny, that nationhood had turned sour, or that the disease that now stalked India, the novel coronavirus, was not so much an aberration as an overdue reckoning for post-independence India's failure to deal adequately with the essential problems of health and well-being. To many in the West the return of pandemic disorders beginning in the 1970s and 1980s—AIDS, SARS, Ebola, and latterly Covid—was an unexpected and unpredictable turn of events after a period of great optimism about the eradication or containment of once world-afflicting contagious diseases.[5] But for India, to invoke Roald Dahl rather than Jawaharlal Nehru, was coronavirus really a 'tale of the unexpected'?[6] Were epidemics and pandemics, however much underplayed or ignored, as much a part of the time of the nation as they had been of the time of empire?

Hiatus

Partition and independence in 1947 came to South Asia at the very moment when a new triumphalism entered global epidemiological discourse. Advances in medical science and public health, the invention of antibiotics and the widespread use of DDT as an insecticide, coupled with the absence of any major pandemic since 1919, encouraged optimism—a false optimism, as it proved—

about the way in which the history of medicine and disease was progressing.[7] The time of pandemics appeared to be over. In the early 1950s Macfarlane Burnet, the Australian Nobel laureate who pioneered modern influenza research, wrote: 'In many ways one can think of the middle of the twentieth century as the end of one of the most important social revolutions in history, the virtual elimination of infectious diseases as a significant factor in social life.'[8] In an updated edition of his book in 1972, Burnet went so far as to conclude that 'the most likely forecast about the future of infectious disease is that it will be very dull.'[9] This triumphalism was shared by the US surgeon-general William Stewart in 1967, who observed that 'the time has come to close the book on infectious diseases. We have basically wiped out infection in the United States.'[10]

Not so 'dull,' in reality, was post-independence India's ongoing struggle with infectious disease. Remarkably, despite the enormous upheaval and mass migration of 1947–8, Partition, while it undoubtedly caused a rise in disease mortality, did not result in a major outbreak of epidemic mortality. With the support and encouragement of the World Health Organization (WHO), India played a vital role in the eradication of smallpox in the 1970s, inoculating an estimated 80 percent of its entire population. It had initial success, too, in attempting to expunge or at least contain malaria. Cholera was resurgent following the war that led to the independence of Bangladesh from Pakistan in 1971, but oral rehydration therapy, cheap, effective, and easily administered, helped curb its spread and has since kept mortality from the disease at relatively low levels.[11] The pandemics of influenza that hit India in the 1950s and 1960s further seemed to suggest that the nightmare mortality of the pandemic age—and the colonial era—was finally over. Between May 1957 and February 1958 there were nearly 4.5 million cases of 'Asian Flu' reported in India but only 1,098 deaths out of 2 million worldwide. With Spanish Flu a fading cultural memory and immunological trace, this pandemic, unlike its deadly predecessor, could be safely characterized as only 'mild' influenza.[12]

In the time of the nation, fighting disease took second place to promoting development, the pursuit of which seemed the most effective riposte to the famines and epidemics that had scarred the colonial age. Kavita Sivaramakrishnan has described how the 1957 influenza epidemic, falling exactly ten years after independence, was received in Nehru's India. The greatest fear was that the epidemic would cause widespread absenteeism and lost productivity, and so stall India's ambitious five-year plans for industrialization and economic regeneration. As in 1918–19, government intervention in 1957 was minimal, if only because this time there was little expectation that India would have to contend with such devastating levels of mortality. Influenza was more an inconvenience than an existential threat. While India was prepared to commit considerable human and financial resources to the eradication of smallpox and malaria, schemes of high national and international importance, influenza did not rate the same degree of attention. Moreover, the language of self-help and self-reliance (of which we saw evidence in the plague and Spanish Flu episodes) was again utilized, only now to remind the public that it was primarily the responsibility of the people to manage their own ill health through 'cooperative citizenship' rather than expecting state assistance. This meant, in practice, a neglect of the poorer classes, who as so often in the past, were left to provide their own healthcare—if, indeed, they were able to do so. Herein lay the recurring ambiguity of self-reliance: was it the laudable self-mobilization of the people in the face of epidemic adversity, or was it the state shrugging off responsibility for public well-being? 'The postcolonial predicament in India,' concluded Sivaramakrishnan, 'brought an awareness and public admission by the state that public health crises needed citizens to act, cooperate, and share risks and vulnerabilities, even though a majority of them had reaped few, if any, benefits from these development projects.'[13]

The fear of epidemics receded as the threat of famine abated. Despite famine or near-famine conditions in some areas, notably Bihar in 1966–7 and Maharashtra in 1970–3, there was immense political determination to escape the horrific famines of the colonial past (while utilizing the administrative expertise gained through the colonial famine codes), and to build a self-sufficient economy able to ensure that India's people were properly fed.[14] Industrialization was one part of this strategy of self-reliance; so, too, was the Green Revolution from the late 1960s which enabled India, at whatever social and environmental cost, to increase its food production massively.[15] Widespread poverty and malnutrition remained, but, without more extreme subsistence crises, the epidemic diseases that had, as late as the Bengal famine of 1943, so closely tracked famine and multiplied its death-toll seemed consigned to an increasingly distant past.[16]

The 1918–19 influenza pandemic has often been taken to mark the end of the pandemic era and a moment of demographic and epidemiological transition. Historians and demographers have advanced various theories to explain why this mortality decline occurred. For Ira Klein, following Kingsley Davis's earlier analysis, the most likely factor was that the Indian population, which had suffered so severely in the nineteenth century from increased exposure to disease and the negative impact of 'imbalanced' modernization, had by the 1920s become immune to leading pathogens, though it is hard to see why this should have happened almost simultaneously with all three of India's principal killers—cholera, plague, and malaria.[17] For Sumit Guha, on the other hand, the primary reason was that the 'weather gods' were kind and India, liberated from the serial droughts and subsistence crises of the nineteenth century, was able to build a new era of agricultural security. In his view, 'climatic change was the most important source of improvement in mortality.'[18] Guha further argued for the importance of an expanding 'information apparatus' that generated reliable data about epidemics and the factors behind their occurrence, and the increasing institutionalization of state health and welfare provision.[19] Tirthankar Roy has similarly reasoned that improved 'water security' from the 1880s onward, and the consequent improvement in crop yields and health conditions for even the poorest sections of society, was also a factor in the elimination of famine and the marked decline in epidemic mortality.[20] Significantly, such arguments suggest that the key factors behind the long-term decline in Indian mortality (apart, catastrophically, from Bengal in 1943) had come into play decades before the end of the colonial era. The advances made in public health after 1900, however piecemeal and insufficient, and the extended use of vaccination against smallpox, cholera, and plague, also help to explain the timing and the parallel decline of mortality from these once-prevalent diseases. Plague and influenza may have declined in intensity as the infectivity and virulence of their pathogens waned, but cholera, smallpox, malaria, and possibly plague as well are likely to have shown some impact from growing public awareness, especially through local health campaigns, from such innovations as the use of DDT against mosquitoes, fleas, and other insect vectors, and from greater scientific understanding of disease causation and transmission. Conceivably, there is no single explanation for the decline in India's epidemic and pandemic mortality but a conjunction of factors, including (among others) climatic stability, the absence of major famines, more effective state policies, improving public health administration, immunization campaigns, and the fading virulence of certain key diseases.

From the 1950s India experienced a number of epidemics (or incipient pandemics) that resulted in only limited mortality, whether due to the mildness of the disease or to the prompt and effective measures taken against them. An outbreak of bubonic plague in Surat in Gujarat in September 1994 briefly revived fears, nationally and internationally, of a return to the dark pandemic days of the 1890s and 1900s—or even the Black Death. Locally, it spread confusion and panic as more than a quarter of the city's 700,000 inhabitants, many of them migrant workers, fled the city: a few cases of plague were thereafter recorded in Delhi, Mumbai, and Kolkata. But, perhaps owing more to good fortune than effective remedial measures, the mortality was low and the epidemic rapidly faded out, though some commentators saw it as a warning of the frailty and unpreparedness of India's public health infrastructure, especially in such a congested, polluted, and fast-growing city as Surat.[21] Overall, though, owing to antibiotics, plague mortality had fallen dramatically in India since the 1950s: only 21 deaths were reported between 1959 and 1966, and none at all between 1967 and 1993. In the 1994 outbreak fewer than 1,200 people were diagnosed with the disease and there were 53 deaths: the whole episode lasted barely two weeks.[22]

In 2009 India was hit by the Swine Flu epidemic emanating from East Asia. In India 2,427 people died out of more than 18,000 worldwide. But the danger posed by this outbreak, declared a pandemic by the WHO in June 2009, was quickly addressed by the

Government of India: 183,027 people were tested, of whom 43,283 proved positive. Despite initial confusion with malaria, dengue, and other diseases, the first cases in Pune were promptly isolated and a public education campaign launched. The antiviral drug oseltamivir was used to treat severe cases, and the outbreak was quickly over.[23] Here, too, was apparent reassurance that India was unlikely to see its pandemic past revisited, and that it could respond promptly and effectively if it did. The past was not likely to be the future. Epidemics of mosquito-borne dengue and chikungunya (originating in East Africa, this disease was first observed in India in the 1960s) struck a number of times—among other places in Delhi in 2016— but, for all the painful and debilitating illness caused, few deaths followed. Such episodes created confidence that the freak mortality of 1918–19 would not be repeated. Indeed, by contrast with cholera and plague in the nineteenth and early twentieth centuries, the limited spread of infectious diseases and their rapid containment within India suggested that the primary danger to global health lay elsewhere—in Africa or China—not in India.

However, India's potential vulnerability was underscored by a disease that has rarely received the attention it deserves in the history of the post-independence nation, a disease that has seldom been brought into comparisons with Covid-19: HIV/AIDS. For example, in his otherwise excellent account of India's pandemic age, Chinmay Tumbe noted that HIV/AIDS 'created a stir in the 1980s and 1990s,' before adding that 'the mode of transmission in that pandemic was entirely different [from the 1918–19 influenza] and, eventually, it did not affect most people in a direct manner.'[24] But it was, above all, AIDS in the 1980s that 'focused attention back onto the global threat posed by infectious diseases.'[25] In the West, the spread of HIV/AIDS not only created renewed fears about epidemic disease; it also led to a new wave of writing about contagion history and the social reception of disease. Sontag's trenchant essay on disease as metaphor; Rosenberg's investigation into the historical nature of epidemics; Nelkin and Gilman's essay on the stigmatization of disease—these were a measure of how this new and fearful disease created a new critical literature.[26] But not in India. The expression 'forgotten pandemic' used by Alfred Crosby and others may apply even more aptly to AIDS in India than to the Spanish Flu seventy years earlier. AIDS was India's missing pandemic, the absent horseman of the Indian apocalypse.

From small beginnings, infection rates from HIV and deaths from AIDS in India rose steeply during the 1990s, with the number of reported cases soon exceeding 250,000 a year: mortality peaked in 2009 at 170,000 (more than the number who died from Covid in 2020). By 2017–18 India had the third largest population of people infected with HIV/AIDS, estimated at 2.1 million, behind only South Africa and Nigeria.[27] Every major disease has its own cultural signature as well as its unique epidemiological profile. In India HIV/AIDS was for long ignored or denied because it was seen as a foreign disease, a 'gay plague,' that could not possibly impact on heterosexual India. In fact, it spread in India mainly through prostitution and intravenous drug use, neither of which attracted substantial levels of health expenditure, but which added greatly to the stigma attached to the disease. The first known cases were among sex workers in Chennai in 1986, and yet the government's National AIDS Control Organization was not set up until 1992. Only gradually did official concern and public awareness grow, helped by antiretroviral drugs and education campaigns. HIV/AIDS is now seen from a global perspective as one of the diseases, along with SARS, Ebola, Zika, and Covid, that have turned the years since the Spanish Flu of 1918–19 into a 'pandemic century.'[28] But for India AIDS seemed to resemble several other entrenched and seemingly intractable contagions rather than the sudden, overwhelming, and deadly onrush of disease associated—in their initial phases—with cholera, plague, and influenza.

But, HIV/AIDS aside, all was not well with India. As we saw at the end of the previous chapter, epidemiologists had long anticipated that India with its one billion or more people, high population densities, widespread malnutrition, and endemic poverty, with its myriad slums and millions of migrant workers, and with a deficient and woefully underfunded public health infrastructure, would be extremely vulnerable to any new pandemic on the scale of the 1918–19 influenza. With less than 1.5 percent of its gross domestic product invested in public health (which is only half of China's expenditure and one of the lowest levels even among 'developing' countries) and decades of underinvestment, India was ill-equipped to meet such a challenge. In the early twenty-first century India had the largest population of undernourished people anywhere in the world. One-fifth of all maternal deaths and one-quarter of child deaths occurred in India. Tuberculosis rates stubbornly remained high. Rabies, a disease that had become rare and treatable in most parts of the world, continued to haunt India, causing an estimated 20,000 deaths a year, a third of the total worldwide.[29] 'India,' to quote Sheetal Chhabria, remained 'one of the worst places in the world to get sick.' More than seventy years after independence, it continued to produce 'an outsized number of deaths per disease outbreak, with illnesses that had all but disappeared from the "developed" world regularly wiping out tens of thousands of inhabitants a year.'[30] One measure of this public health deficiency was the 'abysmally low' number of beds in government hospitals. In 2019 the country had barely 70,000 beds, or 0.55 beds for every one thousand of the population, one of the lowest patient–bed ratios anywhere in the world, lower even than its neighbors Bangladesh, Nepal, and Sri Lanka. This alarming figure masked wide regional variations: the backward and impoverished state of Bihar, for instance, had only 0.11 beds per thousand while Delhi, Kerala, and Tamil Nadu were better provisioned. The WHO's recommendation was one hospital bed for every 300 people: in rural India there was just one bed for 3,125 inhabitants.[31]

There had been two major opportunities to set things right and to correct the underfunding and negligence of the colonial era. One had been the publication of the Bhore Committee report in 1946, which called for a radical overhaul of India's public health system, with greater attention to primary healthcare.[32] A second came with the enunciation of a new National Health Policy by the Government of India in 1982, which 'raised hopes among those concerned with India's poor health' that the government was 'serious about its commitment to provide "health for all"'.[33] But for various reasons—political, economic, professional—those opportunities were allowed to slip away. And there was a fundamental problem (again highlighted in the Covid pandemic) in the way in which, since the constitutional reforms of 1919 and 1935 and continuing with the constitution of independent India in 1950, the primary responsibility for healthcare had been entrusted to the provinces (then, from 1947, the constituent states of the Indian Union). This left the central government relatively powerless, except with respect to broad policy matters, international immunization campaigns, and emergency powers such as the Epidemic Diseases Act. In consequence, the state of India's public health system, wrote Sumit Ganguly in the immediate aftermath of the first wave of the coronavirus pandemic, was 'for the most part, Dickensian. Even under the best of times, it is frequently found wanting.'[34]

To the legacies of colonial neglect and the underfunding of Indian public health since 1947 were added the effects of economic liberalization, begun under the Congress Party administration in 1991, and the heavy reliance on the private sector to meet public need, giving India 'one of the most commercialized health care systems in the world.'[35] The long-term history of neglect, agonizingly brought into focus by the second wave of the coronavirus in 2021, was further accentuated by the rise of the right-wing Hindu nationalist party, the Bharatiya Janata Party (BJP), which took power nationally in 1998, and especially following Narendra Modi's election as prime minister in 2014. While underinvestment in India's public health infrastructure remained chronic, the Modi government spent heavily on showpiece projects such as a lunar space mission and genome sequencing, intended to demonstrate India's global standing as a science superpower and center of technoscientific innovation. But such lavish schemes diverted funding away from urgent public health needs and ignored the poverty, pollution, and deprivation that fueled high sickness and mortality rates. The private healthcare industry, which had grown apace since the 1980s, contributed little to public needs.[36] But, at the same time, it can be said that, until Covid struck, there was little by way of a public outcry or sustained political campaigning against this neglect or the transfer of healthcare responsibility from the state to the private sector. Debate over public health was said to be 'virtually absent' from India's democratic politics.[37]

The Coming of the Coronavirus

The acute respiratory illness caused by the virus SARS-CoV-2, known more simply as Covid, began its global career in late 2019. Like SARS and MERS before it, the virus is thought to have originated among bats, possibly in southern China, before it migrated via some undetermined intermediary to humans. The first known case in India was reported in the southern state of Kerala on 30 January 2020. The patient was a student recently returned from the city of Wuhan, where the pandemic began the previous December, and where, by the end of January 2020, there were an estimated 124,000 cases.[38] At about the same time, in late January and early February, cases of the disease appeared in western Europe and then in the United States, Indonesia and Brazil. The first death in Europe was reported in Paris in mid-February. On 4 March, 22 new cases of Covid were identified in India, including 14 Italian tourists, underscoring the importance of air travel and global tourism to the rapid global dissemination of the virus. 'Airborne' described the virus's mode of transmission in more ways than one. On 11 March, the WHO's director-general, Dr. Tedros Adhanom Ghebreyesus, announced that Covid-19 was now a pandemic: it was bound to spread further and faster, and, unless it could be halted, many more deaths would follow. There were already 118,000 known cases spread across 114 countries and 4,291 deaths. 'If,' Dr. Tedros continued, 'countries detect, test, treat, isolate, trace, and mobilize their people in the response,' those which currently had only a 'handful of cases' could prevent them 'becoming clusters, and those clusters becoming community transmission.'[39] But he did not sound optimistic that prompt, effective, and coordinated action would actually ensue.

India's first Covid fatality followed on 12 March, when a man who had recently visited Saudi Arabia died. India reported 50 coronavirus deaths by 1 April, 100 by 5 April, 500 by 19 April, 1,000 by 29 April, 1,500 by 4 May, and, as the disease escalated ever more rapidly, 10,000 by 15 June.[40] India was no stranger to pandemics, but, having survived SARS relatively unscathed, with only a handful of cases, India's health professionals and the Indian public were less prepared than their counterparts in East Asia for a new and more deadly viral onslaught.[41] As the coronavirus struck in early 2020, horrifically large numbers of casualties were projected for India, one study suggesting that there could be as many as 300 million cases. Of these, 4 to 5 million would be 'severe,' implying that a large percentage would be fatal.[42] A report in April 2020 anticipated that 65 percent of all Indians were likely to be infected with Covid, and, even assuming a low death rate of around 0.3 percent, that would still result in 2 million deaths.[43] Other commentators, like the epidemiologist Siddharth Chandra, were more sanguine. Having previously called for close historical and statistical examination of the Spanish Flu as a likely template for future pandemics, Chandra now argued that Indians were better nourished in 2020 than they had been in 1918, that advances in medical knowledge and technology gave patients with severe respiratory illnesses a much greater chance of survival than a century earlier, and that global information networks now made possible the rapid dissemination of knowledge about new diseases and the sharing of best treatment practices. 'We have come a long way since 1918,' Chandra observed reassuringly. This time around there would be no more apocalyptic scenes of Indian rivers choked with the bodies of the unburied, uncremated dead.[44]

The 'Battle of Life and Death'

As elsewhere around the globe, the pandemic in India rapidly became fuel for both domestic politics and international posturing. Despite the warning given by the outbreak in Wuhan and the first Indian case on 30 January, the Indian government hesitated to act until after the first death on 12 March. The prime minister, Narendra Modi, was still busily hosting public events, including on 24 February the 'namaste Trump' spectacle in Modi's home state, Gujarat, for the visiting US president. As 125,000 cheering (and unmasked) spectators packed into Ahmedabad's vast new cricket stadium, political theatre took precedence over pandemic uncertainty. Covid was declared a national disaster on 14 March, but the government only banned international flights into India eight days later, on 22 March, well after many other countries had taken similar steps. A one-day 'janata curfew' (or 'people's curfew' in the populist language of the Modi regime) was imposed on the country on 22 March, by which time there were 236 known coronavirus cases, but this light-touch gesture, held on a Sunday when many offices, shops, and markets were closed anyway, was widely seen as ineffective. In response to the growing crisis, and without waiting for the central government to act, the cities of Delhi and Mumbai and some of India's constituent states had already taken the initiative and introduced lockdown measures of their own.

Finally, on 24 March 2020, the prime minister made a televised address to the nation, declaring that it was necessary to wage war on the invading virus. The struggle, Modi said, was an existential struggle that India had to win. Around the globe at that point there had been about 17,000 deaths and 400,000 cases, but in India the numbers were still relatively small—519 confirmed cases and 10 deaths—and some commentators believed that only limited measures were required. However, in an unwitting parody of India's 'freedom at midnight' on 14 August 1947, Modi ordered an immediate nationwide twenty-one-day lockdown to start at midnight that day, giving the startled public only four hours' notice. This announcement was made without consultation with India's medical experts, state governments, or even central government ministries.[45] Planes were immediately grounded, with all internal and external flights suspended; passenger trains stopped running, even in suburban areas. Several states closed their borders to prevent travelers and labor migrants, who might be carrying the virus, from heading home. Modi, who had a penchant for sudden, decisive action, struck a determined note, warning that if India did not handle the twenty-one-day lockdown well, 'then our country will go backward by 21 years.'[46] Speaking a week later, a seemingly more contrite prime minister apologized for having given the nation only four hours' notice of the lockdown but insisted there was 'no other way to wage war against coronavirus. For a country like India with a population of 1.3 billion it is a battle of life and death and we have to win it.'[47]

In India, as around the world, military metaphors were used to demonstrate the government's firm resolve to meet the threat posed by the viral 'enemy' and to mobilize public support. This was hardly new: such assertive metaphors had long been used (not least by

India's British rulers) to emphasize the epidemic/pandemic danger and to muster public support.[48] But, in a manner only matched in colonial times by the state's response to plague in 1896–7, Modi's government declared its emphatic ownership of the coronavirus pandemic and its primary responsibility for tackling the disease, while simultaneously presenting the campaign against it as a patriotic duty and even an act of loyalty to the prime minister himself. Unlike some prime ministers and presidents around the world, Modi was clearly on the side of ownership and intervention. In this he seemed to command widespread public support. There may have been some evasion and non-compliance, but there was little outright opposition from the 'more or less disciplined public' to India's lockdown measures, widely regarded as among the most stringent adopted at the time anywhere in the world (figs. 13 and 14).[49] The riots and violent protests that resulted from comparable state measures in the early plague years of the 1890s were not revisited. Aided by a powerful police presence, that 'disturbing' social entity, the urban 'crowd,' had been erased from the suddenly silent streets of Mumbai, Delhi, and Chennai.[50]

There was much, too, about the government's response to the crisis that was new when compared with the pandemics of the late nineteenth and early twentieth centuries. The days when sea travel and 'plague ports' were of paramount concern were largely over: viruses now traveled by air, not on coolie ships and pilgrim steamers. Restricting air travel was central to stopping the importation and spread of the virus, just as television provided a novel medium to address the nation. At the height of the plague and influenza epidemics, as thousands died and thousands more fled, India's major cities had in effect closed themselves down and their normal activity ceased. There was no government lockdown to still the factories and silence the streets. Now, in the new viral age and in lockstep with states across the globe, India's government took the unprecedented step of deliberately shutting down cities, suspending the economy, and restricting individual movement and social interaction.

The time of pandemics had speeded up since 1896 or 1918. Just as modern media—from radio and television to the internet and social media—were able to relay news of, and fears about, the pandemic almost instantly from one part of the globe to another, so measures of public health intervention and prevention that a century earlier took weeks or months to pass from one country to another were now enjoined and implemented in days. One has only to think of Thomas Herriot struggling to learn about the Spanish Flu in his Jullundur hospital in 1918 (see chapter 3) to appreciate the enormous difference a century had made to the global information order. In the past, pandemics had been named after their supposed place of origin—'Asiatic cholera,' 'Oriental plague'—but no longer. Previously pathogens were made visible through their dreaded signs and symptoms—plague buboes, the pustules of smallpox, the violent purging and ghastly hue of cholera victims. The causative viruses and bacilli as such, even when known to science and made visible through a microscope, rarely had much public impact. With Covid that changed. The pathogen became a kind of omnipresent personality, a rogue celebrity. It was a spiky ball, floating in space or hunting in packs, visible almost everywhere, on signs and posters, in news broadcasts and government announcements. The demonic virus was shown, often at first almost playfully, in cartoons, caricatures, and street art, alongside heroic health workers, or in the course of destruction by a strong, vigilant, and many-armed Mother India (fig. 15).[51]

Life under Lockdown

In response to the escalating crisis and in line with decisions taken elsewhere around the world, India ratcheted up its Covid response. The lockdown of 24 March was extended three times and eventually lasted not for twenty-one but for sixty-eight days, until June 1. During that period, case numbers in India grew more than fivefold, reaching over 190,000. For some observers, including many epidemiologists, the prompt declaration of a national lockdown was a bold preemptive move, helping to break the chain of viral transmission at an early stage and so saving many thousands of lives. Conversely, given that the pandemic was still in its infancy in March 2020, and cases were mostly confined to a small number of urban areas, it was argued that a more nuanced and locally responsive strategy to contain the disease within existing 'hotspots' might have been more effective. There were grounds for arguing that the central government in Delhi should have done more to consult with state governments and to allow them the freedom to decide which measures to adopt, how best to mobilize local health services and secure public cooperation. Instead, as already noted, it failed to consult state governments, or even central government departments, before it chose to act.[52]

Aside from the lockdown, Delhi had another formidable weapon in its administrative armory. On 11 March 2020, the day the WHO declared a global pandemic, the Government of India directed all states and union territories to implement the Epidemic Diseases Act, dating from the plague year, 1897. The Act, never rescinded, had been used intermittently and with only minor revisions by state governments since the 1990s but on a purely local scale to tackle temporary emergencies such as outbreaks of plague, cholera, malaria, and dengue.[53] The nationwide resuscitation of the Epidemic Diseases Act was problematic on several fronts. As a hangover from the colonial era and an exceptionally draconian piece of legislation, the Act smacked of colonial authoritarianism. Like the continuing—and equally controversial—use of other items of colonial legislation, such as the sedition laws, the revival of the Epidemic Diseases Act seemed to many opponents to epitomize the Modi government's autocratic style and determination to suppress legitimate criticism of the regime and its handling of the epidemic. The Act, moreover, was designed for a very different pandemic age. It failed to define what constituted 'dangerous epidemic diseases' and, in an age before air travel, it focused heavily on rail and sea passengers. It reflected a nineteenth-century preoccupation with inspection and quarantines but ignored other methods of disease control such as inoculation and alternatives to the state-sanctioned biomedical system. The Act asserted the indisputable right of the state to intervene in all health matters, to carry out (by force if necessary) medical surveillance and physical inspections, to enforce prohibitions on pilgrimages, fairs, and festivals, and to punish non-compliance, and yet it was (not surprisingly for the time) silent on citizens' rights and the state's responsibility for their health and general well-being. As an earlier critic had put it, the Act was 'outdated, merely regulatory and not rights-based, and lacks a focus on the people.'[54]

Writing in August 2020, the historian Dilip Menon observed that 'political crises and epidemic crises are alike in that the sovereign powers of the state are extended, and the exception of emergency becomes the norm.' That said, though, the public response to the pandemic had also demonstrated a widespread 'internalization of deference to governmentality.'[55] The fear of creeping authoritarianism, as well as the lack of sustained opposition to it, was one of the underlying stories of India's Covid-19. There was outrage in April 2021 when the Government of India ordered the removal of Twitter posts critical of its handling of the second wave of Covid on the grounds that they were inaccurate, against the national interest, and likely to cause panic.[56] There were echoes here not so much of colonial repression as of prime minister Indira Gandhi's twenty-one-month-long 'emergency' in 1975–7. To be fair, many governments around the world used the opportunity created by the pandemic crisis in a broadly similar way to advance or entrench their political power and to stifle or quell opposition. But in India these pandemic measures seemed to many critics to represent nothing less than opportune elaboration of a pre-existing strategy to crush opposition and to strengthen the BJP's intolerant and incipiently authoritarian hold over the nation. Covid provided convenient cover for the Modi government to persecute, arrest, detain, and imprison critics and dissenters of all kinds—academics, journalists, intellectuals, and political opponents of every stripe—and to crack down on women's rights activists and minority groups, from Muslims to Dalits, free from the active constraint of the courts (including India's supreme court), the press, and public opinion.[57] This perceived antidemocratic downward spiral caused the US-based Freedom House organization in March 2021 to describe India under Modi as only 'partly free,' one of many international criticisms the government simply brushed aside as ill-informed or hypocritical.[58]

Critics, like the former Congress Party prime minister Manmohan Singh, accepted that a lockdown in some form was unavoidable but deplored the short notice given to the public. The 'shock and awe' tactics of the government were, Singh said, 'thoughtless and insensitive' and caused 'tremendous pain' to the people.[59] Other commentators protested that the action taken by the Modi government was 'shambolic' and they decried the initial three-week lockdown as ill-timed and misjudged, a dramatic but characteristically ill-considered gesture that matched the prime minister's rash and highly detrimental attempt in 2016 to curb 'black money' and corruption by demonetizing the economy.[60] Such criticisms did not, however, appear to significantly dent Modi's popularity. The sentiment 'Modi will take care of us,' which played to the personality cult of the BJP leader, remained widespread among party supporters and even among some of those who had borne the brunt of his communal and economic policies.[61]

As well as its creaky public health infrastructure, India's economy, too, was ill-equipped to stage a quick recovery from the prolonged economic shock of the coronavirus pandemic and the sustained national lockdown. After sustained growth under the initial stimulus of neoliberal reform in the early 1990s, the Indian economy had entered a long period of stagnation well before the pandemic struck. In the general elections of 2014 and 2019 Modi had promised a new age of prosperity, high employment, and reduced red tape, but Asia's third-largest economy repeatedly missed its targets.[62] Exports stalled; growth in 2019 was the lowest in six years. The 2016 currency note ban severely impacted on small businesses; unemployment, already at unprecedented levels, reached new heights during the lockdown. While the Covid crisis temporarily diverted attention away from the government's poor record of economic management, it also limited its capacity to protect citizens from the worst effects of the pandemic and made a more extended or renewed lockdown financially impractical. India was one of many developing nations where leaders felt that they had 'no choice but to prioritize re-openings and accept the risks of surging coronavirus infections.'[63] There were echoes here of the colonial government backpedaling from more extreme and unpopular antiplague measures in the early 1900s.

India's colonial regime offered limited economic support in the wake of famines—agricultural loans, suspension of revenue payments in the worst-hit areas—but nothing at all substantial to the victims of epidemics. There was no recovery program after the

Spanish Flu; the economy and society were left to take their own course. Present-day regimes feel more compulsion to act or to be seen to be acting. In March 2020 Delhi announced a relief package worth US$22.5 billion, followed in mid-May by a further tranche of $308 billion, but to critics neither initiative was anywhere near enough.[64] Nor was a plan to boost growth with a $10 billion injection of funds in October 2020. 'It appears more symbolic rather than anything particularly meaningful,' remarked one commentator.[65] India's 'pandemic budget' in February 2021 gave financial support to the recently launched coronavirus vaccination program and $8.5 billion over six years to upgrade the healthcare infrastructure.[66] But for most Indians that was too little too late.

Stranded

As in the early plague years over a century earlier, it was the measures taken by the state and directed against the incoming contagion, rather than the disease itself, that created the first substantial impact of Covid-19 on India. The 24 March lockdown was enforced without any consideration for the needs and circumstances of the poor, who suddenly found themselves bereft of employment, food, and shelter. The concept of 'social distancing,' adopted around the globe, might make sense to middle-class households in India who could self-isolate, work from home, and order in their food. But for the poor it was an impractical and meaningless idea.[67] The immediate consequence of lockdown was the loss of employment for many millions of migrant workers, triggering a mass exodus from India's cities. Workers in India's huge informal sector—in construction, domestic service, and casual trades—were suddenly left without jobs and wages and began to return, or try to return, to their home villages. For the poor, lockdown was brutally hard. The Delhi government appeared to have bungled, first as panic buying in cities led to long queues outside shops in the few, desperate hours left before the lockdown took effect, and then as vast crowds gathered at rail and bus stations in Mumbai, Delhi, Hyderabad, and other cities, in search of transport to head home, only to find services suspended and state borders closed. In desperation, individuals or small family groups set out on the long trek home on foot, carrying their few possessions with them: for some this involved a journey of hundreds of miles. India, the newspaper headlines declared, was walking home (fig. 16). The 'crowd,' absented from the city streets, had taken to the highway instead. This disastrous outcome could have been foreseen by the government, but clearly it wasn't. As hungry, thirsty, exhausted migrants struggled homeward, as some fell ill or died, as the police stopped, beat, or hosed the hapless travelers with disinfectant, the pandemic became first and foremost a tragedy of the poor.[68]

Here was violence, the violence of the police certainly, but also, as Maria Johns described it in another context, the 'violence of abandonment.'[69] And yet here, too, was a very visual spectacle. As Ramachandra Guha remarked in late April 2020, 'the images of tens of thousands of Indians being brutalized by the police as they sought to walk to their distant villages will remain the enduring visual memory of Covid-19.'[70] For Ranjini Basu, writing in that same sad month, such appalling scenes brought 'under the public eye' the 'otherwise invisibilised population,' estimated at between 30 and 100 million of India's migrant, laboring poor—invisible, that is to the state and to the middle-class public who in normal times would prefer to 'push poverty out of sight.' The unfolding drama reminded many commentators, too, of the colonial state's neglect, amidst the epidemic turmoil of 1896–7 and 1918–19, of the needs of the poor and its 'general absence of sensitivity towards the health and livelihood concerns of the working-class majority.'[71]

Through images that could have been from the 1890s but were actually from 2020, the crisis of a pandemic scrambled up the temporalities of past and present, the scenes of former pestilence—the flight of the laboring poor, the panic occasioned by fear of contagion and antidisease operations, the hosing down of tenements and the burning of hovels, the rough treatment and bodily inspections at railroad stations, the casual brutality of the state, the uncaring disposition of aloof authorities—returning once more to haunt and disquiet the present. Photographs are vivid prompts to the collective pandemic imagination as much as to individual recall: one reason why the absence of such images from the Indian influenza of 1918–19 is so striking. The 2020 exodus put many observers in mind of the black-and-white images of mass migration and the long columns of dispossessed refugees during another time of violence— the Partition of 1947–8.[72] Only now the migrants—hundreds of thousands of them—were not being expelled from their homes by rape, murder, and a tidal wave of communal violence, but through the uncaring disregard of state and capitalism, returning of necessity to the villages they had previously left in search of work. This new partitioning of India was not between Hindus, Muslims, and Sikhs, but between affluent urbanites and the rural, laboring poor.

In the plague past, as in the coronavirus present, the middle classes could protect themselves whether by isolating themselves in their own homes or through the privileged distancing of caste hospitals and gated communities. For the poor, however, self-isolation and social distancing were no more than a fantasy, a mockery. Then in the 1890s, as now in the 2020s, the slum dwellers and the migrant poor were victimized several times over—by the disease that might sicken and kill them, by the loss of their already tenuous livelihoods, and by the abuse and stigmatization they received as the presumed carriers of contagious disease. In such scenes the inconvenient presence of the masses once again asserted itself, as it had done in times of cholera, plague, and influenza, only now in 2020 they were elevated by means of modern technology and the mass media to a new domestic prominence and global visibility. Covid highlighted a half-forgotten truth that for many of these people the city was an alien space—as one participant in a similar exodus from Dhaka in Bangladesh put it, 'the city is not ours.'[73] However integrated the city and the countryside might appear to be, a pandemic (or the stern measures governments decreed in pandemic times) exposed the great economic and social gulf between the two. And yet the disastrous exodus from the cities resolved nothing, as months after their departure the same migrant workers gradually returned there, having found too little work or insufficient food in the villages to support them.[74]

Historians can only visualize the plague scenes of 1896–7 through the iconography of colonial photographs or imagine them by poring over newspaper columns and trawling through official archives and municipal reports. But in March and April 2020, it was possible to witness (though not without some media mediation) similar scenes re-enacted through mobile phones and video cameras, through coverage on prime-time TV and on social media, hourly exposed to national debate and global scrutiny. In India the tradition of disaster journalism goes back at least to William Digby and the many examples of first-hand testimony incorporated into his account of the South Indian famine of the late 1870s.[75] But in 2020, to a degree rare in nineteenth-century reportage, the poor had a name, a face, and a voice: they were not just anonymous 'victims,' the dehumanized, skeletal poor that appear in W. W. Hooper's dismal photographs of that same famine episode.[76] Instead, they spoke now with anger, despair, and impatience to any journalist or bystander willing to listen to them. They—and the calamity they inhabited— existed in real time. The testimony was immediate, impassioned, and direct. Here, in a widely circulated video clip in March 2020, were policemen in Rae Bareilly corralling migrants, as if they were animals, before dousing them with disinfectant. Here was a twelve-year-old tribal girl, Jamla Makhdam, who collapsed and died after walking for three days with her migrant family from Telangana to Chhattisgarh; and here, again, was twenty-five year-old Kundan, who cycled seven hundred miles from Panipat, north of Delhi, to Patna in Bihar, and somehow survived hunger, exhaustion, and police harassment along the way.[77]

Did the immediacy and visibility of such subaltern experiences engender a greater understanding and empathy? Some historians have claimed that epidemic crises bring people together across social divides, arouse compassion, a common sense of humanity, danger, affliction, and purpose.[78] Certainly, we have seen evidence for this benign response from the plague and influenza epidemics. There were similar stories of care and compassion to be told of Covid, too, in the pandemic months of 2020. But more often, the humanitarian gestures failed to match the enormity of the catastrophe and the trend in India, as elsewhere, has been for an epidemic, and still more a pandemic with its far greater capacity for death and disruption, to force social divisions more starkly into the open. Fissures become fault lines.

Coping with Catastrophe

The first Covid cases in India were few in number and widely scattered across the country, suggesting that the disease had arrived through multiple entry points almost simultaneously. Early instances of infection were reported from western India, from Maharashtra and Gujarat, from the southern states of Karnataka and Kerala, and from Mumbai, Delhi, and Chennai. A connection with international air travel was obvious. This was unlike plague in 1896 and influenza in 1918, when the port of Bombay was the primary point of ingress and dissemination, and even the 1957 influenza pandemic, when seaports were still the main entry points. And whereas 1896 and 1918 saw waves of disease emanating outward from Bombay and spreading north, east, and south along rail routes into the hinterland, in 2020 India experienced a splattering of hotspots having seemingly little direct connection with one another, making the disease more difficult to track and contain.

The coronavirus epidemic also unfolded more slowly than influenza had in 1918, especially during its deadly second wave. Despite early fears of rapid mass mortality, in the three months from 31 January to the end of April 2020, there were just over a thousand deaths in India attributed to the virus. In this initial period, India recorded fewer deaths than Ireland and only marginally more than Portugal, though more than its immediate neighbors, Pakistan and Bangladesh; Sri Lanka, with only seven deaths by the end of April 2020, seemed from the start to be relatively immune. However, by early April the number of cases in India began to rise and by 10 May the Covid death-toll had passed 2,000. This remained a small fraction of the 276,421 deaths reported worldwide, but momentum was clearly starting to build.

Unlike in the pandemics of the nineteenth and early twentieth centuries, where morbidity data were scare or fragmentary, Covid case numbers attracted in India, as around the world, almost as much attention as fatalities, giving the disease a new sense of urgency and a new statistical visibility. By 15 July 2020, there were 936,181 cases and 24,309 deaths in India.[79] Barely two weeks later, on 28 July, case numbers had risen to 1,435,616, the third highest after the

United States and Brazil; with 32,771 deaths, India had overtaken France and Spain, and now ranked sixth in the world (such figures were not directly comparable, however, as different countries had different ways of counting Covid deaths). By mid-September India's coronavirus epidemic had begun a 'scary runaway phase,' with new cases touching 90,000, then 100,000, a day.[80] For a while that upward trend seemed set to continue and it looked as though epidemiologists' worst fears were about to be realized. But at that point case numbers and deaths in India slowed down and, apart from a few local surges such as in Delhi, entered a period of sustained decline. On 29 September, the day on which the United States posted 200,000 deaths and 6.9 million cases, India recorded just over 90,000 coronavirus deaths and 5.6 million cases. Despite the large number of cases, India's death-rate remained remarkably, perhaps suspiciously, low (see table 1). With 17 percent of the world's population, India had 10 percent of Covid deaths; the United States, with only 4 percent of the global population, accounted for 20 percent of fatalities. This disparity continued. By early November 2020, India's share of cases worldwide was roughly one-sixth, but barely one in ten of these deaths was in India. On 6 January 2021, India reached the grim milestone of 150,000 coronavirus deaths, but by that date mortality had already fallen dramatically. Many believed that, for India, the worst was now over.[81]

Unlike in Europe and the Americas, there was at this stage no sign in India of a second (or third) wave. In October the country regained some semblance of normality: the Taj Mahal, closed for months, reopened; cricket matches resumed. The fear that the exodus of workers back to their villages would spark a major escalation of the epidemic did not materialize; nor did the somewhat muted celebration of the Hindu festival of Diwali in November 2020 result in a significant surge in cases and deaths. Across India lockdown restrictions were eased, people abandoned social distancing, markets resumed trading, weddings were celebrated, cinemas reopened, and the transport network sprang back to life.[82] India started to feel safe again.

In the first Covid wave no state or union territory was unaffected. But as ever with India's epidemic history, significant regional differences emerged, reflecting the patchwork geographical distribution of the disease, the varying capacity of individual states to combat the virus and enforce lockdowns, and the influence of underlying socio-economic factors, such as poverty levels, population densities, and degrees of urbanization.

Table 1: Covid-19 Cases and Deaths in Leading States, 31 December 2020

	Cases	Deaths	Case fatality ratio
Maharashtra	1,928,603	49,463	2.56
Tamil Nadu	817,077	12,109	1.48
Karnataka	918,544	12,081	1.32
Delhi	624,795	10,523	1.68
West Bengal	550,893	9,683	1.76
Uttar Pradesh	584,966	8,352	1.43
Andhra Pradesh	881,948	7,104	0.81
Punjab	166,239	5,331	3.21
Gujarat	244,258	4,302	1.76
Madhya Pradesh	240,947	3,595	1.50
Chhattisgarh	278,540	3,350	1.20
Kerala	755,718	3,042	0.40
Haryana	262,054	2,899	1.11
Rajasthan	307,554	2,689	0.87
Odisha	329,306	1,871	0.57
Telangana	286,354	1,541	0.54
Uttarakhand	90,616	1,504	1.66
Bihar	251,348	1,393	0.55
Assam	216,139	1,043	0.48
Total India	10,266,674	148,738	1.45

Source: Covid-19 Dashboard, Center for Systems Science and Engineering, Johns Hopkins University, 31 December 2020.

Table 1 gives some indication of this unequal distribution in relation to India's principal states by the close of 2020. The data show the overwhelming impact on Maharashtra and substantial pockets of the disease across southern India, notably in Karnataka and Tamil Nadu. Delhi, Uttar Pradesh, and West Bengal were also badly hit. But the table also suggests a mismatch between cases and deaths. Kerala, for example, registered a large number of cases but relatively few deaths, while some of the more undeveloped and less administratively efficient states (Bihar, Odisha, and Chhattisgarh in particular) showed an improbably low case mortality ratio, probably due to underreporting, poor diagnosis, and misattribution of the cause of mortality.

Several factors may be adduced to explain the differences between states. Kerala, for instance, initially showed much the most successful public health response to the epidemic. Despite the return of 200,000 migrant workers from the Middle East in the early weeks of the pandemic, the state recorded a relatively low incidence and mortality rate. Kerala may have benefited from being a largely rural state without a major international airport or a megacity like Delhi or Mumbai within its borders. This was one state where, in defiance of the central government, Covid was 'locally owned.' It had a robust and effective primary healthcare system, dating back to earlier days of Communist rule, with 30,000 mobile health workers. Keralan Christians were one of the main sources of India's nurses and other medical workers. The state enjoyed a high level of male and female literacy and had a strong culture of secular citizenship. The state's health authorities acted swiftly to contain outbreaks of the virus and ran an effective testing and tracing system. Some commentators pointed to a contrast between Narendra Modi's nationalist rhetoric and the pragmatic approach adopted by the state's health minister, K. K. Shailaja.[83] She had overseen the state's response to an outbreak of Nipah virus in 2018, in which 17 people died, and so was able to apply the lessons of that experience to tackling the coronavirus, much as some East Asian countries profited from their previous encounters with SARS and Swine Flu.[84] Yet even in Kerala there were grounds for believing that many coronavirus deaths had been ignored (especially when the victim came from outside the state) or, owing to comorbidity, were assigned to other causes.[85]

189

By contrast, Maharashtra, overall a more affluent state than Kerala, with a population over three times larger, bore the brunt of Covid-19, registering close to a third of all Indian deaths in the first wave, just as it had been one of the principal sufferers in the plague and influenza epidemics a century before. That the coronavirus should have replicated that earlier pattern is striking: it may be attributed to the prevalence of poor health conditions in Mumbai, now a megacity of over 20 million people. As well as its high-end private hospitals, Mumbai has some of India's largest and most insanitary slums. Further, Maharashtra, run by a Shiv Sena government, also had a less efficient administration and a lower sense of civic responsibility than Kerala, and it was slow to develop an effective tracing system. And it was Maharashtra, Nagpur and Pune especially, that saw a resurgence of cases in February–March 2021, leading to renewed local lockdowns.[86] Delhi, too, another big-city state with a non-BJP administration, also struggled with the high number of Covid cases in the first wave, with the problem posed by large numbers of stranded migrant workers, and with the almost unmanageable demand for hospital accommodation. This provoked the chief minister, Arvind Kejriwal, to insist in June 2020 that the 10,000 beds under his state's jurisdiction be reserved for Delhi residents alone.[87] Covid tested India's federal structure and decentralized health system to the limits. Other states started well and initially recorded relatively low numbers of coronavirus cases and deaths but were then unable to sustain their promising performance. Thus, West Bengal in May 2020 was battered by a cyclone which brought widespread devastation to the state and its capital, Kolkata, causing, in the words of chief minister Mamata Banerjee, 'a bigger disaster than Covid-19.'[88] The cyclone was a reminder of India's susceptibility to multiple and even concurrent disasters, epidemic disease augmenting death and disruption from other causes.

By mid-October 2020 (well before vaccination against the disease had begun), India was able to claim a far lower death-rate than most other countries—just over 83 Covid deaths per million compared to 725 in Brazil, 665 in the United States, and 644 in the UK. India's coronavirus experience was regarded at the time as an enigma.[89] The 150,000 deaths suffered in the first wave was a far from insignificant number and yet India defied immediate expectations that it would suffer millions of deaths. India, it seemed in the early months of 2021, was not to be the great sink of mortality it had been during the 1890s–1900s plague and again during the 1918–19 influenza pandemic. A narrative of Indian exceptionalism emerged. Somehow, one of the most populous nations on earth seemed to be defying global trends. Modi supporters were quick to claim that the government's lockdown in March 2020, for all its severity, had had a significant effect in reducing transmission of the disease and that social distancing and face masks had contributed to keeping the virus under control. But other explanations were also proposed.

As was demonstrated by the new variants that emerged in the UK, South Africa, and Brazil in late 2020, some strains of Covid-19 were more easily transmissible and more lethal than others. India might, it was thought, have been fortunate in the mildness of the strain of the disease it encountered, though there was no clear evidence for this. One possible reason why the exodus of workers from Indian cities in March and April 2020 did not lead to an immediate upsurge in mortality may have been that most of these workers toiled in the open air (as on construction sites): the virus was less easily transmitted outdoors than in enclosed spaces and was unable to survive for long in bright sunlight. Again, India's age profile was very different from that of Western countries like Italy and the UK, where care-home residents and the over-seventies were among the most vulnerable, and most likely to die, in the pandemic's first wave. In India 65 percent of the population was under thirty-five years of age and only 6 percent over sixty-five.[90] A further intriguing theory—the so-called hygiene hypothesis— was that poorer Indians were exposed from birth to a cocktail of pathogens—viruses and bacteria that served to stimulate and strengthen the immune system through repeated but relatively mild or asymptomatic doses of infection. By contrast, people in higher-income countries, cosseted against infection, remained more susceptible. In other words, paradoxically, poor sanitation and crowded living conditions might actual be beneficial in the fight against Covid.[91] While the relative immunity conferred by poor health regimes in developing countries might explain why many affluent Western countries with more comprehensive healthcare systems were susceptible, this hypothesis failed to account for high rates of morbidity and mortality in countries like Brazil, Mexico, and South Africa where similar conditions prevailed.

Perhaps the main reason why Covid mortality appeared so low during the first wave in India was massive underreporting in a country where 80 percent of deaths occurred at home, not in hospital, and where no official notification of cause of death was required before cremation or burial. Apart from a few exceptions, like Kerala and Delhi, testing and contact tracing for the virus were insufficient to provide an accurate picture of the spread of Covid and its level of lethality, and neither the central government nor individual states were overly keen to publicize their deficiencies.[92] In October 2020 India was testing only 69 people out of every thousand, compared with 377 in the UK and 407 in the United States, countries in which, even so, the scale of testing was deemed inadequate.[93] This suggested that India had many more Covid cases and deaths than were officially reported and, in the absence of excess mortality data (one of the more reliable indicators of mortality), cast doubt on the value of the statistics officially issued. As in 1918–19 it was impossible to know with any degree of accuracy exactly how many people had died.

Pandemic Responses

Epidemic accountancy was not the only issue India faced. The hostile stereotyping and scapegoating of past pandemics did not magically cease with the end of the colonial era: indeed, modern mass media gave these responses a new toxicity. In countries around the world the arrival of Covid-19 unleashed a vicious outpouring of Sinophobia, directed against China and the Chinese on the grounds that the virus had originated in that country. Perhaps, it was suggested, the 'Chinese virus' had escaped from a laboratory in Wuhan or been deliberately unleashed by an evil-minded Chinese government. Given India's long history of conflict with China, reawakened by Himalayan border clashes in 2020, the readiness of the media and the public to blame China was perhaps predictable. But in India, this xenophobia was also directed against Assamese and other northeastern students, workers, and residents in Delhi and elsewhere on the grounds that they happened to 'look Chinese.'[94]

In the main, though, India's epidemic scapegoating spewed in a different direction through Islamophobia. Covid followed close on unrest over the Citizenship Amendment Act, one of several measures sponsored by the BJP government which were widely seen as violating the founding principles of the Indian republic, with its promise of religious freedom, and as designed to create a Hindu, faith-based definition of citizenship from which India's largest minority community would in effect be excluded.[95] Hindu–Muslim rioting in Delhi in February 2020, on the eve of the pandemic, in which at least 53 people died, was said to have been fomented by the BJP, and critics feared that Modi's government was intent on using the coronavirus emergency to further marginalize and persecute Muslims and advance its aggressively pro-Hindu (Hindutva) agenda.[96] The history of Hindu nationalism extended far back into colonial history, but the BJP brought to it a new militancy and populist base.[97] In what has been characterized as Hindu nationalism's 'ethnic democracy,' fear of one kind of infection (the coronavirus) was being mobilized to incite and justify hostility to another kind of 'infection' (Islam).[98] As Arjun Appadurai put it, one of the established features of anti-Muslim sentiment in India 'has been the idea that Muslims themselves are a kind of infection in the body politic.' There was, therefore, a kind of toxic affinity between this long-standing image and the newly awakened anxieties surrounding the coronavirus.[99]

An outbreak of Covid at a meeting of the Islamic organization Tablighi Jamaat at Nizamuddin in Delhi in early March 2020 led to wild and furious media claims about this event being the source of thousands of cases and dozens of deaths across India. The incident was blown out of all proportion while the part that Hindu or Sikh gatherings might have had in spreading the disease was barely mentioned or simply ignored.[100] Hatred fueled frantic myth. There were rumors—on a scale and of an intensity perhaps only rarely seen since the plague of 1896–7—that Muslims were deliberately contaminating food and water in order to spread the virus. In a spate of unfounded conspiracy theories that drew upon the caustic language of America's 'war on terror,' as well as home-grown Islamophobia,

Muslims were accused of being 'coronavirus terrorists,' plotting a 'Taliban crime,' and launching a 'corona jihad.' Kapil Mishra, a BJP leader in Delhi, tweeted on 1 April 2020 that the 'Tablighi Jamaat people have started to spit on workers and doctors in quarantine centers. It is clear, their intention is to kill [the] maximum [number of] people. They should be treated like terrorists.'[101] In cities, towns, and villages across the country Muslims were ostracized, boycotted, beaten up, and verbally abused. Muslim street vendors were attacked and told to stop hawking their wares. These incidents fueled the ongoing demonization of the Muslim community, orchestrated by the BJP and its allies, in which Muslims were always 'fanatics,' enemies of the Hindu homeland, and an existential threat to national security.[102] Fortified by its populist appeal and the landslide majority won in the 2019 general elections, the Modi government was slow to rebuke or condemn this vilification of Muslims. Widely criticized for being complicit as chief minister of Gujarat in anti-Muslim riots in 2002, Modi responded to the Covid-inspired round of attacks on Muslims in an anodyne and unapologetic way. He remarked only that the coronavirus did not respect race, religion, color, caste, and creed, and repeated the platitudinous refrain, 'We are [all] in this together.'[103]

Like many an epidemic and pandemic before it, Covid created heroes as well as villains. India's street art celebrated the doctors and nurses who fought the pandemic, glamorizing their service and self-sacrifice. But there were others, too, who cast themselves in a heroic mold. While weaponizing the epidemic against Muslims, the BJP's Hindu nationalist supporters used the onset of the coronavirus to promote their own politico-religious agenda. In reaction against disparaging colonial claims about Hindus' physical weakness, a cult of physical fitness and bodily strength had long been a part of the muscular masculinity of Hindu revivalism. In this, as in other respects, the BJP-led campaign against the virus was a kind of latter-day countercolonialism, an opportunity to demonstrate to India's enemies and detractors the strength and resilience of the Hindutva nation.[104] To show weakness and vulnerability in the face of an invasive disease, especially one identified with the 'enemy'—whether defined as Chinese or Muslim—was unconscionable to the sectarian

Right. Instead, indigenous remedies and patriotic prophylactics had to be trumpeted and deployed to prove the protective power and therapeutic ingenuity of the Hindu tradition.[105] In the first weeks and months of the epidemic it was claimed that the products of the sacred cow, urine (*gaumutra*) and dung (*gaugober*), possessed unique medicinal properties and gave protection against Covid, or that cow urine served as a cheap and effective hand sanitizer.[106] *Gaumutra* parties were held to invoke the protection of the cow and to ask the coronavirus to leave India without killing any more of its people. Suman Haripriya, a BJP member of the Assam legislature, declared unequivocally that the sacred products of the cow could cure the corona sickness.[107] Others went further. Anil Vij, health minister for Haryana, asserted that the disease was a righteous punishment for those Indians who violated Hindu orthodoxy by consuming meat.[108] According to Swami Chakrapani, president of the Akhil Bharat Hindu Mahasabha, 'Coronavirus has come because of the people who kill and eat animals. When you kill an animal, it creates an energy that causes destruction in that place.' Covid was the manifestation of that negative energy.[109] In this way the virus became annexed to the already ferocious (and sometimes life-threatening) attacks on meat-eating Indians, Muslims and Christians among them.

The virus and the campaign waged against it entered into what Banu Subramaniam has described as the 'archaic modernity' of Hindu nationalism, that space of ambivalence, contradiction, and almost infinite possibilities in which modern science and Vedic mythology coexist and combine, where the temporalities of past, present, and mythic time are constantly being scrambled up and imaginatively reconfigured.[110] In rhetoric, if not in actual state policy, Covid was annexed to the mythic time of the Hindu nation rather than to the secular scientific tradition of India's medical modernity. It was characteristic of this mythic entanglement that in March 2020 Modi drew parallels between the fight against Covid-19 and the epic struggle known to all Hindus from the Mahabharata. 'The Mahabharata war,' he declared, 'was won in 18 days, this war the whole country is fighting against coronavirus will take 21 days,' that is, the twenty-one days of the national lockdown.[111] Events soon proved that the coronavirus could not be so speedily vanquished.

As so often in the pandemic past, the coronavirus raised contentious issues about the legitimate role of indigenous healing practices and medical traditions in India and the relationship of the modern, once-secular state to non-biomedical practitioners. Like their precursors during the plague and influenza epidemics a century or so earlier, proponents of Ayurveda claimed a unique efficacy and ancient authenticity for their therapeutic wares, egged on in their claims by Modi and BJP hardliners. A wide range of anti-Covid Ayurvedic drugs were put on sale and publicized domestically and internationally through the press and on YouTube. As in the past, India's medical establishment and the practitioners of modern biomedicine decried this as pseudo-science and ridiculed the wholly unsubstantiated curative and immunological claims, seeing such drugs as useless and possibly dangerous. But no previous pandemic had given Ayurveda such global opportunities. In the new internationalism of alternative and complementary health therapies, its drugs were marketed not only in India but across the globe, especially in countries with diasporic South Asian communities. One example of this was the drug 'Coronil' produced by Patanjali Ayurved, a firm headed by Baba Ramdev, TV yoga megastar and champion of Ayurvedic consumerism. When the drug was put on sale in the UK, there were complaints about its supposed efficacy. It was, the manufacturers reluctantly conceded, an immunity booster rather than an actual cure, though even that more modest assertion remained unproven.[112]

Conflicting claims over Ayurvedic drugs and their efficacy left the Indian state and Modi's populism in an equivocal position: to what extent were public health needs and India's scientific standing in the world being jeopardized by the claims made for these putative remedies? In the new free-market order, was it not legitimate and desirable for private companies and Ayurvedic drug producers, rather than the state, to cater to individual health needs? In 2014 the BJP government had set up a new ministry, known by the acronym AYUSH, to represent the alternative therapies of Ayurveda, Yoga and Naturopathy, Unani, Siddha, and Homeopathy. In practice, the department that skeptics derided as the 'Yoga Ministry' showed a clear preference for Ayurveda and Modi's favored brand of yoga, which he touted, even on the world stage, as a means of achieving individual well-being. Early in the pandemic, on 29 January 2020, AYUSH released an advisory notice listing a number of Ayurvedic and other non-biomedical formulations that could be used against the disease. In particular, arsenicum album 30 (an arsenic derivative) was endorsed as a prophylactic, though the ministry soon afterward backtracked by indicating that this and other prescriptions were recommended only for their immunomodulatory effects, not because they were Covid cures. A subsequent statement at the end of March 2020 retreated still further, urging public caution in assessing claims made for anticoronavirus drugs and declaring its emphatic support for scientific, evidence-based therapeutics.[113]

Shortly after India's lockdown began, Modi spoke in a teleconference with a hundred AYUSH practitioners. He urged them to counter misinformation about the pandemic and to reject unproven drugs—this even while some of the government's own representatives continued to promote cow's urine as an infallible prophylactic or remedy.[114] On 1 March 2021, the prime minister appeared on camera to receive his first anti-Covid vaccination, before taking to Twitter to urge other Indians to follow his example (fig. 17). 'Remarkable,' he tweeted, 'how our doctors and scientists have worked in quick time to strengthen the global fight against Covid-19. I appeal to all those who are eligible to take the vaccine. Together, let us make India Covid-19 free.'[115] (For India's vaccination campaign, see chapter 7.) But, while reiterating India's claim to scientific modernity and his pragmatic advocacy of conventional public health measures, Modi was anxious, for the sake of his domestic support, to keep a hold on mythic as well as modern time. Dressed in the saffron and white robes of the Hindu Right (but wearing a face mask), Modi took time out from the coronavirus crisis in August 2020 to visit Ayodhya. At the site of the destruction of the Babri Masjid mosque by Hindu fanatics in 1992, he laid the foundation stone for the highly controversial, if long-promised, temple to Ram.[116] In the time of the Hindu nation, religion, politics, and pandemic precautions were conjoined, however incongruously.

'It Is Much Worse This Time'

Then, quite suddenly, things went awry and the myth of Indian exceptionalism collapsed. In the early weeks and months of 2021 coronavirus cases and deaths in India had been running at relatively low levels, daily infections having fallen below 9,000 with fewer than 80 deaths. The immunization program, begun in January that year, seemed to be progressing well, and large quantities of locally made vaccine were being exported abroad to countries in apparently greater need. India appeared to be exemplary, not just exceptional. As lockdown restrictions across India eased, normalization gathered pace: everyday life resumed, unmasked. Mass rallies were held in the four states facing elections, in all probability helping to fuel a second pandemic wave.[117] The Kumbh Mela bathing festival at Haridwar on the Ganges, brought forward for obscure astrological reasons from 2022, was allowed to take place in April 2021, supposedly under strict Covid rules, and was attended by millions of worshippers. In one of the most striking of all India's many pandemic parallels, in 1892 the colonial government of the North-Western Provinces had sparked outrage among many Hindus by banning a similar bathing festival at Haridwar on the grounds that a cholera outbreak was imminent (see chapter 2). In 2021 the BJP-led government of Uttarakhand provoked another kind of outrage—among secularists, pragmatists, and physicians—by allowing the Kumbh Mela to go ahead, with minimal health checks, creating a 'super-spreading' event of a magnitude unimaginable in 1892.[118] For the sake of its populist base, the Modi government and its local state representatives put Hindu religious observance ahead of public health.

Meanwhile, the prime minister and members of his government hailed India's extraordinary achievement in beating the deadly demon virus. The home minister, Amit Shah, claimed that Modi and his government were fighting the virus 'on every front,' and expressed confidence that 'we will have a victory over this.'[119] In early March, as the immunization campaign gathered momentum, health minister Harsh Vardhan declared, with inopportune optimism, that India was now entering the 'endgame of the pandemic.'[120] Addressing the World Economic Forum at Davos in January 2021, Modi spoke of India bringing to the global community a 'message of confidence, positivity and hope.' 'It was predicted,' he said, scoffing at the doomsayers, 'that India would be the most affected country' in the whole world, 'that there would be a tsunami of corona infections in India, somebody said 700–800 million Indians would get infected while others said 2 million Indians would die.' None of this had happened. India had not been overwhelmed; on the contrary, India had 'saved humanity from a big disaster by containing corona effectively.'[121]

Many governments around the world—and their public health advisers—began by underestimating the dangers of the Covid pandemic, and, whether from ignorance or arrogance, went on making costly mistakes. But in India in particular, things went catastrophically wrong. From February 2021 Covid cases and mortality began to increase rapidly, and at a much faster rate than in the previous year. The second wave had arrived, and like the influenza of 1918 the second wave proved far more deadly than the first, with several states, including Maharashtra, Karnataka, Delhi, and (despite its earlier success) Kerala severely affected (see table 2). April and May were the deadliest months. From only a few thousand new cases at the start of the year, by late April 2021 the number exceeded 200,000, then 300,000 or 350,000 a day, reaching heights hitherto unimagined and unparalleled, not just in India but around the world. Recorded deaths rocketed up to over 2,000 a day.

Still more so than during the first wave in 2020, there were widespread and well-documented reports, especially from hospitals and crematoria in Delhi and northern India, where the epidemic now raged most fiercely, that the real number of Covid deaths was far, far higher than the official tally. According to the *Financial Times* of 21 April 2021, reports from seven districts in Gujarat, Uttar Pradesh, Madhya Pradesh, and Bihar indicated that at least 1,833 people had died of Covid within recent days; only 228 deaths had been officially recorded. In one district of Gujarat, where only a single coronavirus death was recorded, a hundred people died of the disease. Doubts had been raised during the first wave over the reliability of official data; now the evidence was overwhelming.[122] By late July 2021 an estimate by the Center for Global Development, based on excess deaths rather than reported Covid mortality, put the number of Indians who had died of Covid during the first and second waves at more than 4 million, ten times the 414,000 deaths officially registered at that time.[123] This horrendous figure was no less than what many independent observers had long suspected.

Table 2: Covid-19 Mortality in Leading States, 31 December 2020 and 31 October 2021

	Deaths First wave (to 31/12/20)	Deaths Second wave (to 31/10/21)	Increase
Maharashtra	49,463	140,196	90,733
Tamil Nadu	12,109	36,097	23,988
Karnataka	12,081	38,071	25,990
Delhi	10,523	25,091	14,568
West Bengal	9,683	19,126	9,443
Uttar Pradesh	8,352	22,901	14,549
Andhra Pradesh	7,104	14,369	7,265
Punjab	5,331	16,558	11,227
Gujarat	4,302	10,089	5,787
Madhya Pradesh	3,595	10,524	6,929
Chhattisgarh	3,350	13,576	10,226
Kerala	3,042	31,514	28,472
Haryana	2,899	10,049	7,150
Rajasthan	2,689	8,954	6,265
Odisha	1,871	8,329	6,458
Telangana	1,541	3,955	2,414
Uttarakhand	1,504	7,400	5,896
Bihar	1,393	9,661	8,268
Assam	1,043	5,996	4,953
Total	148,738	459,397	310,659

Source: Covid-19 Dashboard, Center for Systems Science and Engineering, Johns Hopkins University, 31 October 2021.

As the *Guardian* put it on 22 April 2021, this was a 'tragedy of unprecedented proportions.' The newspaper reported 234,000 new coronavirus cases in a single day and 1,341 deaths; hospitals, filled to capacity, turning patients away; a coronavirus positivity rate that had doubled in just twelve days; an increasing number of victims (almost two-thirds in Delhi) under forty years old; and a disease, deadly in the cities, moving inexorably into small towns and villages. This was 'India's descent into Covid hell.'[124] In the first wave in 2020 the enduring images were of the exodus of the laboring poor from the cities and their mistreatment at the hands of the police. As the second wave struck, a very different set of images and reports, more reflective of the fate of the urban middle classes, but also indicative of the suffering of the urban and rural poor, hit the Indian and global media. Here to be seen and heard were the desperate appeals and fruitless quests by relatives in autorickshaws or on mobile phones, searching on behalf of the sick for places in hospitals that were already full, their beds fully (even doubly) occupied, their intensive care units swamped, their oxygen supplies exhausted; the tales of victims, young, old, and middle-aged, struggling for breath, collapsing, or dying before they could receive treatment; reports of oxygen cylinders and essential medical drugs only available on the black market and at wildly inflated prices; the shrouded bodies of the Covid dead piling up at crematoria where the fires never stopped burning, and, with so many dead to dispose of, city parks and waste ground converted into makeshift burning ghats.[125] Comparisons with only a year before seemed stark, death now far more rampant, terrifying, immediate. A nurse in a government medical institute in Lucknow told the *Financial Times*, 'None of us [in 2020] suffered the death and devastation that we are seeing now. It is much worse this time than last year.' She went on: 'The condition is so horrible that so many people are dying in the street, in their houses, before they can see a doctor or even have a test.'[126] Suddenly, predictions made in early 2020 that India might suffer millions of Covid deaths no longer seemed overwrought or unrealistic. The funeral pyres *were*, as in 1890s Bombay, burning non-stop; the corpses *were*, as in 1918, choking India's rivers or lying, washed up and unburied, along their banks; the tsunami *had* happened.

What lay behind this sudden, devastating surge? What had overtaken India's much-publicized near immunity? The simplest explanation was that the measures taken at the start of the first wave in 2020 were thereafter ignored: social distancing had virtually ceased, mask-wearing had become infrequent, and large social gatherings—from weddings and cricket matches, to election rallies, and the Haridwar Kumbh Mela with its millions of attendees—had been allowed to happen, with minimal, if any, anti-Covid precautions. It could be claimed that many of these open-air events carried less danger of infectivity than crowded indoor gatherings, but they contributed cumulatively to a new upsurge in transmissions. Again, for months other mutations of the virus—the English, South African, and Brazilian—had commanded international attention, their greater lethality and possible resistance to vaccines much analyzed and discussed. The double mutation, first known as the 'Indian variant' then quickly renamed the 'Delta variant' to save India offense, had possibly been in circulation in India as early as October 2020, but it was at first little noticed owing to the low level of testing in India. But the new strain of the virus appeared to have the capacity, like the second wave of Spanish Flu in 1918, to spread faster than its predecessor, to be more deadly, and possibly more resistant to vaccines. Overconfidence and complacency, neglect or abandonment of basic disease control measures, a new viral strain, a large and densely populated country in which it could readily circulate and mutate, and a long history of persistently underfunded public health together unleashed a perfect storm.

As a more virulent strain of Covid, the Delta variant revived old fears of the Indian double whammy—a deadly disease rampaging seemingly unchecked in India and spilling over to become a global hazard. Cholera, plague, and even influenza had previously fitted this narrative: now it was Covid's turn. India, once again, as so often in the past, came, by its scenes and by its suffering, to define the pandemic. As countries around the world closed their borders to travelers from India in late April 2021, the old fear of India as the source of infectious diseases, the incubator and disseminator of global pathogens, resurfaced. India's Covid crisis 'mattered to the whole world.'[127] For days, weeks even, India's tragic and seemingly unstoppable affliction made headline news around the world, the exotic but emblematic image of its funeral pyres dominating newspaper front pages and television news bulletins (fig. 18).[128] 'Every night,' reported the *Financial Times*, 'funeral pyres blaze on the banks of the Ganges, a grim symbol of the ferocious Covid-19 wave sparking a health crisis and human tragedy in India that is far surpassing anything seen last year.'[129] The sense of the apocalyptic and the arcane, the Black Death revisited, was palpable. Jonathan Rugman, a reporter for one of the UK's more responsible broadcasters, Channel 4 News, described the funeral pyres as 'medieval looking.'[130] The weight of the world's pandemic past haunted India's twenty-first-century misery. Some observers, not least in the diaspora, recoiled at this constant emphasis on Indian mortality, the graphic images of cremation grounds and funeral pyres, and Western media intrusion into Indians' private grief.[131] The government, too, tried to intervene to prevent the circulation of such damaging and historically resonant images.[132]

Intent on extracting electoral advantage from the rapidly worsening crisis, Narendra Modi and his ministers tried at first to disclaim responsibility for the devastating second wave of the pandemic. Non-BJP administrations in Maharashtra and Delhi were blamed for what had so rapidly and so badly gone wrong, though the same excuse could hardly be used in states like Uttar Pradesh where a BJP government also struggled with soaring numbers of cases and deaths and where, too, oxygen, hospital beds, and even wood for cremation were in desperately short supply. For many critical commentators India felt like a ship that was 'totally adrift,' and it was the Government of India's gross mismanagement of the crisis that was entirely to blame.[133] In the words of a clearly distressed BBC journalist, reporting from Delhi on 23 April 2021, India was 'a broken country, a country in torment.'[134] Covid was not an unauthored misfortune or natural disaster: it was a consequence of political arrogance and human error. From having been widely praised in 2020 for its prompt action, the Modi government now found itself under heavy fire, the prime minister held directly responsible for events that seemed increasingly to spiral out of control.[135] On 24 April London's *Guardian*, reporting 332,730 new Covid cases and over 2,200 deaths in India in the past twenty-four hours, devoted an angry editorial to the subject, declaring, 'Modi's over-confidence lies behind the disastrous Indian pandemic response.' 'Mr Modi's brand of Indian exceptionalism bred complacency,' the article continued; 'an unfounded sense that Indians were somehow more immune to the virus' had been allowed to go unchallenged. Modi was personally to blame. He suffered from 'overconfidence in his own instincts and pooh-poohs expert advice.' However, 'The buck stops with him … Future historians will judge Mr Modi harshly if he continues with the exceptionalist views that have led to a disastrous public health outcome.'[136] Had Covid dealt 'brand Modi' a deadly blow?[137]

* * *

There was much about India's initial response to the Covid pandemic that reflected the global nature of the disease and the almost simultaneous threat it posed to countries around the world. More than a century on from the devastation caused by the Spanish Flu of 1918–19, India seemed unlikely to suffer a comparable disaster. The understanding of epidemics and the science of disease control, the political strength and faith-based populism of the Modi government, India's standing in the world, the material conditions of its population—all appeared substantially different in 2020 from the conditions that had prevailed a century or so earlier. There was little reason to believe, in the first phase of the pandemic, that Covid was, except in some nightmare scenario, India's tryst with destiny. But even so, almost from the outset, it was hard not to see parallels, connections, analogies, and legacies that linked the plague and influenza epidemics (even the earlier cholera pandemics) to their apparent reenactment in Covid-19: the flight from the cities and the rough treatment meted out to the poor, the coercive and intolerant disposition of a state which rapidly redeployed the Epidemic Diseases Act of 1897, the ethnic and religious scapegoating, the tension between state-sponsored public health and the claims made for alternative medical practices—all these resonated with the history of earlier pandemics.

But the arrival of a more powerful and deadly second wave of Covid in early 2021, while in some respects replicating or reimagining the horrors of India's previous pandemic experiences, also changed, or threatened to change, the relationship with that past. In a situation in which the immediacy of suffering, grief, and loss was so overwhelming, the search for historical comparisons and analogies, even lessons, that was so marked in the first Covid wave became supplanted by the urgent press of events as they rapidly unfolded. This, it seemed to many of those who observed or were caught up in these tumultuous events, was unlike anything that had happened before. It is at such moments that history can shift on its axis. New traumas usurp the old. New pasts, new memories, are waiting to be born.

7

CORONAVIRUS AND THE USES OF HISTORY

One of the immediate responses to the outbreak of Covid in India in 2020, as in many countries around the world, was to turn to history, to look to past pandemics in the expectation that they would provide precedents, lessons, warnings, perhaps even reassurance for the present. SARS-CoV-2 might be a novel coronavirus to the epidemiologist, but for the historian—or the historically minded journalist and media commentator—there was much about the nature of the disease and its socio-political impact that made it appear decidedly lacking in novelty. At the heart of this response was the familiar idea that history repeats itself or that, at the least, one pandemic was sufficiently like another to make it possible to draw lessons on what to do, or what not to do, from an earlier pandemic—even one as apparently remote in time and human experience as the fourteenth-century Black Death. For India, though, more immediate parallels were conveniently to hand—cholera from the early nineteenth century, bubonic plague in the 1890s, the Spanish Flu of 1918–19. But how useful or meaningful was this revisiting of India's pandemic past? What purpose, or purposes, did it serve? Was the past in any sense a retrievable entity or was it simply being used as a metaphor or analogy for the present? In a situation of such monumental catastrophe as Covid presented, what use is history?

Recollection of Plagues Past

There is nothing new about revisiting past pestilences in order to illuminate or inform the pandemic present. Indeed, over the last century or so this has been a common response, as the repeated references to the Black Death in connection with the Bombay plague of the 1890s and 1900s have shown earlier in this book. But the invocation of the past can be more subtle and purposeful than a few crude analogies and headline comparisons might suggest. In 1898, for example, the Bombay journalist and historian R. P. Karkaria published an article in which he compared 'two years of calamities,' exactly sixty years apart, 1837 and 1897, seeing in them 'a remarkable parallelism.' Just as in 1897, the year of Queen Victoria's diamond jubilee, so in 1837, the year of her accession, there had been a series of 'equally dire and crushing' disasters. 'Nearly every calamity under which the country is groaning at present,' he wrote, 'or has been lately groaning, may be paralleled from the records of that year [1837].'[1] Conspicuous among the many disasters Karkaria cited (famine, fires, floods, insurrection) was bubonic plague. In 1837 it was the Pali plague in Rajasthan and northern India; in 1897 it was the Bombay plague in western India. Aligning these 'heavy and widespread natural calamities' with the 'serious political troubles' that accompanied them, he found further parallels in state responses and public unrest, linked in both instances to plague policies. In reflecting on the assassination in 1897 of W. C. Rand, Poona's plague commissioner, Karkaria looked beyond the mere coincidence of two epidemic events sixty years apart to issue a warning to the embattled colonial regime of his own day about the risks it ran by pursuing unpopular policies. The past was not a remote abstraction, but a worthy vehicle for critical reflection on the present. 'There is nothing new under the sun,' he concluded; 'history repeats itself with strange persistency.'[2]

Karkaria died in May 1919, possibly from the after-effects of the influenza that had devastated the city, Bombay, about which he wrote so extensively and with such affection.[3] But the notion of a recurring pandemic past and the relevance or 'persistency' of its message did not die with him. Indeed, this search for meaning in parallel historical episodes was particularly marked at the time of the 1957 influenza pandemic, at a time when memories of its 1918–19 precursor were still relatively fresh. In May 1957 a doctor by the name of B. G. Vad, writing to the *Times of India*, remarked: 'Having forgotten the lessons of the 1890 epidemic [of influenza] we were caught unawares in the 1918 epidemic which took such a catastrophic toll.' Citing a mortality of 'more than seven million lives,' he reminded readers that at the peak of the epidemic in Bombay deaths were running at 800 a day and 'long queues were awaiting their turns at the burning place and burial ground.' He saw this past calamity as a warning of the need to take the current epidemic seriously and for the public health authorities to prepare for a 'probable catastrophe before it is too late.'[4] Two months later the *Times of India* returned to the same story. 'Will history repeat itself?' an unnamed correspondent asked. This question 'readily poses itself to those who lived through the influenza pandemic of 1918 and carry memories of the dreadful dimensions of the mortality it caused.'[5]

As these articles from the *Times of India* demonstrate, the 1918–19 pandemic had *not* been forgotten, even four decades later. For many, including those in the medical profession, it remained a vivid memory, a horrific episode people still talked about and needed to reflect on. But recalling the Spanish Flu had a clear contemporary purpose as well. In the middle months of 1957 influenza was again rampaging across India and many observers were alarmed by the 'parallels' and 'resemblances' between the current epidemic and 'the one which struck the country just forty years ago.' As the *Times of India* declared in bold type: 'The 1918 Flu Epidemic Holds a Lesson for Us.' But at stake now was not the prestige or arrogant folly of a colonial regime but the success of post-independence nation-building. 'Prostration of so large a section of the population today' would, the writer cautioned, 'seriously hinder, if not jeopardise,' the execution of the Government of India's five-year plan. 'We have been forewarned; now we must be forearmed.' The Bombay government had convened a conference of officials and municipal authorities to discuss measures to fight the epidemic: a repetition of history could be evaded 'if we avoid the mere formality of the usual warnings to the public without energetic propaganda,' and instead adopted the active 'observance of elementary sanitary and hygienic practices.' 'Appropriate and vigorous measures' needed to be taken without delay and 'at the least sign of danger.'[6] Past experience highlighted the current need for action.

Karkaria's 1898 essay and the *Times of India* article of July 1957 serve as representative responses to the arrival or threatened return of a pandemic, in India or anywhere else. History, whether that of the professional historian or of personal recollection and popular memory, has an authority that those who wield power in the present are expected to acknowledge. History has heft. It can speak truth to power, even where there is censorship or circumspection about uttering direct criticism and outright condemnation of the current regime. History is invoked as a remembered past shadowing an emergent present, as the narrative of a disaster that might be repeated with similarly distressing and destructive results, but that can be avoided if prompt and effective measures are taken. The past doesn't just inform the present; it gives it meaning. It yields timely warnings and persistent lessons; it posits a way forward. Still more, it conveys criticism of the inertia, complacency, or arrogance of present-day authorities by proposing parallels with a more distant past. History *may* repeat itself, but, if we are sensible, it doesn't have to. History communicates reassurance in the sense of knowing that the present need be no worse than the past and, forearmed by past experience, might conceivably turn out better.

The Past Lives of Covid-19

In 2020 the history of India's pandemic past hung heavily over the ongoing Indian experience of the coronavirus pandemic. Current events so often reminded commentators of the pandemics that issued from or impacted upon the subcontinent over the previous two hundred years that it became predictable, even facile, to repeat the mantra that history was (albeit with some qualifications) repeating itself. 'When,' one irate academic asked in June 2020, 'will we learn our lessons from previous pandemics?' Even a cursory examination of the subject would, Mohammad Sajjad averred, suggest 'eerie similarities' in the 'anti-people response' of the 'ruling elites' to the three modern Indian epidemics of 1896, 1918, and 2020.[7] It was, observed another writer, the function of the colonial-era epidemics 'to teach us about society's response' to such calamities.[8] Black-and-white photographs of India's plague years or, for want of equivalent Indian material, scenes from the influenza in the United States were juxtaposed with color pictures of present-day health workers in hazmat suits spraying disinfectant or policemen corralling migrant workers. While some writers took as their guide one particular historical episode, such as the Rand assassination or the plague riots in Bombay and Calcutta, others chose to emphasize the living legacy of earlier pandemics. Common themes were the reintroduction of the Epidemic Diseases Act of 1897 (dubbed British India's 'medical surveillance tool'), how the state's draconian intervention against plague had provoked popular resistance and ultimately had to be modified in favor of greater popular involvement, and how colonial inaction had allowed millions to die from influenza in 1918–19. Other writers took a more original approach, demonstrating how, for example, the onset of plague and the government's anti-plague measures in Calcutta in 1898 gave workers there 'their first opportunity to organise themselves and to build the city's labour movement.'[9]

Taking a wider perspective and reflecting on contemporary episodes of Covid-linked ethnic discrimination in the United States, other writers outlined how the British representation of cholera in the nineteenth century had fueled 'anti-Asian racism.' The message here, according to Sagaree Jain, was that 'we should learn from, instead of repeating, the racist assignations of the past.'[10] The backstory to Covid-19 was seen as one of decades-long poverty, hunger, and ill health, dating back to colonial times but substantially unchanged in the post-independence era. The history of past epidemics thus offered instructive insights into understanding the 'structural roots' of India's 'poor public health infrastructure' and the continuities, rather than the contrasts, that flowed from that common neglect. 'Pathogens need poverty,' Sheetal Chhabria observed, and neither the British nor their successors had done enough to address the fundamental issue. Through the persistence of hardship, poverty, and malnutrition, epidemics were still being 'manufactured' in

India much as they had been made in the colonial past.[11] There was nothing natural or inevitable about the situation in which India found itself. The responsibility of governments, past and present, was real and apparent. Drawing on pandemic history, the Bombay plague in particular, made the message simple and stark: 'It is crucial that the Indian government learns from the historical mistakes that its colonial predecessors had committed. The present authorities must act with patience and sagacity. The ongoing [coronavirus] crisis can only be won with the active co-operation of the masses and by taking community leaders into confidence.'[12]

There were in effect two critiques of the exercise or misuse of power at work here. One used the opportunity presented by the coronavirus pandemic to remind readers of the searing iniquities of colonial rule; the other employed that same history as a vehicle to attack the present government of India or to warn of the dangers of autocratic rule and communal extremism by highlighting the 'colonial character' of Modi's regime.[13] In one example of the former, Maura Chhun drew upon her recent doctoral research to identify the influenza pandemic of 1918–19 with the 'British overlords' indifference' to a disease which caused little hardship to Europeans in India but which by their disdain 'became one more example of British injustice that spurred Indian people on in their fight for independence.'[14] Covid provided an occasion, in a suitably epidemic idiom, to 'unmask the empire.'[15] By contrast, an opinion piece for Kolkata's *Telegraph* in April 2020 by the historian and media commentator Ramachandra Guha followed the second strategy— using the past as a means of attacking current trends and policies. Under the somewhat misleading heading 'Repeating the Past,' Guha briefly explored the history of colonial India's plague and influenza episodes before observing: 'The outbreak of Covid-19 in India brings to mind both the Black Death in fourteenth-century Europe and epidemics at the time of the British *raj*. Religious minorities have been targeted; while the working classes … have experienced enormous suffering.' But, he noted, more judiciously than many commentators, there were also significant differences. 'Unlike medieval Europe, whose states were fanatically devoted to Christian supremacy, India is in theory a secular state. Unlike the British *raj*, which was authoritarian to the core, independent India is a democratic republic, whose elected leaders are in theory accountable to their voters, the poor and vulnerable among them.' He then criticized the stance taken by Narendra Modi and his BJP supporters, and the class-based and communally biased response to the pandemic by much of the Indian media. More openly and courageously censorious of the current regime than Karkaria had been with respect to the British in 1898, Guha ended by reiterating his earlier indictment: 'our professedly democratic government has been as callous towards the poor as the authoritarian British *raj*, while our allegedly modern society has displayed the sort of venomous hatred towards religious minorities once characteristic of medieval Europe.'[16]

Guha's dual thematic—colonial autocracy reincarnated in a communalist and undemocratic BJP government—was matched, if hardly bettered, by several other commentaries published in the Indian press in the early and middle months of 2020. Significantly, as during the early plague years, in many of these accounts the disease itself bore less significance than the manner in which its arrival and spread were handled by the colonial authorities, the historical legacies of their actions (or inaction), and the expression of popular dissent, whether to the disease itself or, more commonly, to measures deployed by a negligent or oppressively autocratic state.

A few, but not many, media commentators undertook a more detailed historical investigation into past pandemics before offering their critical analysis of the present. The most thorough of these came not from India, but from a Pakistani historian, Yaqoob Khan Bangash. From May through September 2020 he published a series of articles in Lahore's *News on Sunday* on 'epidemics in South Asia.' His aim was not to address the wider pandemic question, but to investigate how, with particular reference to his home province, Punjab, British India had responded to successive crises of contagion and how the public had reacted alike to the disease and to the state's public health measures. These insights, Bangash wrote, would then 'enable us to understand and assess current government policy and people's responses across the different governments of South Asia in the coronavirus pandemic.' While stressing that 'every issue needs to be understood in and from its context' and should not simply be viewed on the basis of present-day knowledge, Bangash held that 'Given an uncertain future, the past has become the main avenue of inquiry, comment and judgment.'[17]

It is unnecessary to repeat his detailed and nuanced account of specific epidemics—smallpox, cholera, plague, influenza—but in his final and concluding article Bangash proposed eight lessons that might be drawn from the past and applied to the present. These are worth summarizing, if only because they demonstrate the extent to which (in the hands of a professional historian) historical parallels and contrasts can be made and used to inform and appraise the present. First, Bangash noted, 'there is no real way in which a government can control the spread of an epidemic.' In the current coronavirus pandemic, as in former times, 'diseases are easily spread, regardless of education levels, better sanitary conditions, and government measures.' Second, 'the government must devise clear and concrete plans to contain the disease.' The British handling of plague exhibited commendable transparency of purpose but 'such clear and planned measures are sorely lacking in Pakistan today.' Third, experience showed the efficacy of modern medicine in the containment and treatment of epidemic diseases. 'While Ayurveda and Unani medicine did have some remedies for epidemics, they were very limited in their efficacy.' Fourth, any amount of government coercion, 'no matter how well founded and well-meaning, is bound to backfire'— as it had in heavy-handed British attempts to control plague in the 1890s. Fifth, government measures 'must include adequate ration provision for the affected.' In the current pandemic 'the failure of the government [in Pakistan] is most stark in the lack of ration support to the people, which forces them to go out in search of work, further exacerbating the situation.' Sixth, government measures can only be successful if the people are properly educated about their benefits and are 'co-opted by the government to aid the process,' a strategy the British had been slow to adopt in their antiplague campaign. Seventh, both the government and private organizations must make a concerted effort to 'dispel rumours and panic during an epidemic.' Experience showed that 'panic has always exacerbated the disease, while rumours have barred people from seeking help.' Eighth, given past pandemic experience, public health reform must be adequately financed to ensure a 'safe and healthy population.' Epidemics 'lay bare the meagre financing of healthcare, be it under colonial or independent rule.' Bangash's final conclusion was that 'harsh government measures never succeed … Without clear measures to prevent and cure a disease by the government, the epidemic will only cause widespread misery and death.'[18]

Bangash's lucid analysis is of interest from several angles. It showed how, in a relatively early stage of the pandemic, history appeared not only relevant but accessible and how a detailed scholarly critique could be extracted from a close analysis of the historical record without resorting to crude polemic or empire-bashing for its own sake. The conclusions he drew from his survey were more appreciative of some aspects of colonial policy and public health intervention and more antagonistic to vernacular medicine than many Indian commentators appeared to be. As the coronavirus epidemic became more established, especially with the terrifying second wave in April–May 2021, the perceived value of the historical experience diminished. The overwhelming scale and horrific immediacy of the present crisis took precedence over past analogies—though the Modi government's failure to ban the Haridwar Kumbh Mela prompted some renewed discussion of the contrast between this and more interventionist British policies.[19] Bangash's articles demonstrated how historians and media commentators in other parts of South Asia besides India—in Pakistan, Bangladesh, even Nepal, though it was never a colonial territory—also looked back to the past of British India as a shared heritage and a fitting source of parallels and lessons for the Covid-19 pandemic.[20] By contrast, more recent epidemics and pandemics, including HIV / AIDS, seldom entered this analysis, as if colonial time and the lessons it bore had leapfrogged into present-day consciousness, overtaking more immediate and arguably more unsettling events that happened in the time of the nation.

Lessons and Anti-lessons

These newspaper sources and online commentaries have not been cited in order to disparage them. Rather, they help bring to our attention the unease some historians felt about the way in which, in the time of Covid, history was being almost randomly plundered, especially by the media, in search of soundbite lessons and precooked precedents. They were concerned at the way in which events, specific to their own time and place, were being wrenched out of context to provide ready-made stories—more often alarming than reassuring—for mass consumption. In the first phase of the coronavirus pandemic many historians as well as epidemiologists found themselves called upon to provide instant expertise. They were expected to pronounce authoritatively on the Spanish Flu especially, and to predict how the current crisis would unfold, how many casualties there would be, how it would ultimately end, and how soon 'normal' life would return. To this abrupt demand for expertise some professional historians responded by stressing the complexity and contextuality of history and the absence of any meaningful lessons. In such a view an 'over-reliance on the allure of "pandemic precedents" needed to be replaced with an enhanced understanding of present crises to resist historical interpretation.' In other words, 'history has no lessons.'[21] Or, to quote Robert Peckham, 'A lessons approach to the past, which usually comes from outside the discipline of history, reinforces an idea of the past as a series of interlinked crises that offer instructive insights into cause and effect.' It was, by contrast, the task of historians 'to push back against easy analogies and examine the specific contexts of outbreaks, asking, for example, in what ways [in the context of China's pandemics] SARS and COVID-19 are in fact comparable.'[22]

There is, though, a danger in being too negative or too restrictive about the activism of history and the political, social, and literary possibilities of the historian's craft. Certainly, history does not directly repeat itself: the world, we know, is in constant flux. Changing scientific knowledge, techniques of disease control, the end of empire, the rise of globalization—these and a host of other factors have created in the age of Covid a very different world from the one in which the Spanish Flu rampaged a century earlier. And yet it is an understandable instinct—and a legitimate authorial strategy—in moments of crisis to look back to the past for instruction or reassurance. Such a utilization of the past helps to keep history alive, responsive to current needs and concerns. One doesn't decolonize the past or best serve the present by closing that past off from critical scrutiny or by ignoring the present-day analogies, legacies, and reenactments that keep that history vital and alive.

Moreover, as this book has tried at several points to suggest, although the past may not deliver neatly packaged 'lessons,' it does present some remarkable and instructive parallels. The flight of migrant workers from India's cities during the first Covid lockdown of 2020 and its parallels with the Bombay plague exodus of 1896–7 tell us much about the nature and consequences of public health intervention and the ongoing plight of the laboring poor. The banning of the Haridwar mela and the dispersal of pilgrims in the North-Western Provinces in 1892 from fear of an imminent cholera outbreak provide a striking parallel and an informative contrast with the failure of the government of Uttarakhand to prohibit a comparable, but far larger, bathing festival in 2021 during the emerging second wave of the coronavirus pandemic. The manner in which epidemics and pandemics across the colonial and postcolonial periods have created existential crises for the state system of medicine and, conversely, opportunities for indigenous systems of therapeutics offers another set of engaging parallels and contrasts. The language used to describe the pandemic disasters of the past, even the language of colonial sanitary officers, can be employed to anticipate and further inform the present—'the burning ghats and burial grounds … swamped with corpses,' 'the depleted medical service … incapable of dealing with more than a minute fraction of the sickness requiring attention,' and 'every household … lamenting a death,' when 'everywhere terror and confusion reigned.'[23] Who, then, can doubt the ability of the past to speak to the present?

Certainly, we need to question exactly what it is that we are seeking to recuperate when we look back on an episode like the influenza pandemic of 1918–19. State policies, disease narratives, public reactions, personal experiences, international responses—all may constitute different kinds of historical parallels and analogies rather than offer one single 'lesson.' We need to consider the nature of different kinds of source materials available to us, who authored them and for whose consumption; we need to reflect on absences as well as presences. We need to be sensitive to the nuances and complexities of history as well as open and self-critical about the uses to which we are putting that history. Historians make poor prophets, but, given due diligence, that does not deny them the ability to relate the past to the present in a meaningful and insightful way.

The media response to the Covid pandemic clearly showed beyond question that history *is* important to modern South Asia, and that an awareness of, and appetite for, history are by no means confined to university departments and practicing academics. The coronavirus crisis encouraged a healthy desire to recover a lost or underutilized past. Why, asked Mohammad Sajjad of Aligarh Muslim University in June 2020, do we know so little about the major epidemics of modern India? 'Why do we avoid putting the histories of the origin, spread, human sufferings, [and] administrative response ... into our syllabi?' India's history textbooks barely mentioned these calamities, or, if they did, they dealt with them in 'just [a] few words.' 'Why have we not been letting such studies enter the popular, public domain?'[24] While one may question whether the epidemics and pandemics of modern India have been quite as neglected as this comment suggests, there must be a case for making their history, in India and elsewhere, a more prominent part of both university teaching and the public awareness of history. Even when they appear to have been forgotten, pandemics are recoverable histories. They come laden with an abundance and diversity of meaningful human experience, and the global shock of Covid-19 will have had laudable effect if it provokes a more informed understanding of how epidemics and pandemics have impacted on and, still more, help constitute the modern history of South Asia.

But this recuperative quest can have its perversions and political misuses. In June 2020 India's University Grants Commission (UGC) was quick to recognize the polemical opportunity the coronavirus pandemic created. It invited the vice-chancellors and principals of the country's universities and colleges to investigate the handling of the Spanish Flu pandemic by the British, to assess what measures were taken thereafter to boost the Indian economy, and to compare this with the BJP government's response to Covid. A questionnaire was drawn up for the purpose, though it failed to explain how the replies were to be assessed and analyzed. The political purpose behind this exercise was transparent. The central government's 'diktat' and its clearly political attempt to gain kudos by invoking the colonial regime and its demonstrable public health failings were clearly designed to flatter the achievements and bolster the prestige of the current BJP regime (it was less eager to do so when the second wave struck and deaths spiraled out of control). The UGC's intervention was seen by some academics as a 'moronic' exercise, if only because, in the words of the president of the Federation of Central Universities Teachers' Associations, in 1918–19 India 'was under a colonial government which treated the Indian masses as cannon fodder to die in the pandemic.' 'After 102 years and 72 years of Independence,' he added, 'with unprecedented development in science to boot, if the 1918 Spanish flu still becomes a benchmark to work on, one does not know whether to laugh or cry!'[25] Crying might not help.

Imperial Contagion and the Pathogenic Empire

Pandemics are a global phenomenon, but their impact and ascribed meaning are seldom identical from one country to another. Nowhere perhaps around the globe has a recent pandemic—Covid-19— been so closely associated with an imperial past as in India. Many countries might attribute their underlying vulnerability to the virus, and their limited capacity to mobilize the resources needed to fight it effectively, to the enduring consequences of colonial rule and the gross inequalities between rich and poor nations that empire instituted in the first place. But in India, especially during the first wave of the coronavirus pandemic, there was an immediacy as well as an intensity to this perceived connectivity between empire and disease that was unmatched anywhere else. Why, more than seventy years on from India's independence, was this so?

There are several possible reasons. If empire figured so prominently in the Indian coronavirus narrative, it was in part because so much past mortality in the subcontinent happened on empire's watch. India's experience of disease, and especially of epidemic/pandemic disease, during the colonial era was (as previous chapters have indicated) exceptionally gruesome, destructive, and protracted, even by the standards of other colonial territories, and reflects in an extremely negative manner on the nature of British rule. By Chinmay Tumbe's calculation, of an estimated 72 million deaths worldwide from just three pandemic diseases—cholera, plague, and influenza—in the period 1817–1920, 40 million of those deaths occurred on Indian soil. More than 90 percent of deaths from bubonic plague in the third pandemic were in India; half of the total influenza mortality worldwide in 1918–19 happened in India.[26] This was death on a colossal, horrific, and, from a global perspective, highly disproportional scale. And yet, what is striking is how little critical attention and detailed analysis this appalling tally, sustained or 'manufactured' over many decades and not the result of a single, atypical occurrence, received until relatively recently. The nationalist critique of British rule focused far more on the misery and destruction wrought by famines, while epidemic mortality, from cholera but also from malaria and plague, was largely subsumed within famine's dark penumbra. Even now famine, encompassing almost the entire period of the British occupation of India from Bengal in the 1770s and back again to Bengal in the 1940s, has been the ultimate indictment of colonial misrule. Perhaps deaths from starvation appeared more directly the consequence of human callousness and misjudgment; perhaps deaths from epidemic disease appeared somehow more 'natural' and less obviously the consequence of the brutalization of colonial subjects. There are sound epidemiological reasons for connecting death from disease with starvation and hunger, but the elision of one with the other, the confluence of pandemic and famine mortality, detracted from closer attention to the phenomenal disease burden India endured during the nineteenth century and well into the twentieth. It was famines that were listed, their course narrated, their geography mapped, their mortality counted. Epidemics, by and large, were only assigned a secondary role.

It is hard to say quite why it has taken so long for the colonial record on disease to be brought to account. But it has. The almost complete neglect of India's influenza (as discussed in chapter 5) is only the most striking example of this historical amnesia. As recently as 2005, Mike Davis (who earlier characterized India's famines as 'late-Victorian holocausts') remarked of the influenza pandemic that 'shockingly little attention has been paid to the disease's ecology in its major theater of mortality in 1918–19: British India.' He likened this lacuna to writing a history of the First World War which concentrated on campaigns in the Balkans and Gallipoli while relegating the mass slaughter on the Western Front to a mere footnote. 'The enormity of influenza's impact on India has never been questioned.'[27]

The sources for such a history, including the published reports and the extensive colonial archive, were there all the time, but perhaps their utilization had to wait until there were medical historians and historians of empire disposed to address such issues and willing to trawl through the vast quantities of available data. The sheer size and volume of the colonial archive and its bureaucratic intricacies and deceits have sometimes served as one of empire's most powerful defenses. Only since the 1980s has the full extent of India's appalling and sustained disease tally begun to be brought to light and exposed to critical scholarly scrutiny. AIDS, Ebola, and SARS, and the growth of global concern about the next possible pandemic, and then the eruption of Covid-19, at last brought India's long and bitter disease experience to the fore and helped highlight the connectivity between epidemics and empire. The Covid pandemic was thus the first opportunity for this historical research to be brought to public attention and to be mobilized in, and through, its association with a current disaster. And Covid itself came at a time of renewed criticism of empire, a searching reexamination of its impact and legacies, and amidst calls to decolonize history. The crisis of 2020–1 suddenly made India's pandemic past seem hugely urgent and relevant.

At its most casual and polemical, the invocation of empire serves as a convenient metaphor for evil, violence, and oppression. Seen thus, empire, itself a kind of pathogen, requires little investigation because its crimes are self-evident. Used with greater subtlety and dexterity of purpose, the imperial charge-sheet on epidemics and pandemics becomes a more useful tool of contemporary analysis, less metaphor than analogy. History has the leverage to pry open present-day politics, to provide a ready-made critique of how— not least in a pandemic emergency—rulers misuse their powers, mislead, neglect, or abuse the people they should serve, and seek to stifle legitimate dissent and opposition. And yet, this alone is not enough of an explanation for why empire figured so prominently in the Covid pandemic. For many Indians and, more especially, for many people of South Asian descent in the West, empire never ended. It has remained constantly present, a shadow presence that never went away, a specter from the past that has continued to haunt the temporality of the now. Empire is revived, not least in Britain, by every act of racial abuse and discrimination, by every crass celebration of imperial greatness, by every literary and cinematic invocation of imperial nostalgia, by every denial of, and attempt to expunge from history, the crimes that empire callously, consistently, and often casually committed. In memory, in imagination, in experience, empire is not dead: far from being merely metaphor or myth, it remains alive, resilient, and oppressive.[28]

For India itself, the history of pandemics is more than a history neatly corralled within the chronological confines of the long colonial epoch; it is an indicative history that still lives on. Things that happened in the past don't remain in the past; they continue to fashion and inform the present. India's pandemic experience encapsulates, replicates, and perpetuates what many writers have seen as the 'trauma' of empire.

In *Wronged by Empire*, Manjari Chatterjee Miller argued that colonialism constituted a form of 'collective historical trauma' for societies, like India, that experienced it. She quoted Jeffrey Alexander's definition of 'cultural trauma' as occurring 'when members of a collectivity feel that they have been subjected to a horrendous event that leaves indelible marks upon their group consciousness, marking their memories forever and changing their future identity in fundamental and irrevocable ways.'[29] To examples like the Holocaust and African American slavery, Miller added colonialism and its historical legacies. 'The core of anti-colonial nationalism that emerged in colonized states was an emphasis on the sufferings and injustices of colonial rule and the search for redress,' she remarked, but that sense of grievance and loss, and the search for redress have persisted into the postcolonial era too.[30] The historian Sunil Amrith similarly observed that British colonialism was a 'source of enduring trauma for many Indians, including for the educated elite that led India's nationalist movement in the first half of the twentieth century. Beyond the outright violence that the British government of India deployed, this trauma resided in a profound sense of social and economic destabilization.' Amrith related this to such specific events as the famines that 'killed millions' (but not to the epidemics). He likened India's experience to China's 'century of humiliation' at the hands of the European powers from the 1840s onward. At the core of such an enduring ordeal was a determination that the nightmare humiliations of the past should not be allowed to recur. There was a clear message: 'never again.'[31]

That colonialism can be labelled 'traumatic' implies more than a historical loss of political sovereignty and economic autarky. The term articulates a collective and personal loss of selfhood, of cultural and social autonomy, a snatching away of the proud and independent place India once held in the world, and an enduring sense of humiliation and exploitation that has persisted long after the formal ending of an 'inglorious empire.'[32] As the pandemic unfolded and the British government, the ex-imperial power, appeared to act prejudicially—in introducing discriminatory bans or quarantine measures against Indian travelers or in questioning the validity of Indian-made vaccines and Indian 'vaccine passports'—so one of the effects of Covid-19 was to revive that never quite quiescent trauma and endow it with a renewed sense of frustration and anger.

The coronavirus pandemic and its colonial antecedents have served, as we have seen, as a vehicle for criticisms of present-day regimes across South Asia. But the repeated invocation of empire simultaneously echoed this deep sense of colonialism as a still-living trauma, a crime for which there has been no recompense, a catastrophe in terms of lives lost and suffering endured whose repetition must be avoided. An article by Md Toriqul Islam in a Bangladeshi journal in November 2020 on the topic of the coronavirus captured the historical depth and emotional intensity of this anticolonial anguish and rage. 'The colonial history of this land,' he wrote, 'is ... the history of famine, plague and epidemic.' Each chapter of the colonial history of Bengal was 'tainted with [the] miseries of the people from deadly disasters. From Sultanate era to the British Raj, foreign rulers ... were unresponsive and apathetic to the people. They never cared about [the] wellbeing of the populace, while they hungered for power and possessions.' With the coronavirus pandemic specifically in mind, Islam concluded that history 'always has two things to offer—recapitulation of the past and lessons for the future.' A century on from the 1890s plague, 'the colonial ghosts still play pranks on us as we see ... the repetition of [the] same past mistakes during another pandemic.' However, 'we now live in a different era ... These mistakes must not recur.'[33]

There is perhaps one further reason why empire figured so prominently in the Indian media during the first coronavirus wave. India still finds itself torn between past and present or, to be more precise, divided between different versions of past and present, and the multiple or shifting temporalities of its 'archaic modernity,' to use Banu Subramaniam's phrase, with its characteristic braiding of science, religion, and capitalism, history and myth.[34] On the one hand India has aspired to be a superpower, in the premier league of nation-states and, as the coronavirus pandemic showed, to be in the forefront of scientific measures both to contain the virus and to curb its onward spread. But, on the other hand, the government of Narendra Modi sought to distance itself from the secularism of the Nehru–Gandhi dynasty that had once dominated Indian politics, and to use the colonial era as an area of irredeemable darkness the better to shine light on its own world. Muslims and the rule of Islam in South Asia were not the BJP's only targets. Colonial representations of India as a land of superstition and disease, the implication of Hinduism in the origin and spread of nineteenth-century epidemics, the manner in which Indians were portrayed as physically weak and morally lax and in which Ayurveda and vegetarianism were derided—these derogatory slurs and racist accusations were now inverted to show instead the British colonialists as weak, intolerant, ignorant, and duplicitous, and as the real reason behind India's devastating history of famines and epidemics.

As the UGC's memorandum requiring universities and colleges to compare the British handling of influenza in 1918–19 with the Modi government's response to Covid may remind us, the pandemic past offered a timely opportunity to eulogize the present. The colonial era, like Muslim rule before it, was to be seen as a dismal hiatus, between the long and glorious era of ancient Hindu science and medicine, eclipsed by foreign rule, and a second dawning in the modern age of Hindutva. In this 'golden age' mythology, Hindus, before their colonization first by the Muslims and then by the British, lived in a land of health and plenty, innocent of epidemics. Within the ideology of the Hindu Right the pathogenesis of foreign rule served a useful polemical purpose.

Alternative Histories

Whether by looking back to the colonial past in order to extract practical 'lessons' for the pandemic present, as a means of castigating empire and its legacies, or as a method of critiquing contemporary politics, the past has clearly had its uses. But history doesn't replicate itself, especially with such complex and polyvalent events as pandemics. As Richard Evans observed, 'history never repeats itself; nothing in human society, the main concern of the historian, ever happens twice under exactly the same conditions or in exactly the same way.'[35] Even by invoking the past, we are affected by that past and either strenuously avoid its repetition or are unable (even if we so wished) to replicate it. Given the immense changes that have taken place in science and society even since the influenza of 1918–19, it should have been clear that no easy lessons or straightforward analogies with Covid-19 were really possible. As Adam Kucharski noted from the epidemiologist's perspective: 'If you've seen one pandemic, you've seen … one pandemic.'[36] In writing of the 'anti-lessons of history,' Robert Peckham remarked that the 'history-as-lessons approach pivots on the assumption that epidemics are structurally comparable events, wherever and whenever they take place.' While the Covid pandemic provided 'a compelling argument for why history matters,' analogical views of the past 'constrain our ability to grasp the complex place- and time-specific variables that drive contemporary disease emergence.' Historians, he concluded, need to 'challenge efforts to corral and straightjacket the past into summary lessons.'[37]

Certainly, there is a counterargument to be made about the novelty of the present over the resonances of the past. The lockdown and the scenes of migrant workers fleeing Mumbai in 2020 might look like a replay of the plague in that same city in 1896–7 or recall the long lines of Partition refugees in 1947. The resurrection of the Epidemic Diseases Act in 2020 might make us see the response of the Modi government as analogous to that of the British to plague in 1897. With Covid we may fear the return of the mass mortality of 1918–19 or see parallels between the stigmatizing and scapegoating of nineteenth-century cholera epidemics and the more recent treatment of Muslims and other minorities. Even the scenes of the burning pyres of the dead in 2021 may recall similar images from 1890s Bombay and send similarly mixed sentiments of repugnance, fear, and pity around the world. These and other episodes and images from the pandemic past help to supercharge the present, to direct our attention and concentrate our scrutiny, fuel our anger or alarm. But they don't actually repeat the past.

If there were echoes in 2020 of the rumors and violence of the early plague years, we should also remind ourselves that the target of such acts and suspicions was a colonial regime whose often arbitrary conduct and Olympian unconcern for the culture and well-being of the people provoked a backlash across classes and communities. Very different was the situation in 2020 when the pandemic was seized upon to mobilize majoritarian hostility not to an alien colonial regime but to a perceived 'enemy' within or 'unpatriotic' criticism of the ruling regime. Colonial India was an alien bureaucratic autocracy, albeit one increasingly tempered by Indian participation; India in the 2020s was, in a cherished phrase, 'the world's largest democracy,' even if tarnished by increasing intolerance of difference and dissent.[38] The BJP government in Delhi might fear a popular backlash, especially in the wake of the mishandling of the pandemic's second wave, but it had more ideological weapons and political tools at its command, including a resilient populist base and a proven capacity to win state and national elections, than the British ever had in the 1890s or 1918.

In the late 1890s and early 1900s, at the height of the colonial era, India was beset by famine and recurrent epidemics of cholera, malaria, and still-unextinguished smallpox. Infant and maternal mortality rates were staggeringly high. Food shortages and hunger were rife again in 1918. The pandemics of the late nineteenth and early twentieth centuries were played out against a backdrop of starvation, war, and a public health system still in its infancy, underfunded and ill-equipped to deal with the multiple challenges it faced. India was not in that extreme position in 2020, even though poverty and malnutrition remained widespread and levels of infant and maternal health remained among the worst anywhere in the world. One effect of Covid-19, the nationwide lockdown, the loss of employment, and the inadequacy of state support schemes was to push millions of Indians once more to the brink of destitution and hunger, to render them still more liable to infection, or unable (unless they were wealthy or privileged) to access even basic healthcare. But famines, as experienced under colonial rule, are unlikely to recur, if only because the political cost of failing to feed the nation is so high.

But, if we don't look back to the colonial past, where should we look? Where do we find a different narrative, an alternative history of India, pandemics, and public health, one less governed by imperial templates? There is, of course, the record of India since independence in 1947. Since the Spanish Flu, India has ridden out a host of lesser or greater epidemics, from cholera and plague to dengue and chikungunya, from Asian Flu in 1957 to Nipah virus in 2018, without suffering morbidity and mortality on anything like, or vaguely comparable to, 1918's apocalyptic scale. Western countries may have begun by the 1950s to think of themselves as immune to pandemics and consigned them to a half-forgotten past. India did not have that luxury. With help from the WHO, the country played a major part in the eradication of smallpox in the 1970s and in the immunization campaign against polio; it had hopes of eliminating malaria by 2030.[39] Despite widespread poverty and illiteracy, in spite of the vastness of the country and the size of its population, India had the experience and the confidence of knowing how to contain or eliminate major infectious diseases. India's public health system might have been defective, frail, and woefully underresourced, and the second wave of Covid again exposed its alarming fragility, but did more affluent and medically better-served countries like the United States, Britain, France, and Germany fare very much better? Surely not.

The story of India's Covid-19 vaccination program provides a fascinating historical case study, both for what it achieved (or failed to achieve) and for the light it casts on the country's epidemic and pandemic past. It demonstrated, on the one hand, the extent to which modern India, with its advanced medical and manufacturing sectors, had broken away from its colonial forebears and could mobilize the skills and resources not only to address its own health crisis but also to export surplus vaccines overseas. It showed how India, colony no longer, could seize the opportunity of the pandemic to demonstrate its rightful place in the global economy and the international public health order. Here was an alternative history in the making. At the same time, that colonial past had its resonances. It was, after all, in colonial times that prophylactic vaccines were pioneered in India and the first, albeit tentative, steps taken toward mass immunization. Some of the difficulties that beset the colonial health regime (producing enough vaccine, ensuring its safety, overcoming resistance) still existed in 2020–1; and even some of the doubts raised internationally about the reliability of India's vaccine manufacture and criticism of its inability, during the second wave of the pandemic, to keep up with the demand seemed to smack of postimperial arrogance.

In common with governments around the world, and in keeping with its own colonial and postcolonial public health strategies, in 2020 India turned to vaccines as the most likely route out of the coronavirus crisis. Just as he had taken political ownership of the nationwide lockdown, so Modi explicitly identified himself with the vaccination campaign, even to the extent of having his photograph prominently displayed on India's Covid vaccine certificates.[40] Setting aside its earlier endorsement of Ayurvedic remedies and flirtation with cow-urine parties, the government began an ambitious vaccine rollout on 16 January 2021 with the aim of delivering 300 million inoculations by the end of July 2021. This was to be immunization on a scale that utterly dwarfed colonial vaccination against smallpox, cholera, and plague. Among developing nations, India had, at least in theory, certain advantages in combating a modern pandemic. It had the experience of past mass immunization campaigns and had shown, despite some resistance, or 'vaccine hesitancy' as it might now be called, that such prophylactics were largely acceptable to, and even widely sought after by, the general public. In the main, the doubts about the effectiveness and acceptability of vaccination that plagued colonial India in the 1890s and 1900s had largely (though not entirely) disappeared.[41] Again, in the nineteenth century India's pharmaceutical industry was still in its infancy and the country remained heavily reliant on imported drugs (many of which were preferred by colonial physicians over viable local alternatives). Dubbed 'the pharmacy of the developing world,' India has become one of the world's leading producers of generic drugs and has annually exported billions of doses of vaccines to other countries. Pharmacology, serology, and immunology, and the technical expertise and productive capacity that underpin them, form a substantial part of India's claim to be, in medical terms, a 'science superpower.'[42] India's manufacture of the antimalarial hydroxychloroquine even had President Donald Trump threatening India with unspecified 'retaliation' unless it agreed to continue exporting the drug as a (soon to be discredited) prophylactic against the coronavirus. In this instance, India duly complied.[43]

By late 2020 several Indian drug manufacturers were either developing their own anti-Covid vaccines or collaborating with foreign firms to do so under license, confident that, once they were approved for use, India had the capacity to produce millions of doses a month for its own use and also to supply other countries. One of India's leading firms and the world's largest vaccine producer, the Serum Institute in Pune, reached an agreement with the Anglo-Swedish pharmaceutical giant AstraZeneca to conduct trials in India with its new anti-Covid vaccine and then manufacture millions of doses of the vaccine locally. Marketed as 'Covishield,' the vaccine was officially approved in January 2021, alongside an Indian-originated vaccine 'Covaxin' made by Bharat Biotech.[44] Doubts surfaced as to whether Covaxin had completed the necessary trials and suspicions arose that a rash, politically motivated decision had been made by the prime minister to approve the drug in an overeager attempt to show Indian prowess. In a characteristic defense, Modi's supporters were quick to retort that even doubting the efficacy of an Indian vaccine was unpatriotic.[45] For Modi, who adopted 'Make in India' as one of his favored slogans, the mass production of Indian vaccines was a shining example of Indian ingenuity and postimperial self-reliance. Since the vaccines were also destined for export, principally to India's neighbors and other low-income countries, they were seen as enabling India to exercise its 'soft power' and 'vaccine diplomacy' (or 'vaccine friendship,' as the government preferred to describe it) in competition with China, Russia, and other rival producers.[46] By mid-March 2021, India had distributed 58 million doses of vaccine to sixty-five nations, mostly through the international vaccine-sharing COVAX scheme.[47]

Difficulties lay ahead. Mercifully, India did not suffer a repeat of the 'Mulkowal disaster' of 1902 in which nineteen Punjabi villagers died of tetanus and confidence in the immunization program was badly, if only temporarily, affected (see chapter 3). Reports of 'adverse events' remained reassuringly low. And, though the old rumors about vaccines causing sterility, infertility, and even death resurfaced in 2020–1, in general India encountered less by way of sustained opposition than many other nations, including the strident anti-vaxxers and conspiracy theorists of Western countries like the United States, Britain, and Germany.[48] India's vaccination program began impressively, with more than 600,000 people (mostly health workers) vaccinated in the first three days, but it soon fell behind schedule. By late April 2021, 135 million doses of vaccine had been delivered but, for a country of over 1.3 billion people, that figure (equivalent to less than 2 percent of the population) was nowhere near enough.[49] As its own death-toll climbed during the second wave of infection, there was no longer enough vaccine for India's own requirements. From having been an exporter of millions of vaccine doses at the start of 2021, India was now forced to retract, first canceling exports (including to the UK) and then asking for ventilators, surplus vaccines, and emergency oxygen-making equipment from overseas, and even from the archenemy, China.[50] The doctor had become the patient.

Although the government announced that all Indians over eighteen were eligible for inoculation, in reality even the needs of the over-forty-fives could barely be met.[51] Vaccine manufacturers, led by the Serum Institute in Pune, had to admit that they could not meet demand or were running short of essential ingredients. The central government added to the confusion and shortages in April 2021 by transferring responsibility for the purchase of vaccine to individual states, creating an internal market where vaccines went to the highest bidder, leaving poorer states less able to compete for supplies or complaining of hoarding by wealthier states.[52] This decision was subsequently reversed in late June 2021. By October 2021, as the second wave of India's Covid epidemic subsided, the situation had greatly improved. The numbers vaccinated (and double-vaccinated) were relatively high: by the end of that month India had administered more than a billion doses of vaccine, nearly half of the eligible population had received one dose, and nearly 20 percent had been given both, though this performance still compared poorly with vaccination rates in many other countries, including China where twice as many vaccine doses had been administered. On the positive side, distribution of the locally made Covishield far exceeded both its domestic rival (Covaxin) and Russia's Sputnik V.[53] Production and supplies had so far improved that overseas exports could be resumed. But the continuing emergence of new variants and the short-term (six-month) immunity given even by two doses of the vaccine posed problems for the future. Like the British earlier, the Indian government needed to recognize that, vital though immunization was in meeting an immediate health crisis, vaccination alone could not offer a long-term solution. More radical and sustained answers had to be found to the underlying problems of poverty, ill health, and a seriously defective public health system.

A Third Narrative

There is a third possibility, another kind of 'tryst with destiny.' Beyond the historical narrative that related India's experience of Covid-19 back to the age of empire, and an alternative story of the post-1947 nation and its new global standing, it is possible to imagine an emerging or anticipatory history, a scenario that draws upon the past to look forward into a highly uncertain future and that locates both empire and nation in a longer-term context. The political scientist Adam Roberts remarked in 2020 that 'the well-documented history of pandemics suggests that we do not live in uniquely dangerous times.'[54] It is, on the face of it, a reassuring statement, a rational call to temper present fears with a balanced view of the past. We should not be too hasty in calling in the apocalypse. But the possibility exists that we *do* live in 'uniquely dangerous times,' and that the coronavirus pandemic cannot be viewed in isolation from a wider and still more alarming narrative of planetary degradation and environmental crisis.

Each pandemic is different and has different characteristics even when, like cholera or influenza, it involves the same recurrent pathogens. Diseases mutate or present themselves in very different circumstances from their predecessors. Human behavior changes; science moves on. There are too many contingent factors to allow us to derive simple lessons from the pandemic past. Each pandemic is played out against a kaleidoscope of varied and shifting factors, as the example of India since 1817 has shown. Covid-19, though terrifying and deadly enough in India, especially in its second wave, was not quite the holocaust forecasters had expected, and, besides, before 2019 their fears had been concentrated not on a coronavirus but on avian flu or the return of a highly lethal strain of influenza. Not just the fear but the likelihood of a new pandemic, and possibly repeated or overlapping pandemics, occurring over a short space of time rather than divided by a century-long hiatus, now appears more than ever likely. And while the production of anti-Covid vaccines was an undoubted success story in 2020–1, it may not be possible to replicate that remarkable scientific achievement in future pandemics and with new, more vaccine-resistant variants, or to maintain the effective, worldwide delivery of such a vaccine. Modern medical science has proved remarkably effective, but the Covid-19 pandemic also showed the difficulty of producing and distributing enough vaccine to inoculate the whole world and to combat new viral strains and mutations.

Science, adept though it has been so far at contagion catch-up, cannot be infinitely inventive; nor do the resources or, it would seem, the political will exist to encompass rich and poor, every country and every need. Meanwhile, as South Asia should remind us, older diseases, like malaria, cholera, polio, and tuberculosis, become forgotten or marginalized in public health, only for new drug-resistant strains to reemerge and return to reap their grim human harvest. Or, as international attention and medical resources are diverted to firefighting coronavirus, the containment and treatment of other, older 'plagues' are neglected, allowing them to regroup and regrow.

Covid-19 gave pandemicity a new template and a new temporality, one much closer to our own time and experience than the increasingly distant Spanish Flu on which, until 2020, so much epidemiological modeling and pandemic prediction were predicated. This comes on top of the evidence we have already seen for the emergence of new, mostly viral infections over recent decades—HIV/AIDS, SARS, Ebola, Swine Flu, Avian Flu. Most of the killer diseases of the so-called pandemic century since 1918 have erupted only since the 1970s—one reason why the WHO definition of a pandemic has shifted from recurrent or residual diseases like cholera to new and emerging contagions.[55] Measured on a pandemic timescale, time seems to be rapidly contracting. Perhaps, too, this means that the colonial past and the pandemic age of empire are no longer quite so proximate and relevant to our contemporary experiences, and that the current conduct of independent nation-states and the leading powers in the modern world will supersede some of the ageing empire experience. Or they may simply be overtaken by a world in which anthropogenic environmental change and the climate crisis present a still greater and more imminent danger.

Few pandemics in the past have been as truly global as Covid, and even the few that were (such as the influenza of 1918–19) passed relatively quickly. We exist in an age of unprecedented global consciousness, thanks to contemporary media and the almost universal access to information it provides, but also in an age of 'fake news' and 'misinformation' that exceeds or radically transforms the unsettling role of rumor in earlier pandemics. There has been an unmatched simultaneity, as well as a remarkable lack of preparedness in most countries, about responses to the coronavirus, such as in the timing of lockdowns and the rollout of vaccination programs across the globe. But consciousness and knowledge alone have not been enough to stem the tide of disease or prevent repeated pandemic waves. Perhaps, in this respect as in others, we are in unprecedented ('uniquely dangerous') times, times in which the past, any past, can be of only limited utility. Covid may come to be seen not as the most recent in a long series of pandemics, but as the first pandemic of a new pathogenic and environmental order rather than the last of a disappearing breed.

In its timing as much as in its nature, the coronavirus pandemic of 2020–1 occurred against a backdrop of unprecedented planetary crisis, a point that the meeting of the UN climate change conference COP26 at Glasgow in November 2021, even while Covid still raged, made eloquently clear. The regional, as well as global, consequences of global warming and rapid climate change were evident to anyone who cared to see them. While doctors, nurses, vaccinators, and virologists battled the coronavirus across India, firefighters struggled, amidst drought and soaring temperatures, to contain rampant forest fires in Uttarkhand, the same state that had hosted the Kumbh Mela at the start of the country's second coronavirus wave.[56] West Bengal was hit by a devastating cyclone early on in the pandemic; a plague of locusts ravaged fields in drought-ridden Rajasthan in May 2020; Kerala suffered severe monsoonal floods in 2018 and again in 2021, said to be the worst for a hundred years; further flooding hit Andhra Pradesh in November 2021. Zika virus, too, returned to Kerala and Uttar Pradesh. Perhaps, with hindsight, colonial physicians and medical topographers were not entirely wrong in the attention they gave to the connection between climate, landscape, and disease, though they could hardly have anticipated the scale on which that environmental relationship is now playing out.

At the same time as Covid swept the globe, world leaders meeting at Glasgow were meant to be turning their thoughts to how to curb the use of fossil fuels and prevent the remorseless rise in global temperatures beyond 1.5 degrees above pre-industrial levels. For many commentators India (along with Bangladesh and the island nation of the Maldives) was in the front line of anthropogenic climate change. And yet, just as in early 2021 the Indian government turned a blind eye to the likelihood of a second, still more deadly wave of the coronavirus virus and claimed national near-immunity, so that same government's energy minister decried international attempts to cut carbon emissions. He called it 'pie in the sky,' arguing that low-income or developing nations like his own wanted to continue to use fossil fuels, and the rich nations 'can't stop it.' This view was reiterated at the COP26 meeting in November 2021 to the dismay of many delegates.[57] And this despite the fact that India and South Asia at large were among the areas of the world already most drastically affected by climate change and extreme weather events—by soaring temperatures, rising sea levels, droughts, floods, landslides, erratic monsoons, and shrinking Himalayan glaciers. The kindly 'weather gods' that may have helped India escape famine in the early twentieth century and the colonial-era irrigation projects that helped to relieve 'water stress' and so ensure better health conditions (see chapter 6) could no longer be relied upon in the twenty-first century to avert the growing threat of water shortages, drought, and ultimately, perhaps, mass migration and starvation. In an earlier time, as during the Spanish Flu of 1918–19, 'storms,' 'floods,' 'lightning strikes,' and 'avalanches' had been metaphors for epidemic disaster; now they were the reality of contemporary climate-related catastrophe.[58] In this context it is hard not to see how the pandemic history with which this book has been concerned may itself become swamped by and subsumed within a still-greater environmental narrative. The coronavirus pandemic, not least as it impacted on India, can be understood as an outlier or precursor to what Amitav Ghosh termed 'the Great Derangement,' that immense tide of environmental degradation and climatic change that is visibly and catastrophically wrecking the entire planet on which we live.[59] This is an ecological and, for many species as well as our own, existential crisis, in a way that even the Spanish Flu pandemic never was.

'Pandemic,' that now overused word, barely describes the interlocking causes and multiple manifestations of the crisis in which we find ourselves. By focusing on one disease, politicians, epidemiologists, historians, and the public they serve may be in danger of marginalizing or ignoring the monumental nature of that much greater crisis that threatens to overtake us. Or they are guilty of believing that somehow, once the immediate threat of the coronavirus pandemic is over, and the monstrous genie has been tricked back into its bottle, we will fly less, eat less, burn less, breathe freer air. It was for a while confidently hoped that the global shutdown caused by Covid-19 in 2020 would result in lasting change. In the new 'normal,' the skies over Delhi would stay clear and smog-free; the waters of the Ganges would remain unpolluted. But this did not happen. As Diwali came around again in October 2020 and still more in November 2021, Delhi was once more choked by the thick fog caused by festival fireworks, the burning of crop stubble in nearby states, and coal-burning power stations.[60] As with some past pandemics, little or nothing had changed for the better.

Half a century ago it was possible for historians and epidemiologists to envisage the end of a long and arduous journey from a world repeatedly racked by pandemic 'plagues' and epidemic diseases to one in which such contagions had been systematically eradicated or confined to a few isolated and dwindling locations. That Panglossian view of the human relationship with disease was always hubristic. But it is now possible to see a rather different journey, one that does not end in so triumphalist a fashion. Following AIDS, SARS, Ebola, Swine Flu, and Covid-19, we can now discern a different trajectory. Individual diseases may be contained. But the prospect remains of other diseases, new viruses especially, rushing in to replace those that have been medically constrained, posing ever more intractable problems for medical science and for the resourcefulness and adaptability of states and societies around the world to cope with. More than that, we are beginning to see pandemics as happening against the backdrop of climate change and rapid ecological crisis, the anthropogenic disordering of our only planet. Where this new pandemic journey ends is far from clear; but, if our history is to be of value, it has to engage not just with the past but also with the new world in which, unhappily, we find ourselves.

CONCLUSION

From cholera to Covid-19, from its obscure and contested origins in the mid-nineteenth century to unquestioned authority in the twenty-first, the idea of the pandemic has become universal. Through a series of devastating events and deadly epidemiological encounters, pandemics have come to be understood as truly global phenomena, threatening or in some way affecting virtually every person on the planet. Once thought, in the wake of scientific discoveries and medical advances, to be destined for extinction, pandemics have returned, revenant, to haunt our modern lives, and to define, in a uniquely terrifying way, the perils and the hubris of our globalized existence.

But if 'pandemic' is the familiar label we use to describe this planetary phenomenon, what is it that makes the modern pandemic? Infection—and more especially death—on a massive scale is one of the most obvious characteristics. Pandemics are played out in terms of numbers. It is through the accountancy of cases and deaths that we gain a sense of the human tragedy and devastating consequences of mass contagion. Statistics provide a vital means by which we can examine the rise and fall of a disease, identify waves and troughs, unpack the impact of past pandemics, or try to imagine how a future pandemic might unfold. But statistics have their limitations. As seemingly authoritative statements of fact, they can be wildly unreliable, as the example of both influenza in 1918–19 and Covid-19 in India, episodes a century apart, attest. By their sheer scale and anonymity, statistics preclude or anesthetize individual suffering, or make matters appear reassuringly orderly and under control, when in fact (as is the way with pandemics) they remain chaotic and unpredictable. And, while there is undoubtedly a politics in numbers and in weighing one country's death-toll against another, what does it actually mean in human terms to say that 20 rather than 6 or 12 million people died in India in the Spanish Flu of 1918–19, or that as many people died in one Indian province as in the whole of the United States and Britain? How do we imagine death on such a scale? How do we evaluate one life as against another? What we can know, however, is that historically all lives are not treated equally, and that, for instance, the fatalities that occurred among Indians under colonial rule were not judged by the same criteria as lives lived in the West. Mortality alone does not define the modern pandemic. Around a million people a year were dying of malaria in India in the late nineteenth and early twentieth centuries, but no one thought to designate that a pandemic, if only because the disease was endemic within the subcontinent and not seen to threaten societies beyond India. By contrast, SARS was declared a pandemic by the WHO in 2003 and yet it resulted in fewer than 800 deaths worldwide: here 'pandemic' better represents the fear of a new or emerging contagion and its deadly potential rather than the actual number of casualties caused.

Pandemics need a pathogen, a specific disease-causing microorganism, one that stands out from the jostling crowd of competing pathogens. In the modern world, viruses like influenza, SARS, and Covid-19 have best captured the infectivity, and demonstrated the speed and spread, as well as the lethality, that we now associate with the pandemic phenomenon. But pandemics are social and political constructions as much as they are pathogenic happenings. As in the case of colonial India from cholera's emergence in 1817 onward, pandemics need an information order by which to identify new and recurring diseases, to trace their origins and track their onward dissemination. They need public health experts to name them, to advise on their prevention, containment, and treatment, and to pass on to other medical professionals and the public information about the pathogenic danger to life. This individual and collective decision-making process involves many layers of expertise, of social subjectivity as well as the presumed objectivity of science. It reflects the political context in which critical judgments are made, and health policies devised and implemented.

As Alex de Waal remarked with respect to famine in Africa: 'Who defines an event as a "famine" is a question of power relations within and between societies.'[1] Modern pandemics are likewise highly political events. This is evident from the political considerations that impelled India's colonial government to act, or not to act, in relation to epidemics of cholera, plague, and influenza. This politicization was especially marked when local outbreaks fed, or threatened to feed, into global pandemics and so acquired wider international significance. The same is true in more recent times. The Chinese government was initially reluctant to admit to the world the pandemic danger posed by Covid when it first erupted in Wuhan in December 2019. Equally the WHO was extremely cautious about calling it a pandemic before the evidence of global danger and its international spread was established beyond reasonable doubt—and, with hindsight, it acted later than it should have done. Pandemics require politicians and administrators to accept, in whole or in part, the advice their public health experts give them, to take ownership of that knowledge, and to authorize the kinds of measures (so evident with Covid-19, but with precedents in India going back to cholera and plague in the 1890s) by which the disease threat is to be met and its further spread contained. Pandemics in the modern world have not only involved colonial or national governments; they have also been a stimulus to international governance—the international sanitary conferences that met from 1851 onward; the WHO from its founding in 1948.

The pathogens that cause pandemics are real, and the history of pandemicity over the past two centuries has in no small part been a history of scientific investigation—the quest to identify new pathogens or better determine the character of old ones, to devise ways to analyze and explain their infectivity and spread, to marshal the means to prevent, cure, or contain them. The investigations into the etiology of cholera and plague, the development of prophylactic vaccine against those same contagions—these are examples of what science could achieve. But pathogens, as they act in human society, are also hyperreal. They come encumbered with trauma, enshrouded with myth; they are vehicles for fear, loathing, compassion, and visceral hate. They engender a violence—of state and society, of persecution or abandonment—that extends far beyond the violence of the causative pathogen itself. Socially, pandemics represent far more than the scientifically defined physical nature and pathological effects of individual infection; they speak louder than statistics. And it is this social context and social construction that have given modern pandemicity so much of its universality and its potency. Pandemics don't just exist; they have been made.

However they may be defined by epidemiologists, to historians pandemics are inseparable from the social and cultural milieu in which they exist. As the chapters in this book have tried to suggest, pandemics are multi-sited phenomena, embodied in texts and narratives (in fiction and non-fiction, in memoirs, medical journals, official reports, and government records). They are kept alive, reworked, and re-presented through paintings and photographs, in street art and moving images, just as they are embedded in personal memories and recollections. They reflect and inhabit the human emotions. Their elaborate architecture incorporates rumor, gossip, metaphor and myth, even what we would now call 'fake news' and the 'misinformation' order. These are also the means by which an awareness of pandemic danger is socially processed and stored in the collective memory. And though historically much of the making of the pandemic idea has been done in the West, by and for the West, there are various ways in which pandemics, or their epidemic outliers and endemic residues, have been locally owned, reimagined, and reenacted according to the culture, politics, and location of the society concerned. No two pandemics are ever the same, even when they involve identical, or nearly identical, pathogens. Quite apart from changes to science and the technologies of public health, their social, political, and cultural contexts shift not only over time, but from one region to another. Covid was but the latest example of how a pandemic can have a global identity while simultaneously exhibiting an extraordinarily diverse set of local characteristics.

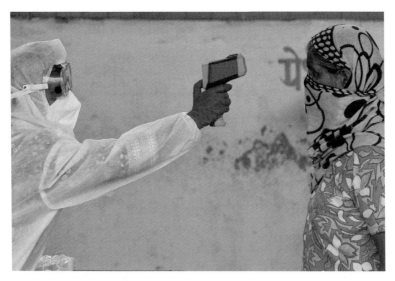

13. A Doctor in Personal Protective Equipment Taking a Woman's Temperature as Part of Covid-19 Testing, Mumbai, 18 May 2020.

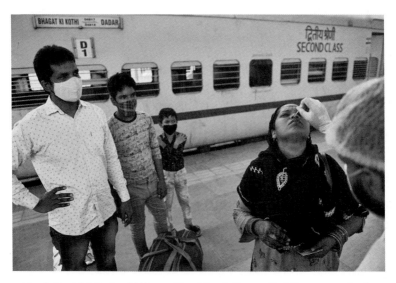

14. A Health Worker Taking a Nasal Swab from a Rail Passenger, Dadar Station, Mumbai, 29 October 2021.

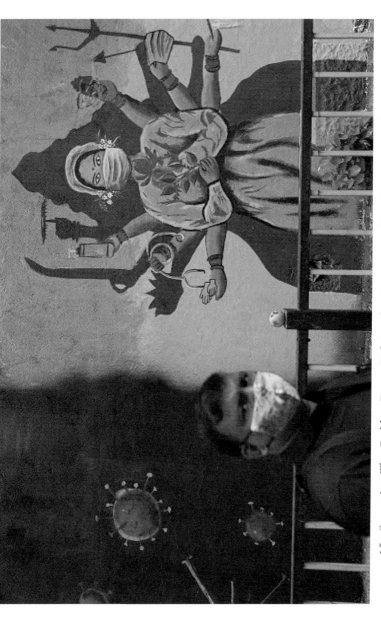

15. Street Art: The Goddess Durga Fighting the Coronavirus, Mumbai, 17 November 2021.

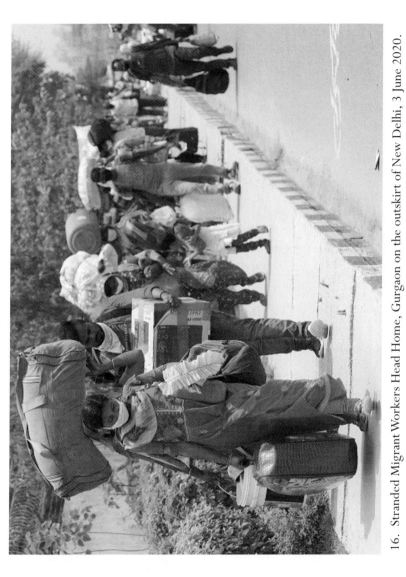

16. Stranded Migrant Workers Head Home, Gurgaon on the outskirt of New Delhi, 3 June 2020.

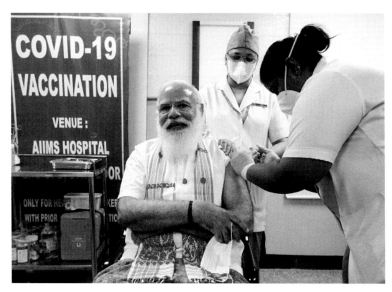

17. Prime Minister Narendra Modi Receives His First Dose of Covid-19 Vaccine, 1 March 2021.

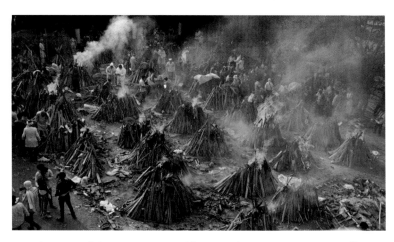

18. Funeral Pyres Burning at Ghazipur Crematorium, New Delhi, During Second Wave of Covid-19, 28 April 2021.

India, this book has argued, played a central part in the unfolding pandemic narrative. Under colonial rule it provided a crucial site of epidemiological observation and investigation, beginning with the cholera outbreak of 1817. As the perceived 'home' of that disease, and as an epicenter of plague, it epitomized what the West most feared in the serial invasion of 'foreign' contagion in the nineteenth and twentieth centuries, a role in part revisited with the 'Indian' or 'Delta' variant in the second wave of the coronavirus pandemic in 2021. By the size and poverty of its population, by its repeated and often concurrent experience of famine, by its centrality to global networks of trade and communication, it had long shown both a chronic vulnerability to pandemic infections and an alarming propensity to disseminate them abroad. But India also endured to an exceptional degree the strains of empire, epitomized by the way in which the Spanish Flu of 1918–19 latched on to the wartime shortages, the effects of wholesale recruitment, the prevalent 'distress' (more frankly, famine), and the long-term debility of a large section of the population. Pandemics everywhere were cruel, but in some places their cruelty was more evident, more intensive, and longer-lasting than in others. While in many areas of the West pandemics came and went in distinctive waves and through short-term invasions, in India many of the very same diseases remained, obdurate and entrenched, exacting their deadly toll over many generations.

And yet, while weighing up the exploitation and negligence of empire, it is also pertinent to note how India was the site, too, of medical investigations and experiments (again, cholera and plague provide the most notable examples) that were of benefit not just to the subcontinent but to the world beyond. Despite the arrogance and racism of the colonial administration and many in its medical establishment, Indians gained invaluable expertise in the investigation of disease and in public health administration, just as since independence India has become a crucial arena for implementing mass vaccination campaigns and in developing one of the world's leading pharmaceutical industries. There are significant lines of continuity here rather than a simple tale of colonial–postcolonial rupture. Less successfully, perhaps, India grappled with the problem of trying to reconcile modern scientific medicine with vernacular alternatives

241

and the role of religion in public health. Empire dispossessed and empire disparaged, but it also left legacies that remain at the heart of India's medical modernity and the dilemmas that still perplex it.

It has been a central argument of this book, in focusing on India, that the pandemic idea has had an intimate connection with the history of empire. This is doubly so. The idea of a pandemic grew up in the nineteenth and early twentieth century, at the height of empire. Imperial territories, especially India with its 'Asiatic cholera' but also the Caribbean, Africa, Southeast Asia, and China, were the perceived source of the contagions that most threatened Europe, against which Western powers needed to erect barriers and build defenses, against which the empires of Europe (and later America) had to deploy their medical science and public health expertise. Then, in the time of empire, but still also now, pandemicity defined an external threat to Western health. Disease, on the march into Europe and North America, articulated a powerful sense of civilization in danger. This was the barbarism lurking at the gates of Elysium that ever threatened a fall from progress and modernity back into primitivism, squalor, and death. Whenever, as in the mid- and late nineteenth century, or again in the middle and late decades of the twentieth, the West saw or predicted an end to such atavistic horror, somehow or other that threat was revived, the vulnerability relived.

From a reverse perspective, as seen from the India that has been at the center of this work, it was the era of British colonial rule that stood at the core of the pandemic issue—the colonialism that impoverished and weakened India and facilitated the invasion or incubation of lethal pathogens, the colonialism that from its laissez-faire languor or from its racialized arrogance or indifference failed to address the problem of epidemic disease and the socio-economic causes that underlay it. Colonialism stigmatized the sufferers while lauding the self-interested actions of the colonizers. The time of empire was *the* time of epidemics, and empire, for many who live in India or who write about India, remains the default position, the essential reference point in seeking to appraise all that happened before and that has happened since in the long career of subcontinental disease. Empire casts a long, dark shadow, even— decades on from independence—in the time of Covid. Conceivably, one legacy of the coronavirus pandemic may be to force a rethinking of how far empire can still be held responsible when an autonomous Indian government, with its own very different agenda, showed itself almost as inept and blameworthy.

It is important to recognize how pandemics, perhaps more than any other manifestation of disease with which historians concern themselves, are used. They have variously served as an instrument of political and social power, as an agent of exculpation and denial or of self-reliance and self-affirmation, as a means of reinterpreting the past and reordering the present. Pandemics are sometimes viewed as game-changers, as monumental events that changed the course of history. India's plague years can, in some respects, be viewed in this affirmative or consolatory manner, even though its experience of influenza surely cannot. In time, Covid-19 may come to be seen, for all the immense suffering it occasioned, as having had a positive effect, providing a portal into a new India. But there is also the depressing possibility that pandemics in actuality change remarkably little, or that they only add incrementally to processes already in train. Rather than providing lessons or recycling the past, they are 'anti-lessons,' not just in the sense that they possess no clear, didactic message but in the manner in which they distract attention away from issues that are still more profound and intractable—how we deal with mass poverty, with global inequality, with the systemic crisis of a rapidly degrading environment and an overheating planet. Pandemics can be, and historically have been, explained away. They are labeled 'natural disasters'; they are seen as the consequence of a rogue virus or the outcome of a regrettable confluence of war, famine, and flood. But if pandemics have a value, if the history of pandemics has a use, that may lie in forcing us to look at what is wrong, structurally, socially, politically, with the world we have made.

A NOTE ON PLACE NAME CHANGES

Since 1947 a number of Indian cities and towns have been renamed or their spelling has been changed from that of the colonial era. Although the changes have occurred at various times since independence, for the sake of consistency they are treated here as if they all date from that time. Changes include:

Allahabad	Prayagraj
Bangalore	Bengaluru
Benares	Varanasi
Bombay	Mumbai
Calcutta	Kolkata
Cawnpore	Kanpur
Hardwar	Haridwar
Madras	Chennai
Poona	Pune
Simla	Shimla

Many former British provinces have been renamed. Hence:

Central Provinces	Madhya Pradesh
Orissa	Odisha
Rajputana	Rajasthan
United Provinces, formerly the North-Western Provinces	Uttar Pradesh

Others have been divided up to form new states. They include Andhra Pradesh, Tamil Nadu, and parts of Karnataka, from the former Madras Presidency; Gujarat, Maharashtra, and parts of Karnataka from the Bombay Presidency; Telangana from Mysore; Kerala from the princely states of Travancore and Cochin, plus Malabar from the Madras Presidency; Chhattisgarh and Jharkhand from Bihar and Orissa; Haryana from Punjab; and Uttarakhand from Uttar Pradesh.

NOTES

INTRODUCTION

1. Soutik Biswas, 'Covid-19: India Excess Deaths Cross Four Million, Says Study,' BBC News, 20 July 2021, https://www.bbc.co.uk/news/world-asia-india-57888460.
2. Kingsley Davis, *The Population of India and Pakistan* (Princeton: Princeton University Press, 1951), 42.
3. Chinmay Tumbe, *The Age of Pandemics, 1817–1920: How They Shaped India and the World* (Noida: HarperCollins, 2020), 1.
4. Dipesh Chakrabarty, *Provincializing Europe: Postcolonial Thought and Historical Difference* (Princeton: Princeton University Press, 2000), 111–12.
5. Arundhati Roy, 'The Pandemic Is a Portal,' *Financial Times*, 3 April 2020, https://www.ft.com/content/10d8f5e8-74eb-11ea-95fe-fcd274e920ca.

1. WHAT IS A PANDEMIC?

1. Christian W. McMillen, *Pandemics: A Very Short Introduction* (Oxford: Oxford University Press, 2016), 1.
2. Mark Honigsbaum, *The Pandemic Century: A History of Global Contagion from the Spanish Flu to Covid-19* (London: Penguin, 2020), xi.
3. Chloe Sellwood, 'Brief History and Epidemiological Features of Pandemic Influenza,' in *Introduction to Pandemic Influenza*, ed. Jonathan Van-Tam and Chloe Sellwood (Wallingford: CAB International, 2010), 41; David M. Morens, Gregory K. Folkers, and Anthony S. Fauci, 'What Is a Pandemic?' *Journal of Infectious Diseases*, 200: 7 (2009), 1018–21.
4. Mike Davis, *The Monster at Our Door: The Global Threat of Avian Flu* (New York: New Press, 2005).
5. Charles E. Rosenberg, 'What Is an Epidemic? AIDS in Historical Perspective,' in *Explaining Epidemics and Other Studies in the History of Medicine* (Cambridge: Cambridge University Press, 1992), 278.

pp. [15–25]

6. Ibid., 279.
7. Ibid., 279, n. 1.
8. Jeremy A. Greene and Dora Vargha, 'How Epidemics End,' *Boston Review*, 30 June 2020, https://bostonreview.net/science-nature/jeremy-greene-dora-vargha-how-epidemics-end.
9. Clare Anderson, David Arnold, Juanita de Barros, Luka Bair, and Robert Peckham, 'Epidemics in the Past and Now: A Roundtable on Colonial and Postcolonial History,' *Journal of Colonialism and Colonial History*, 22 (2021), doi: 10.1353/cch.2021.0003.
10. Mark Harrison, 'Pandemics,' in *The Routledge History of Disease*, ed. Mark Jackson (London: Routledge, 2016), 141.
11. Erica Charters and Richard A. McKay, 'The History of Science and Medicine in the Context of COVID-19,' *Centaurus*, 62: 2 (2020), 223.
12. David Arnold, 'Cholera and Colonialism in British India,' *Past and Present*, 113 (1986), 151.
13. Susan Sontag, 'AIDS and Its Metaphors,' *New York Review of Books*, 27 October 1988, https://www.nybooks.com/articles/1988/10/27/aids-and-its-metaphors/. For Europe's fear of 'exotic' diseases, see Alan Bewell, *Romanticism and Colonial Disease* (Baltimore: Johns Hopkins University Press, 1999), especially chapter 7.
14. As in Mircea Eliade, *Patterns in Comparative Religion* (London: Sheed and Ward, 1958), chapters 11 and 12.
15. Richard J. Evans, *In Defence of History* (London: Granta, 1997), 151.
16. Wendy Doniger, *The Hindus: An Alternative History* (New York: Penguin, 2009), 23. On Ranke, see Evans, *Defence*, 17.
17. Doniger, *Hindus*, 23–4.
18. 'WHO Director-General's Remarks at the Media Briefing on 2019-nCOV on 11 February 2020,' https://www.who.int/dg/speeches/detail/who-director-general-s-remarks-at-the-media-briefing-on-2019-ncov-on-11-february-2020.
19. 'WHO Director-General's Opening Remarks at the Media Briefing on COVID-19 – 11 March 2020,' https://www.who.int/director-general/speeches/detail/who-director-general-s-opening-remarks-at-the-media-briefing-on-covid-19--11-march-2020.
20. Thus, in R. N. O. Moynan and D. C. Meneses, 'The Influenza Pandemic,' *IMG*, 54: 1 (1919), 14–17, the authors used 'pandemic' only in the title of their article; in their text they referred to the 'two epidemics' of 1918.
21. Nükhet Varlik, 'The Plague That Never Left: Restoring the Second Pandemic to Ottoman and Turkish History in the Time of COVID-19,' *New Perspectives on Turkey*, no. 63 (2020), 176–89.
22. William H. McNeill, *Plagues and Peoples* (Harmondsworth: Penguin, 1979), 163–4.
23. Elsewhere, the McNeills describe the influenza of 1918–19 as 'the first truly global pandemic in history.' J. R. McNeill and William H. McNeill,

The Human Web: A Bird's-Eye View of World History (New York: W. W. Norton, 2003) 295.

24. Alfred W. Crosby, *America's Forgotten Pandemic: The Influenza of 1918* (2nd ed., Cambridge: Cambridge University Press, 1989).

25. James Cantlie, 'Plague and Its Spread,' *Journal of the Royal Society of Arts*, 59: 3042 (1911), 434–41. Cantlie co-founded the London School of Tropical Medicine with Patrick Manson and was a founding editor of the *Journal of Tropical Medicine and Hygiene* in 1898.

26. The colonial spelling of Indian place names is retained in this book when referring to the British period; the more recent names that have replaced them are used for India after 1947: see 'Note on Place Name Changes'.

27. Cantlie, 'Plague and Its Spread,' 438–40.

28. James Longrigg, 'Epidemic, Ideas and Classical Athenian Society,' in *Epidemics and Ideas: Essays on the Historical Perception of Pestilence*, ed. Terence Ranger and Paul Slack (Cambridge: Cambridge University Press, 1992), 21–44.

29. *Irish Times*, 21 April 1873, 2.

30. Michel Foucault, *The Order of Things: An Archaeology of the Human Sciences*, trans. Alan Sheridan (London: Tavistock Publications, 1970); Michel Foucault, *The Archaeology of Knowledge*, trans. Alan Sheridan (London: Tavistock Publications, 1972).

31. For the genealogy of a related concept, see Paul James and Manfred Steger, 'A Genealogy of "Globalization": The Career of a Concept,' *Globalizations*, 11: 4 (2014), 417–34.

32. J. F. C. Hecker, *The Epidemics of the Middle Ages*, trans. B. G. Babington (2nd ed., London: George Woodfall and Son, 1835), ix–xi, 4, 52.

33. August Hirsch, *Handbook of Geographical and Historical Pathology*, vol. I: *Acute Infective Diseases*, trans. Charles Creighton, London: New Sydenham Society, 1883), 394. In the 1859 edition Hirsch used the term pandemic seventeen times to cover malaria, yellow fever, dengue, and typhoid, as well as cholera and influenza: August Hirsch, *Handbuch der Historisch-Geographischen Pathologie*, 2 vols. (Erlangen: Verlag von Ferdinand Enke, 1859), vol. 1.

34. Hirsch, *Handbuch*, 1: 111–48.

35. J. D. Rolleston, 'The Smallpox Pandemic of 1870–1874,' *Proceedings of the Royal Society of Medicine*, 27: 2 (1933), 177–92. See the speech by the MP Lyon Playfair in the House of Commons on 19 June 1883, reported in *The Times*, 20 June 1883, 8. By the 1890s diphtheria, too, was being described as pandemic: Arthur Newsholme, *Epidemic Diphtheria: A Research on the Origin and Spread of the Disease from an International Standpoint* (London: Swan Sonnenschein, 1898).

36. Mark Harrison, *Medicine in an Age of Commerce and Empire: Britain and Its Tropical Colonies* (Oxford: Oxford University Press, 2010); Mark Harrison, *Contagion: How Commerce Has Spread Disease* (New Haven: Yale University Press, 2012).

37. Michael Worboys, 'The Emergence of Tropical Medicine: A Study in the Establishment of a Scientific Specialty,' in *Perspectives on the Emergence of Scientific Disciplines*, ed. Gerard Lemaine, Roy Macleod, Michael Mulkay, and Peter Weingart (The Hague: Mouton, 1976), 75–98; David Arnold, ed., *Warm Climates and Western Medicine: The Emergence of Tropical Medicine, 1500–1900* (Amsterdam: Rodopi, 1996).

38. Cantlie, 'Plague,' 438.

39. W. J. R. Simpson, 'Plague,' *The Lancet*, 29 June 1906, 1758.

40. W. J. R. Simpson, *A Treatise on Plague: Dealing with the Historical, Epidemiological, Clinical, Therapeutic and Preventive Aspects of the Disease* (Cambridge: Cambridge University Press, 1905); Merle Eisenberg and Lee Mordechai, 'The Justinianic Plague and Global Pandemics: The Making of the Plague Concept,' *American Historical Review*, 125: 5 (2020), 1632–67.

41. W. J. R. Simpson, 'Plague,' *The Lancet*, 13 July 1907, 73–4.

42. Similarly, Clifford Allchin Gill, 'The Epidemiology of Plague,' *The Lancet*, 25 January 1908, 213–16.

43. Erwin H. Ackerknecht, *History and Geography of the Most Important Diseases* (New York: Hafner Publishing, 1965), 9.

44. Emmanuel Le Roy Ladurie, 'A Concept: The Unification of the Globe by Disease,' in *The Mind and Method of the Historian*, trans. Sian Reynolds (Brighton: Harvester Press, 1981), 28–91; Valeska Huber, 'The Unification of the Globe by Disease? The International Sanitary Conferences on Cholera, 1851–1894,' *Historical Journal*, 49: 2 (2006), 453–76.

45. *Manchester Guardian*, 23 May 1919, 6.

46. *Manchester Guardian*, 19 February 1923, 6, emphasis added. On China, see Christopher Langford, 'Did the 1918–19 Influenza Pandemic Originate in China?,' *Population and Development Review*, 31: 3 (2005), 473–505.

47. *Manchester Guardian*, 19 February 1923, 6.

48. For a refutation of the Malthusian argument that epidemics in India were 'a necessary evil designed by Nature to eliminate the unfit' and a check on 'an inordinate increase of population,' see Clifford Allchin Gill, *The Genesis of Epidemics and the Natural History of Disease* (London: Ballière, Tindall, and Cox, 1928), ix.

49. *The Times*, 20 October 1919, 9; 28 November 1919, 13; 29 November 1919, 6.

2. THE TIME OF CHOLERA

1. Gabriel García Márquez, *Love in the Time of Cholera*, trans. Edith Grossman (London: Penguin, 1989), 105–16, 292.

2. E.g., Iona Heath, 'Love in the Time of Coronavirus,' *BMJ*, 6 May 2020, https://doi.org/10.1136/bmj.m1801.

3. Irwin W. Sherman, *The Power of Plagues* (Washington, D.C.: ASM Press, 2006), 167.

4. Kelley Lee and Richard Dodgson, 'Globalization and Cholera: Implications for Global Governance,' *Global Governance*, 6: 2 (2000), 219.

5. William Campbell Maclean, *Diseases of Tropical Climates* (London: Macmillan, 1886), 217–19; James Ranald Martin, *The Influence of Tropical Climates on European Constitutions* (London: Churchill, 1856), 293–6.

6. Mark Harrison, 'A Dreadful Scourge: Cholera in Early Nineteenth-Century India,' *Modern Asian Studies*, 54: 2 (2020), 502–53.

7. John Macpherson, *Annals of Cholera from the Earliest Periods to the Year 1817* (London: Ranken, 1872), 172–3.

8. John F. Richards, *The Unending Frontier: An Environmental History of the Early Modern World* (Berkeley: University of California Press, 2003), 33.

9. Rhoads Murphey, 'The City in the Swamp: Aspects of the Site and Early Growth of Calcutta,' *Geographical Journal*, 130: 2 (1964), 241–56; Debjani Bhattacharyya, *Empire and Ecology in the Bengal Delta: The Making of Calcutta* (Cambridge: Cambridge University Press, 2018).

10. Rita R. Cowell, 'Global Climate and Infectious Disease: The Cholera Paradigm,' *Science*, 274: 5295 (1996), 2025–31; Salvador Almagro-Moreno and Ronald K. Taylor, 'Cholera: Environmental Reservoirs and Impact on Disease Transmission,' *Microbiology Spectrum* (2013), https://doi.org/10.1128/microbiolspec.OH-0003-2012.

11. Shahid Jameel, 'On Ecology and Environment as Drivers of Human Disease and Pandemics,' *ORF Issue Brief*, no. 388 (July 2020).

12. Almagro-Moreno and Taylor, 'Cholera,' 8–9.

13. Leonard Rogers, *The Incidence and Spread of Cholera in India: Forecasting and Control of Epidemics* (Calcutta: Thacker, Spink, 1928), 5.

14. Collector, Masulipatnam, to Board of Revenue, 31 May 1819, Madras Board of Revenue, 7 June 1819, IOR; Magistrate, Jessore, to Secretary, Bengal, 25 August 1817, Bengal Judicial, 9 September 1817, F/4/610: 15058, IOR.

15. Robert Peckham, 'Symptoms of Empire: Cholera in Southeast Asia, 1820–1850,' in *The Routledge History of Disease*, ed. Mark Jackson (London: Routledge, 2016), 183–201.

16. Anon., 'The Asiatic Cholera,' *Fraser's Magazine*, December 1831, 614.

17. Frank G. Clemow, *The Geography of Disease* (Cambridge: Cambridge University Press, 1903), 88–106.

18. Sheldon Watts, *Epidemics and History: Disease, Power and Imperialism* (New Haven: Yale University Press, 1997), 167.

19. Richard J. Evans, *The Pursuit of Power: Europe, 1815–1914* (London: Penguin, 2017), 400.

20. Marcos Cueto, Theodore M. Brown, and Elizabeth Fee, *The World Health Organization: A History* (Cambridge: Cambridge University Press, 2019), 13.

21. W. W. Hunter, *Orissa*, 2 vols., (London: Smith, Elder, 1872), 1: 156, 166–7.

22. W. F. Bynum, 'Policing Hearts of Darkness: Aspects of the International Sanitary Conferences,' *History and Philosophy of the Life Sciences*, 15: 3 (1993), 427.

23. Norman Howard-Jones, *The Scientific Background of the International Sanitary Conferences, 1851–1938* (Geneva: WHO, 1975), 9; Valeska Huber, 'The Unification of the Globe by Disease? The International Sanitary Conferences on Cholera, 1851–1894,' *Historical Journal*, 49: 2 (2006), 453–76.

24. *Proceedings of the International Sanitary Conference Opened at Constantinople on the 13th February 1866* (Calcutta: Superintendent of Government Printing, 1868), 8.

25. *ToI*, 21 July 1892, 4.

26. Ibid.

27. August Hirsch, *Handbuch der Historisch-Geographiscen Pathologie*, 2 vols. (Erlangen: Verlag von Ferdinand Enke, 1859), 1: 111–48.

28. Editorial, 'Cholera: A Forecast and Forewarning,' *The Lancet*, 25 May 1867, 632.

29. William R. E. Smart, 'On Cholera in Insular Position,' *The Lancet*, 14 April 1873, 522–4.

30. Editorial, 'The Teachings of the Late Epidemic of Cholera,' *BMJ*, 9 May 1868, 456.

31. Arthur Ransome, 'On the Form of the Epidemic Wave, and Some of Its Probable Causes,' *Transactions of the Epidemiological Society of London*, 1: 1 (1883), 96–107.

32. *BMJ*, 7 February 1863, 149–51; 25 July 1863, 98–9; 27 May 1871, 567.

33. M. C. Furnell, *Cholera and Water in India* (London: J. and A. Churchill, 1887).

34. *ToI*, 21 August 1895, 4. For the controversy, see Ira Klein, 'Cholera Therapy and Treatment in Nineteenth Century India,' *Journal of Indian History*, 58 (1980), 35–51.

35. *BMJ*, 15 October 1892, 867.

36. *BMJ*, 10 December 1892, 1288.

37. Charles C. J. Carpenter, William B. Greenough, and Robert S. Gordon, 'Pathogenesis and Pathophysiology of Cholera,' in *Cholera*, ed. Dhiman Barua and William Burrows (Philadelphia: Saunders, 1974), 129–31.

38. Benjamin Kingsbury, *An Imperial Disaster: The Bengal Cyclone of 1876* (London: C. Hurst, 2018), 128–31.

39. I. H. Rosenberg, W. B. Greenough, J. Lindenbaum and R. S. Gordon, 'Nutritional Studies in Cholera: The Influence of Nutritional Status on Susceptibility to Infection,' in *Proceedings of the Cholera Research Symposium, January 24–29, 1965, Honolulu, Hawaii*, ed. O. A. Bushnell and S. Brookhyser (Washington, D.C.: US Government Printing Office, 1965), 68–72.

40. This is not to deny the complex causation behind famine mortality: see Elizabeth Whitcombe, 'Famine Mortality,' *Economic and Political Weekly*, 5 June 1993, 1169–79; Ira Klein, 'When the Rains Failed: Famine, Relief, and Mortality,' *Indian Economic and Social History Review*, 21: 2 (1984), 185–214.

41. David Arnold, *Colonizing the Body: State Medicine and Epidemic Disease in Nineteenth-Century India* (Berkeley: University of California Press, 1993), 161–8.

42. *ARSC Madras, 1877*, 85, lxiii; Alexander Porter, *The Diseases of the Madras Famine of 1877–78* (Madras: Government Press, 1889), 57.

43. *ARSC Madras, 1897*, 41; *ARSC Madras, 1898*, 37.

44. Christopher Hamlin, *Cholera: The Biography* (Oxford: Oxford University Press, 2009).

45. Kama Maclean, *Pilgrimage and Power: The Kumbh Mela in Allahabad, 1765–1954* (Oxford: Oxford University Press, 2008); Ritika Prasad, *Tracks of Change: Railways and Everyday Life in Colonial India* (Cambridge: Cambridge University Press, 2015), 171–9.

46. John Murray, 'Report on the Hurdwar Cholera of 1867,' in *Report Regarding the Control of Pilgrimages in the Madras Presidency* (Madras: Gantz, 1868), app. B, 25–32; 'History of the Cholera Epidemic of 1867 in Northern India,' Sanitary Commissioner, India, July 1868, IOR.

47. David B. Smith, *Report on Pilgrimage to Juggernauth in 1868* (Calcutta: Lewis, 1868).

48. *Report of the Cholera Committee* (Madras: Gantz, 1868), 2–3.

49. *ToI*, 27 November 1869, 3.

50. James Jameson, *Report on the Epidemick Cholera Morbus, as It Visited the Territories Subject to the Presidency of Bengal in the Years 1817, 1818 and 1819* (Calcutta: Government Gazette Press, 1820), 110–11.

51. William Scot, *Report on the Epidemic Cholera as It Has Appeared in the Territories Subject to the Presidency of Fort St George* (Madras: Asylum Press, 1824), 13.

52. Ian J. Kerr, *Building the Railways of the Raj, 1850–1900* (Delhi: Oxford University Press, 1995), 97–8.

53. Ibid., 163.

54. Christian Wolmar, *Railways and the Raj: How the Age of Steam Transformed India* (London: Atlantic Books, 2017), 44.

55. Jayeeta Sharma, *Empire's Garden: Assam and the Making of India* (Durham, N.C.: Duke University Press, 2011), 81; *ARSC Assam, 1899*, 25.

56. Satya Swaroop, 'Endemiology of Cholera in the Madras Presidency,' *IJMR*, 39: 2 (1951), 185–96.

57. Jameson, *Report on the Epidemic*, 12–17.

58. *Rules Regarding the Measures to Be Adopted on the Outbreak of Cholera or the Appearance of Small-Pox* (Calcutta: Office of Superintendent of Government Printing, 1870), 9.

59. *Report of the Commissioners Appointed to Inquire into the Cholera Epidemic of 1861 in Northern India* (Calcutta: Cutter, 1864), 6.

60. 'Cholera in the Punjaub,' *ToI*, 6 September 1861, 4.

61. *ToI*, 12 August 1861, 3.

62. John Murray, *Report on the Attack of Cholera in the Central Prison at Agra in 1856* (Agra: Secundra Orphan Press, 1856); Arnold, *Colonizing*, 102–13.

63. Joseph Ewart, *A Digest of the Vital Statistics of the European and Native Armies in India* (London: Smith, Elder, 1859), 2, 147–63.

64. [Julia Maitland], *Letters from Madras, during the Years 1836–1839, by a Lady* (London: John Murray, 1846), 43.

65. *ToI*, 10 September 1892, 4.

66. C. P. Lukis and R. J. Blackham, *Tropical Hygiene for Anglo-Indians and Indians* (Calcutta: Thacker, Spink, 1911), 3.

67. Judith N. Shklar, *The Faces of Injustice* (New Haven: Yale University Press, 1990), 1.

68. Ibid., 67, 70.

69. Ralph W. Nicholas, 'The Goddess Sitala and Epidemic Smallpox in Bengal,' *Journal of Asian Studies*, 41: 1 (1981): 21–44; Arnold, *Colonizing*, 121–5.

70. Sunder Lal Hora, 'Worship of the Deities Ola, Jhola and Bon Bibi in Lower Bengal,' *Journal of the Asiatic Society of Bengal*, 29: 1 (1933), 1–4.

71. Nandini C. Sen, 'Corona Mata and the Pandemic Goddesses,' *The Wire*, 25 September 2020, https://thewire.in/culture/corona-mata-and-the-pandemic-goddesses; Sumathi Ramaswamy and Ravinder Kaur, 'The Goddess and the Virus,' in *The Pandemic: Perspectives on Asia,* ed. Vinayak Chaturvedi (Ann Arbor: Association for Asian Studies, 2020), 75–94.

72. William Crooke, *Religion and Folklore of Northern India* (3rd ed., London: Oxford University Press, 1926), 114; cf. R. E. Enthoven, *The Folklore of Bombay* (Oxford: Clarendon Press, 1924), chapter 9.

73. T. S. Weir in P. C. H. Snow, *Report on the Outbreak of Bubonic Plague in Bombay, 1896–97* (Bombay: Times of India, 1897), 71.

74. R. H. Kennedy, *Notes on the Epidemic Cholera* (Calcutta: Baptist Mission Press, 1827), ix–xiii.

75. Dorothy Nelkin and Sander L. Gilman, 'Placing Blame for Devastating Disease,' *Social Research*, 55: 2 (1988), 362.

76. Kennedy, *Notes*, viii.

77. *ToI*, 25 July 1865, 2.

78. Nelkin and Gilman, 'Blame,' 362–3.

79. James Annesley, *Sketches of the Most Prevalent Diseases of India* (London: Underwood, 1829), 15–112; William Twining, *Clinical Illustrations of the Most Important Diseases of Bengal* (Calcutta: Baptist Mission Press, 1832), chapter 4.

80. Mark Harrison, 'A Question of Locality: The Identity of Cholera in British India, 1860–1890,' in *Warm Climates and Western Medicine: The Emergence of Tropical Medicine, 1500–1900*, ed. David Arnold (Amsterdam: Rodopi, 1996), 133–59.

81. A. T. Christie, *Observations on the Nature and Treatment of Cholera* (Edinburgh: Maclachlan and Stewart, 1828), 97; Mark Harrison, *Climates and Constitutions: Health, Race, Environment and British Imperialism in India, 1600–1850* (New Delhi: Oxford University Press, 1999), 177–91.

82. H. Young to Magistrate, Calcutta, 31 August 1818, F/4/617: 15372, IOR.

83. James L. Bryden, *Epidemic Cholera in the Bengal Presidency* (Calcutta: Superintendent of Government Printing, 1869), 91–2, emphasis added.

84. H. W. Bellew, *The History of Cholera in India from 1862 to 1881* (London: Trübner, 1885), v, 5–7.

85. *ARDPH Madras, 1921*, 13.

86. Rogers, *Incidence*, 4, 8.

87. Michael Zeheter, *Epidemics, Empire and Environments: Cholera in Madras and Quebec City, 1818–1910* (Pittsburgh: University of Pittsburgh Press, 2015), 9.

88. J. L. Ranking, *List of Fairs and Festivals Occurring within the Limits of the Madras Presidency* (Madras: Government Press, 1868), 2.

89. *Report of the Pilgrim Committee: Bihar and Orissa, 1913* (Simla: Government Central Branch Press 1915), 57–9.

90. *ToI*, 21 July 1892, 4; 1 August 1892, 4.

91. Sandhya Polu, *Infectious Disease in India, 1892–1940: Policy-Making and the Perception of Risk* (Basingstoke: Palgrave Macmillan, 2010), 27–38.

92. Biswamoy Pati, 'Ordering "Disorder" in a Holy City: Colonial Health Interventions in Puri during the Nineteenth Century,' in *Health, Medicine and Empire: Perspectives on Colonial India*, ed. Biswamoy Pati and Mark Harrison (New Delhi: Orient Longman, 2001), 270–98.

93. India Home (Public), nos. 24 to 29, December 1892, NAI. On the Hardwar episode, see Katherine Prior, 'The British Administration of Hinduism in North India, 1780–1900,' unpublished PhD, University of Cambridge, 1990, 203–12.

94. India Home (Judicial), no. 94, January 1893, NAI; Home (Sanitary), nos. 316–20, July 1905, NAI; Home (Sanitary), no. 314, January 1906, NAI.

95. Bombay, General, vol. 34, no. 416, 1900, Maharashtra State Archives, Mumbai; India Home (Medical), no. 10, April 1900, NAI; Home (Sanitary), nos. 78–83, August 1909, NAI.

96. *ARSC Assam, 1895*, app. C.

97. *ARDPH United Provinces, 1928*, 8; *ARDPH United Provinces, 1929*, 11; *ARDPH United Provinces, 1935*, 12, 26.

98. A. C. Banerjea, 'Note on Cholera in the United Provinces,' *IJMR*, 39: 1 (1951), 17–40.

99. Leonard Rogers, 'Thirty Years' Research on the Control of Cholera Epidemics,' *BMJ*, 23 November 1957, 1193–7.

100. S. Kanungo et al., 'Cholera in India: An Analysis of Reports, 1997–2006,' *Bulletin of the World Health Organization*, 88: 3 (2010), 185–91.

101. Jeremy A. Greene and Dora Vargha, 'How Epidemics End,' *Boston Review*, 30 June 2020, https://bostonreview.net/science-nature/jeremy-greene-dora-vargha-how-epidemics-end.

102. Chinmay Tumbe, *Pandemics and Historical Mortality in India* (Ahmedabad: Indian Institute of Management, 2020), 64.

103. W. M. Haffkine, *Anti-cholera Inoculation* (Calcutta: Thacker, Spink, 1895), 46.

3. A MODERN PLAGUE

1. Marc Bloch, *The Royal Touch: Sacred Monarchy and Scrofula in England and France*, trans. J. E. Anderson [originally published as *Les rois thaumaturges*] (London: Routledge and Kegan Paul, 1973).

2. Jane Munro, 'The Pesthouse at Jaffa,' in *The Orientalists, Delacroix to Matisse: European Painters in North Africa and the Near East*, ed. Mary Anne Stevens (London: Royal Academy of the Arts, 1984), 65; L. Fabian Hirst, *The Conquest of Plague: A Study of the Evolution of Epidemiology* (Oxford: Clarendon Press, 1953), 77.

3. Nükhet Varlik, 'Rethinking the History of Plague in the Time of COVID-19,' *Centaurus*, 62: 2 (2020), 285–93.

4. Jacqueline Rose, 'Pointing the Finger: *The Plague*,' *London Review of Books*, 7 May 2020, https://www.lrb.co.uk/the-paper/v42/n09/jacqueline-rose/pointing-the-finger.

5. James M'Gregor, *Medical Sketches of the Expedition to Egypt from India* (London: J. Murray, 1804), 100–46.

6. Patrick Russell, *A Treatise of the Plague: Containing an Historical Journal, and Medical Account, of the Plague, at Aleppo, in the Years 1760, 1761, and 1762* (London: Robinson, 1791).

7. Aparna Nair, "An Egyptian Infection': War, Plague and the Quarantines of the English East India Company at Madras and Bombay, 1802,' *Hygiea Internationalis*, 8: 1 (2009), 7–29.

8. George D. Sussman, 'Was the Black Death in India and China?,' *Bulletin of the History of Medicine*, 85: 3 (2011), 319–55; Enayattulah Khan, 'Visitations of Plague in Mughal India,' *Proceedings of the Indian History Congress*, 74 (2013), 305–12.

9. I. J. Catanach, 'The "Globalization" of Disease? India and the Plague,' *Journal of World History*, 12: 1 (2001), 140–1.

10. C. Renny, *Medical Report on the Mahamuree in Gurhwal in 1849–50* (Agra: Secundra Orphan Press, 1851).

11. J. F. C. Hecker, *The Epidemics of the Middle Ages*, trans. B. G. Babington (2nd ed., London: George Woodfall and Son, 1835); August Hirsch, *Handbook of Geographical and Historical Pathology*, vol. I: *Acute Infective Diseases*, trans. Charles Creighton (London: New Sydenham Society, 1883), 495–7, 541–2.

12. R. P. Karkaria, '1837 and 1897: Two Years of Calamities,' *Calcutta Review*, 106 (1898), 4–9.

13. Clifford Allchin Gill, 'The Epidemiology of Plague,' *The Lancet*, 25 January 1908, 213.

14. James Cantlie, 'Plague and Its Spread,' *Journal of the Royal Society of Arts*, 59: 3042 (1911), 438; W. J. R. Simpson, 'Plague,' *The Lancet*, 29 June 1906, 1758.

15. Alfred Russel Wallace, *The Wonderful Century: The Age of New Ideas in Science and Innovation* (2nd ed., London: Swan Sonnenschein, 1903), 468–9.

16. Victor Heiser, *An American Doctor's Odyssey: Adventures in Forty-Five Countries* (New York: W. W. Norton, 1936), chapter 7.

17. Hirst, *Conquest*, 300.

18. Myron Echenberg, *Plague Ports: The Global Urban Impact of Bubonic Plague, 1894–1901* (New York: New York University Press, 2007).

19. *ToI*, 9 May 1900, 8.

20. W. Glen Liston, *The Cause and Prevention of the Spread of Plague in India* (Bombay: Times Press, 1908).

21. Merle Eisenberg and Lee Mordechai, 'The Justinianic Plague and Global Pandemics: The Making of the Plague Concept,' *American Historical Review*, 125: 5 (2021), 1632–67.

22. *ToI*, 24 February 1909, 15.

23. *ARMCB, 1901–2*, 151.

24. Echenberg, *Plague*, chapter 1.

25. Ibid., 47–8.

26. *ARMCB, 1896–7*, 593–779; M. E. Couchman, *Account of the Plague Administration in the Bombay Presidency, from September 1896 till May 1897* (Bombay: Government Central Press, 1897), 2.

27. Ibid., 5.

28. David Arnold, *Colonizing the Body: State Medicine and Epidemic Disease in Nineteenth-Century India* (Berkeley: University of California Press, 1993), 201–2.

29. P. C. H. Snow, *Report on the Outbreak of Bubonic Plague in Bombay, 1896–97* (Bombay: Times of India, 1897), 6–7.

30. J. M. Campbell, *Report of the Bombay Plague Committee on the Plague in Bombay, 1st July 1897 to the 30th April 1898* (Bombay: Times of India, 1898), 34.

31. Rajnarayan Chandavarkar, 'Plague Panic and Epidemic Politics in India, 1896–1914,' in *Epidemics and Ideas: Essays on the Historical Perception of Pestilence*, ed. Terence Ranger and Paul Slack (Cambridge: Cambridge University Press, 1992), 203–40; David Arnold, 'Touching the Body: Perspectives on the Indian Plague, 1896–1900,' *Subaltern Studies V*, ed. Ranajit Guha (New Delhi: Oxford University Press, 1987), 55–90; Samuel K. Cohn, *Epidemics: Hate and Compassion from the Plague of Athens to AIDS* (Oxford: Oxford University Press, 2018), chapter 14.

32. Sandhya L. Polu, *Infectious Disease in India, 1892–1940: Policy-Making and the Perception of Risk* (Basingstoke: Palgrave Macmillan, 2012), chapters 1 and 2.

33. India Legislative, nos. 37–46, app. 21, February 1897, NAI.

34. India already had a Contagious Diseases Act, dating back to the 1860s, but this was solely concerned with sexually transmitted diseases and the regulation of prostitution.

35. Ibid.

36. Ira Klein, 'Plague, Policy and Popular Unrest in British India,' *Modern Asian Studies*, 22: 4 (1988), 729; J. K. Condon, *The Bombay Plague: Being a History of*

the *Progress of Plague in the Bombay Presidency from September 1896 to June 1899* (Bombay: Education Society, 1900), 132.

37. Mike Davis, *Late Victorian Holocausts: El Niño Famines and the Making of the Third World* (London: Verso, 2001), 141–75.

38. Campbell, *Report*, 32.

39. R. A. Gopalaswami, *Census of India, 1951, 1: 1A, Report* (Delhi: Government of India, Manager of Publications, 1957), 127–8.

40. Campbell, *Report*, 52.

41. P. C. Tallents, *Census of India, 1921, VII: 1, Bihar and Orissa, Report* (Patna: Superintendent of Government Printing, Bihar and Orissa, 1923), 168. Also E. A. H. Blunt, *Census of India, 1911, XV: 1, United Provinces, Report* (Allahabad: Government Press, United Provinces, 1912), 43.

42. *ARSC India, 1899*, 149–50.

43. Couchman, *Account*, 10, 21, 44.

44. Snow, *Report*, 20.

45. *ToI*, 18 January 1899, 5.

46. *ARSC North-Western Provinces, 1899*, app. C, 6A–8A.

47. C. H. James, *Report on the Outbreak of Plague in the Jullundur and Hoshiapur Districts of the Punjab during the Year, 1898–99* (Lahore: Punjab Government Press, 1902), 9.

48. Aidan Forth, *Barbed Wire Imperialism: Britain's Empire of Camps, 1873–1903* (Oakland: University of California Press, 2017), chapters 3 and 4.

49. James, *Report*, 205–9.

50. Nick Lombardo, 'Controlling Mobility and Regulation in Urban Space: Muslim Pilgrims to Mecca in Colonial Bombay, 1880–1914,' *International Journal of Urban and Regional Research*, 40: 5 (2016), 983–99.

51. *ARSC India, 1899*, 151.

52. Plague Commission Report, 'Measures for the Suppression of Plague,' India Home (Sanitary), no. 250, July 1900, NAI.

53. Ibid.; *ARSC Bengal, 1897*, 8; Ritika Prasad, *Tracks of Change: Railways and Everyday Life in Colonial India* (Cambridge: Cambridge University Press, 2015), 179–90.

54. Secretary, Bengal, to India Home, 1 November 1897, India Home (Sanitary), no. 197, December 1897, NAI.

55. Harald Fischer-Tiné, *Shyamji Krishnavarma: Sanskrit, Sociology and Anti-imperialism* (London: Routledge, 2014), 31–2, quoting from *Indian Sociologist*, 9 (1913), 13–14.

56. Government of Punjab, 11 January 1898, India Home (Sanitary), no. 293, February 1898, NAI.

57. Bengal Municipal and Medical, 8 February 1898, India Home (Sanitary), no. 482, March 1898, NAI.

58. W. C. Rand, *Supplement to the Account of Plague Administration in the Bombay Presidency from September 1896 till May 1897* (Bombay: Government Central Press, 1897).

59. Ibid., 34.

60. Ibid., 7.

61. I. J. Catanach, 'Poona Politicians and the Plague,' *South Asia*, 7: 2 (1984), 1–18.

62. India Home (Public), June 1900, nos. 291–302, NAI.

63. Campbell, *Report*, 113; Mridula Ramanna, *Health Care in Bombay Presidency, 1896–1930* (Delhi: Primus, 2012), chapter 1.

64. Campbell, *Report*, 137–55.

65. Rand, *Supplement*, 22.

66. W. B. Bannerman, *The Plague Prophylactic: What It Is, How It Is Prepared, and What Its Uses Are* (Bombay: Government Central Press, 1905), 24.

67. As in Punjab: John C. Hume, 'Rival Traditions: Western Medicine and Yunan-i Tibb in the Punjab, 1849–1889,' *Bulletin of the History of Medicine*, 51: 2 (1977), 214–31.

68. On the treatment of plague by Unani physicians, see Guy N. A. Attewell, *Refiguring Unani Tibb: Plural Healing in Late Colonial India* (Hyderabad: Orient Longman, 2007), chapter 2.

69. *Punjab Plague Manual* (Lahore: Punjab Government Press, 1909), 10.

70. I. J. Catanach, 'Plague and the Tensions of Empire, 1896–1918,' in *Imperial Medicine and Indigenous Societies*, ed. David Arnold (Manchester: Manchester University Press, 1988), 161–2.

71. Nicholas H. A. Evans, 'Blaming the Rat? Accounting for Plague in Colonial Indian Medicine,' *Medicine, Anthropology, Theory*, 5: 3 (2018), 20.

72. *Punjab Manual*, 1.

73. Charles E. Rosenberg, 'Framing Disease: Illness, Society, and History,' in *Explaining Epidemics and Other Studies in the History of Medicine* (Cambridge: Cambridge University Press, 1992), 318.

74. Rose, 'Pointing.'

75. W. J. R. Simpson, 'Plague,' *The Lancet*, 13 July 1907, 74–6; James, *Report*.

76. E.g., Alok Sheel, 'Bubonic Plague in South Bihar: Gaya and Shahabad Districts, 1900–1924,' *Indian Economic and Social History Review*, 35: 4 (1998), 421–2.

77. Arthur Crawford, *Our Troubles in Poona and the Deccan* (Westminster: Constable, 1897), 78.

78. S. N. Paul, *Public Opinion and British Rule: A Study of the Influence of Indian Public Opinion on British Administration and Bureaucracy (1899–1914)* (New Delhi: Metropolitan Book Co., 1979), chapter 5.

79. *Mahratta*, 5 September 1897, quoted in Echenberg, *Plague*, 56.

80. On women's changing role in public life, see Geraldine Forbes, *Women in India* (Cambridge: Cambridge University Press, 1996), chapter 3.

81. Sister Nivedita, 'The Plague,' in *The Complete Works of Sister Nivedita*, 2 vols. (Calcutta, 1967), 2: 340–7.

82. Lakshmibai Tilak, *Smritichitre: The Memoirs of a Spirited Wife*, trans. Shanta Gokhale (New Delhi: Speaking Tiger, 2017), 172, 184.

83. Ibid., 189–93.

84. Ibid., 207, 259–64.

85. Ibid., 264–5.

86. David Arnold, 'Picturing Plague: Photography, Pestilence and Cremation in Late Nineteenth- and Early Twentieth-Century India,' in *Plague Image and Imagination from Medieval to Modern Times*, ed. Christos Lynteris (London: Palgrave Macmillan, 2021), 111–39.

87. R. W. Hornabrook, *Report on the Dharwar Plague Hospital, August 28th – December 18th 1898* (Dharwar: Dharwar Plague Hospital, 1899).

88. Haffkine, 'Report on Bacteriology of Plague,' 1 October 1897, in Snow, *Report*, 40; W. B. Bannerman, *Statistics of Inoculations with Haffkine's Anti-plague Vaccine, 1897–1900* (Bombay: Government Central Press, 1900).

89. Harvey, 'Note on Anti-plague Inoculations,' 19 April 1898, India Home (Sanitary), no. 76, May 1898, NAI.

90. Harvey, 5 July 1898, India Home (Sanitary), nos. 766–71, August 1898, NAI.

91. J. Neild Cook, *Report of the Epidemics of Plague in Calcutta during the Years 1898–99, 1899–1900 and up to 30th June 1900-01* (Calcutta: Municipal Press, 1900), 14, 23–5.

92. E. Wilkinson, *Report on Plague in the Punjab from October 1st, 1901, to September 30th, 1902* (Lahore: Punjab Government Gazette, 1904), 28.

93. E. Wilkinson, *Report on Plague and Inoculation in the Punjab from October 1st, 1902, to September 30th, 1903* (Lahore: Government Press, 1904), 7–13.

94. India Home (Medical), nos. 43–80, January 1904, NAI; Home (Sanitary), nos. 51–64, January 1905, NAI; Home (Sanitary), nos. 151–62, December 1906, NAI.

95. Joel Gunter and Vikas Pandey, 'Waldemar Haffkine: The Vaccine Pioneer the World Forgot,' BBC News, 11 December 2020, https://www.bbc.co.uk/world-asia-india-55050012.

96. Pratik Chakrabarti, *Bacteriology in British India: Laboratory Medicine and the Tropics* (Rochester, NY: Rochester University Press, 2012), 58.

97. Bannerman, *Plague*; *ToI*, 28 January 1905, 7.

98. *Punjab Manual*, 44–8.

99. Bannerman to Secretary, General, 14 August 1905, India Home (Sanitary), no. 329, February 1906, NAI.

100. Hirst, *Conquest*, 259.

101. Wilkinson, *Plague, 1902–03*, 37; I. J. Catanach, '"Fatalism"? Indian Responses to Plague and Other Crises,' *Asian Profile*, 12: 2 (1984), 183–92.

102. For a critical view of the Plague Commission's findings, see Catanach, 'Plague,' 158–9.

103. R. Nathan, *The Plague in Northern India, 1896, 1897*, 2 vols. (Simla: Government Central Printing Office, 1898), 1: 48; *The Etiology and Epidemiology of Plague: A Summary of the Work of the Plague Commission* (Calcutta: Superintendent of Government Printing, 1908), 61.

104. Chakrabarti, *Bacteriology*, chapter 2.

105. Adam Kucharski, *The Rules of Contagion: Why Things Spread—and Why They Stop* (London: Profile Books, 2020), 3.

106. S. C. Seal, 'Epidemiological Studies of Plague in India,' *Bulletin of the World Health Organization*, 23: 2–3 (1969), 283–92.

107. Vempalli Raj Mahammadh, 'Plague Mortality and Control Policies in Colonial South India, 1900–47,' *South Asia Research*, 40: 3 (2020), 323–43.

108. H. H. King and C. G. Pandit, 'A Summary of the Rat-Flea Survey of the Madras Presidency,' *IJMR*, 19: 2 (1931), 357–92; Plague Advisory Committee, 'On the Seasonal Prevalence of Plague in India,' *Journal of Hygiene*, 8: 2 (1908), 266–301.

4. WAR FEVER

1. Christopher McKnight Nichols, Nancy Bristow, E. Thomas Ewing, Joseph M. Gabriel, Benjamin C. Montoya, and Elizabeth Outka, 'Reconsidering the 1918–19 Influenza Pandemic in the Age of Covid-19,' *Journal of the Gilded Age and Progressive Era*, 19: 4 (2020), 642.

2. The description of the Spanish Flu as 'forgotten' originated with Alfred W. Crosby, *America's Forgotten Pandemic: The Influenza of 1918* (2nd ed., Cambridge: Cambridge University, 1989). It has been repeated many times since. See, too, Nancy K. Bristow, *American Pandemic: The Lost Worlds of the 1918 Influenza Epidemic* (Oxford: Oxford University Press, 2012).

3. August Hirsch, *Handbook of Geographical and Historical Pathology*, vol. I: *Acute Infective Diseases*, trans. Charles Creighton (London: New Sydenham Society, 1883), 18.

4. Frank G. Clemow, *The Geography of Disease* (Cambridge: Cambridge University Press, 1903), 191–2.

5. Editorial, 'Influenza,' *IMG*, 25: 4 (1890), 112–13; W. Glen Liston, 'Influenza Epidemics: History and Experience,' *ToI*, 11 October 1918, 8.

6. F. Norman White to Secretary, India, 15 October 1918, India Education (Sanitary), no. 7, October 1918, IOR; *ToI*, 1 July 1918, 6.

7. Niall Johnson and Juergen Mueller, 'Updating the Accounts: Global Mortality of the 1918–20 "Spanish" Influenza Pandemic,' *Bulletin of the History of Medicine*, 76: 1 (2002), 105–15; Prema-Chandra Athukorala and Chaturica Athukorala, 'The Great Influenza Pandemic of 1918–20: An Interpretive Survey at the Time of Covid-19,' discussion paper, Centre for Economic History, Australian National University, Canberra, 2020, 9.

8. Cited in Liston, 'Influenza,' 8.

9. F. Norman White, *A Preliminary Report on the Influenza Pandemic of 1918 in India* (Simla: Government Monotype Press, 1919), 7; Malcolm Hailey to Lord Chelmsford, 19 October 1918, cited in John W. Cell, *Hailey: A Study in British Imperialism, 1872–1969* (Cambridge: Cambridge University Press, 1992), 57.

10. Koilas Chandra Bose, 'Epidemic Influenza in and around the City of Calcutta,' *IMG*, 55: 5 (1920), 169.
11. Edwin O. Jordan, *Epidemic Influenza: A Survey* (Chicago: American Medical Association, 1927), 100.
12. *ToI*, 3 July 1918, 6; 24 July 1918, 6.
13. *ARSC India, 1918*, 56–67.
14. Jordan, *Influenza*, 100; S. P. James in Ministry of Health, *Report on the Pandemic of Influenza, 1918–19* (London: HMSO, 1920), 383–4.
15. *ARSC Bombay, 1918*, 23.
16. N. H. Choksy, 'Influenza,' in *ARMCB, 1918–19*, 79.
17. For the global impact of influenza, see Crosby, *Pandemic*; Niall Johnson, *Britain and the 1918–19 Influenza Pandemic: A Dark Epilogue* (Abingdon: Routledge, 2006); *The Spanish Influenza Pandemic of 1918–19: New Perspectives*, ed. Howard Phillips and David Killingray (London: Routledge, 2003); Laura Spinney, *Pale Rider: The Spanish Flu of 1918 and How It Changed the World* (London: Jonathan Cape, 2017).
18. *ARSC India, 1918*, 58–63; *ARSC Madras, 1918*, 8.
19. *ARMAC, 1918–19*, 21, 60, 63.
20. Ibid., 81.
21. *ARSC Central Provinces and Berar, 1918*, 8.
22. Ibid.
23. *ARSC Punjab, 1918*, app. D, xi.
24. Collector, Satara, to Secretary, Bombay, 2 November 1918, Bombay Revenue (Famine), no. 100, 20 January 1919, IOR.
25. *ARSC United Provinces, 1918*, app. D, 11A.
26. *ARSC India, 1918*, app. C, 61.
27. White, *Report*, 1.
28. For Calcutta, see *ARSC Bengal, 1918*, 23.
29. *Young India*, 2 October 1918, *RNP*; White, *Report*, 78; *ARSC India, 1918*, 59.
30. *Praja Mitra*, 10 October 1918, *RNP*; *Sunday Chronicle*, 16 October 1918, *RNP*.
31. Jim Corbett, *The Man-Eaters of Kumaon* (London: Oxford University Press, 1952), xvi.
32. M. S. Leigh, *The Punjab and the War* (Lahore: Superintendent, Government Printing, Punjab, 1922), 25; *Paigham-i-Sulah*, 25 July 1918, *RNP*.
33. *Kesari*, 12 November 1918, *RNP*.
34. Crosby, *Pandemic*, 124, 216.
35. White, *Report*, 1–2.
36. E. H. H. Edye, *Census of India, 1921, XVI: 1, United Provinces, Report* (Allahabad: Government Press, United Provinces, 1923), 13.
37. L. Middleton and S. M. Jacob, *Census of India, 1921, XV: 1, Punjab, Report* (Lahore: Civil and Military Gazette, 1923), 61.
38. Edye, *United Provinces*, 35.
39. *ARSC Madras, 1918*, 8.
40. *ARMAC, 1921–2*, 63–4.

41. *ARMCB, 1921–2*, 21; *ARMCB 1924–5*, 1.

42. Kingsley Davis, *The Population of India and Pakistan* (Princeton: Princeton University Press, 1951), app. B, proposed a figure of around 20 million. I. D. Mills, 'The 1918–1919 Influenza Pandemic: The Indian Experience,' *Indian Economic and Social History Review*, 23: 1 (1986), 1–40, calculated about 18 million; K. David Patterson and Gerald F. Pyle, 'The Geography and Mortality of the 1918 Influenza Pandemic,' *Bulletin of the History of Medicine*, 65: 1 (1991), 18, 12.5 to 20 million; Kenneth Hill, 'Influenza in India in 1918: Excess Mortality Reassessed,' *Genus*, 67: 2 (2011), 9–29, revised this downward to between 10.9 and 13.5 million. More recently, Chinmay Tumbe, *The Age of Pandemics, 1817–1920: How They Shaped India and the World* (Noida: HarperCollins, 2020), 140–1, suggested 'close to or upwards of 20 million.'

43. *ABP*, 13 February 1919, 3.

44. Edye, *United Provinces*, 13.

45. Crosby, *Pandemic*, 97; John M. Barry, *The Great Influenza: The Story of the Greatest Pandemic in History* (London: Penguin, 2004), 223.

46. Ira Klein, 'Death in India, 1871–1921,' *Journal of Asian Studies*, 32: 4 (1973), 639.

47. Ibid., 641–3.

48. *ARMAC, 1917–18*, 14, 54–7.

49. *ARMAC, 1918–19*, 21.

50. *ARMCB, 1923–24*, 5.

51. *ToI*, 19 July 1918, 7; White, 'Retrospect,' 442.

52. On the importance of 'war conditions' for the incubation and spread of the influenza globally, see Athukorala and Athukorala, 'Influenza,' 7–8.

53. India was not alone in this. In Mexico, too, the pandemic encountered a 'war-weary and hungry population.' Benjamin C. Montoya in Nichols et al., 'Reconsidering,' 648.

54. DeWitt C. Ellinwood, 'The Indian Soldier, the Indian Army, and Change, 1914–1918,' in *India and World War I*, ed. DeWitt C. Ellinwood and S. D. Pradhan (New Delhi: Manohar, 1978), 183–4.

55. *Tribune*, 13 February 1919, *RNP*.

56. White, 'Retrospect,' 441.

57. Barry, *Influenza*; Crosby, *Pandemic*.

58. *ToI*, 12 July 1918, 9; 16 July 1918, 8.

59. *ToI*, 26 July 1918, 9; 29 July 1918, 8; *ARSC United Provinces, 1918*, app. D, 8A; Ruby Bala, 'The Spread of Influenza Epidemic in the Punjab (1918–1919),' *Proceedings of the Indian History Congress*, 72 (2011), 989.

60. L. Middleton and S. M. Jacob, *Census of India, 1921, XV: 1, Punjab, Report* (Lahore: Civil and Military Gazette, 1923), 51; Leigh, *Punjab*, 14.

61. White, *Report*, 6; E. S. Phipson, 'The Pandemic of Influenza in India in the Year 1918,' *IMG*, 58: 11 (1923), 516. Of the 54,675 Indian soldiers hospitalized in India with influenza in 1918–19, roughly one in ten (5,805) died: *ARSC India, 1919*, 30–1.

62. *ASRC India, 1918*, 30, and accompanying graphs.

63. White, *Report*, 5.

64. Jordan, *Influenza*, 207.

65. Middleton and Jacob, *Punjab,* 51.

66. Leigh, *Punjab*, 1–12.

67. George Lloyd to Edwin Montagu, 10 January 1919, cited in Rajnarayan Chandavarkar, *The Origins of Industrial Capitalism in India: Business Strategies and the Working Classes in Bombay, 1900–1940* (Cambridge: Cambridge University Press, 1994), 115. Similar complaints about acute fodder shortages came from other provinces, including Punjab and the United Provinces: India Revenue and Agriculture (Famine), no. 52, December 1918, IOR.

68. Phipson, 'Pandemic,' 515; *ARSC Punjab, 1918*, app. D, xvi.

69. 'Statistical Abstract for India, 1917–18 to 1926–27,' *Parliamentary Papers*, Cmd 3291, table 296, 628.

70. David Arnold, 'Looting, Grain Riots and Government Policy in South India, 1918,' *Past and Present*, 84 (1979), 111–45.

71. E.g., Leela Visaria and Pravin Visaria, 'Population (1757–1947),' in *The Cambridge Economic History of India*, vol. 2, ed. Dharma Kumar (Cambridge: Cambridge University Press, 1983), 528–31.

72. Mills, 'Influenza,' 35.

73. Tumbe, *Pandemics*, 166.

74. Athukorala and Athukorala, 'Influenza,' 18.

75. *ToI*, 16 July 1918, 7; 30 September 1918, 6.

76. *ARSC Punjab, 1918*, app. D, xvi.

77. On the difficulty of distinguishing influenza from malaria deaths, see R. C. MacWatt, *Report on Malaria in the Punjab during the Year 1918* (Lahore: Superintendent of Government Printing, Punjab, 1919), 1–2.

78. Lord Chelmsford to Secretary of State for India, 30 April 1919, India Revenue and Agriculture (Famine), no. 3, April 1919, IOR.

79. India Revenue and Agriculture (Famine), no. 51, November 1918, IOR.

80. White, *Report*, 1, 7, 11.

81. Willingdon to Viceroy, 10 October 1918, Willingdon Papers, MSS Eur. F. 93/1, IOR.

82. Cited in Cell, *Hailey*, 58.

83. *ARSC United Provinces, 1918*, app. D, 15A.

84. *ARSC Bengal, 1918*, 9.

85. Tallents, *Bihar and Orissa*, 14.

86. Middleton and Jacob, *Punjab*, 41; *Season and Crop Report of the Madras Presidency for the Agricultural Year, 1918–19*, 1.

87. *ARSC Central Provinces, 1918*, app. C, 1.

88. Nancy Bristow, in Nichols et al., 'Reconsidering,' 655.

89. As among the Mangs of Maharashtra: Bombay Revenue (Famine), no. 16, 4 January 1919, IOR. See also G. T. Boag, *Census of India, 1921, XIII: 1, Madras, Report* (Madras: Government Press, 1923), 68.

90. David Hardiman, 'The Influenza Epidemic of 1918 and the *Adivasis* of Western India,' *Social History of Medicine*, 25: 3 (2012), 644–64.

91. Lakshmibai Tilak, *Smritichitre: The Memoirs of a Spirited Wife* (New Delhi: Speaking Tiger, 2017), 410–11. Lakshmibai's husband died in 1919, but not it seems from influenza.

92. Tallents, *Bihar and Orissa,* 13.

93. Bose, 'Influenza,' 171; cf. Barry, *Influenza*, 224, 236.

94. For the advice issued by the Government of India, see J. A. Turner and B. K. Goldsmith, *Sanitation in India* (3rd ed., Bombay: Times of India, 1922), 688–700.

95. *ToI*, 19 July 1918, 4.

96. *ToI*, 30 December 1915, 5; 13 January 1890, 4.

97. Phipson, 'Pandemic,' 515.

98. Bengal Municipal (Sanitation), no. 15, January 1920, IOR.

99. India Education (Sanitary), nos. 6–19, November 1918, IOR.

100. *ABP*, 13 February 1919, 4.

101. Phipson, 'Pandemic,' 520–1.

102. Tallents, *Bihar and Orissa*, 13.

103. *ARSC Bengal, 1918*, 24.

104. Cited in Turner and Goldsmith, *Sanitation*, 693.

105. James, *Report*, 13–14; H. R. Dutton, 'Note on a Recent Outbreak of Influenza,' *IMG*, 56: 2, (1921), 56.

106. On the vaccine question, see Barry, *Influenza*, 356–8.

107. *The Army in India and Its Evolution* (Calcutta: Superintendent, Government Printing, 1924), 117–18.

108. James, *Report*, 385.

109. Thomas P. Herriot, 'The Influenza Pandemic, 1918, as Observed in the Punjab, India,' unpublished MD thesis, University of Edinburgh, 1920, 1–2.

110. *ARSC Punjab, 1918*, app D, xv.

111. Middleton and Jacob, *Punjab*, 58.

112. *ARMAC, 1918–19*, 1, 83; Bhupal Singh, 'Influenza,' *IMG*, 55: 1 (1920), 15.

113. Herriot, 'Influenza,' 4.

114. Leigh, *Punjab*, 11.

115. Herriot, 'Influenza,' 6.

116. Ibid., 8–11, 50. Pneumonia cases were more concerning than simple influenza ones, with death-rates twice as high: U. N. Brahmachari and S. N. Ghosh, 'The Bacteriology of the Blood and Treatment of Influenza Occurring Epidemically in Calcutta,' *IMG*, 54: 3 (1919), 90–2; Debendra Nath Sen, 'Influenza Observed in the Sambhu Nath Pandit Hospital, Calcutta,' *IMG*, 55: 3 (1920), 89–92.

117. Herriot, 'Influenza,' 16, 39.

118. *Bombay Chronicle*, 16 October 1918, *RNP*.

119. *ARSC Central Provinces and Berar, 1918*, 8.

120. *ARMCB, 1918–19*, 39–40; *ARMAC, 1918–19*, 81–9. On Indian responses, see Mridula Ramanna, 'Coping with the Influenza Pandemic: The Bombay Experience,' in *Spanish Influenza*, ed. Phillips and Killingray, 86–98; Samuel K. Cohn, Jr., *Epidemics: Hate and Compassion from the Plague of Athens to Aids* (Oxford: Oxford University Press, 2018), 522–9; Madhu Singh, 'Bombay Fever/Spanish Flu: Public Health and Native Press in Colonial Bombay, 1918–19,' *South Asia Research*, 41:1 (2021), 35–52; T. V. Sekher, 'Influenza Pandemic of 1918: Lessons in Tackling a Public Health Catastrophe,' *Economic and Political Weekly*, 22 May 2021, 32–8.

121. *ToI*, 27 September 1918, 9.

122. *ToI*, 11 October 1918, 8.

123. On the Social Service League, see *ToI*, 3 October 1918, 8; on the rise of Indian philanthropy, see Georgina Brewis, '"Fill Full the Mouth of Famine": Voluntary Action in Famine Relief in India, 1896–1901,' *Modern Asian Studies*, 44: 4 (2010), 887–918.

124. *ToI*, 9 November 1918, 12.

125. *ABP*, 16 February 1919, 2.

126. Leigh, *Punjab*, 12.

127. *ToI*, 3 December 1919, 7.

128. *ToI*, 19 August 1924, 8.

129. Cited in Argha Kumar Banerjee, 'Tagore and Pandemics,' *Statesman*, 27 December 2020, https://www.thestatesman.com/opinion/tagore-and-pandemics-1502942965.html.

130. *ABP*, 30 January 1919, 8; *Tribune*, 13 November 1918, *RNP*; *ToI*, 2 April 1920, 6; 5 April 1920, 5.

131. *Deccan Ryot*, 31 October 1918, *RNP*; Rajendra Kumar Sen, *A Treatise on Influenza* (North Lakmipur: R. K. Sen, 1923); *Praja Mitra*, 23 October 1918, *RNP*.

132. *ABP*, 16 February 1919, 4; *Hamdan*, 20 May 1919, *RNP*. For the evolving relationship between Ayurveda and the colonial state, see Rachel Berger, 'From the Biomoral to the Biopolitical: Ayurveda's Political Histories,' *South Asian History and Culture*, 4: 1 (2013), 48–64.

133. Patterson and Pyle, 'Geography,' 18.

5. ORPHANS OF THE STORM

1.   *ToI*, 29 December 1923, 9.

2.   *ToI*, 16 October 1926, 6.

3.   F. Norman White, *A Preliminary Report on the Influenza Pandemic of 1918 in India* (Simla: Government Monotype Press, 1919).

4.   E.g., Maria Misra, *Vishnu's Crowded Temple: India Since the Great Rebellion* (New Haven: Yale University Press, 2008), 149. For the 5 million figure, see J. A. Turner and B. K. Goldsmith, *Sanitation in India* (3rd ed., Bombay: Times of India, 1922), 689.

5.   *ToI*, 8 November 1918, 8.

6.   J. T. Marten, 'The Census of India of 1921,' *Journal of the Royal Society of Arts*, 71: 3672 (1923), 362.

7.   Sam Higginbottom, Allahabad, to Secretary, Viceroy of India, n.d., India Revenue and Agriculture (Famine), no. 22, October 1919, IOR.

8.   Quoted in India Revenue and Agriculture (Famine), no. 17, October 1919, IOR; see also Peter Harnetty, 'The Famine That Never Was: Christian Missionaries in India, 1918–1919,' *Historian*, 63: 3 (2001), 555–75.

9.   As quoted in Higginbottom to Secretary, Viceroy of India, n.d., India Revenue and Agriculture (Famine), no. 22, October 1919, IOR.

10. J. Hullah to Higginbottom, 28 August 1919, in ibid., no. 27.

11. The entire episode is absent from Higginbottom's autobiographical account: *Sam Higginbottom, Farmer: An Autobiography* (New York: Charles Scribner's Sons, 1949).

12. Marten, 'Census,' 356.

13. L. J. Sedgwick, *Census of India, 1921, VIII: 1, Bombay, Report* (Bombay: Government Central Press, 1922), 23.

14. L. Middleton and S. M. Jacob, *Census of India, 1921, XV: 1, Punjab, Report* (Lahore: Civil and Military Gazette, 1923), 60.

15. G. T. Lloyd, *Census of India, 1921, III: 1, Assam, Report* (Shillong: Government Press, 1923), 19–20.

16. The orphaning effects of Covid-19 were, however, much noted in media reports of the pandemic in 2021: e.g., Vikas Pandey and Andrew Clarance, 'Coronavirus: The Indian Children Orphaned by Covid-19,' BBC News, 31 May 2021, https://www.bbc.co.uk/news/world-asia-india-57264629.

17. *ToI*, 27 March 1919, 9.

18. *ToI*, 12 November 1918, 9.

19. Bombay Revenue (Famine), no. 16, 4 January 1919, IOR.

20. *Report on the Administration of Bihar and Orissa, 1919–1920* (Patna, 1921), iii. There is reference elsewhere to private charity for orphans and the old: e.g., P. C. Tallents, *Census of India, 1921, VII: 1, Bihar and Orissa, Report* (Patna: Government Printing, Bihar and Orissa, 1923), 49–50.

21. *ToI*, 1 December 1919, 6.

22. Sedgwick, *Bombay Presidency*, 70–2; Margaret F. Kennedy, *Flame of the Forest: Canadian Presbyterians in India* (Ontario: Board of World Missions, c.1980), 65–9; George W. Clutterbuck, *In India, the Land of Famine and of Plague* (London: Ideal Publishing Union, 1897), chapter 10.

23. Mills gives some data for the increase in widows and widowers in the Bombay Presidency between 1911 and 1921: I. D. Mills, 'The 1918–19 Influenza Pandemic: The Indian Experience,' *Indian Economic and Social History Review*, 23: 1 (1986), 29.

24. *ToI*, 3 June 1919, 8; 1 December 1919, 6; 19 March 1920, 14; 30 July 1935, 11.

25. *Leader*, 15 January 1920, 17.

26. *ToI*, 30 March 1919, 16.

27. James Fenske, Bishnupriya Gupta, and Song Yuan, 'Demographic Shocks and Women's Labor Market Participation: Evidence from the 1918 Influenza Pandemic in India,' discussion paper 15077, Centre for Economic Policy Research, London, 2020.

28. *The Times*, 11 April 1919, 24.

29. *Report on the Administration, Bihar and Orissa*, 5.

30. Commissioner, Sind, 7 January 1919, Bombay Revenue (Famine), no. 2435, 14 March 1919, IOR.

31. E. H. H. Edye, *Census of India, 1921, XVI: 1, United Provinces, Report* (Allahabad: Government Press, United Provinces, 1923), 12.

32. *ToI*, 15 July 1918, 8.

33. Tallents, *Bihar and Orissa*, 14.

34. H. A. Antrobus, *A History of the Assam Company, 1839–1953* (Edinburgh: T. and A. Constable, 1957), 201.

35. *The Times*, 25 June 1919, 22.

36. *The Times*, 22 July 1920, 21.

37. India Education (Sanitary), no. 17, December 1918, IOR; R. H. Malone, 'A Bacteriological Investigation of Influenza Carried Out under the Indian Research Fund Association,' *IJMR*, 7: 3 (1919–20), 495–518.

38. Koilas Chandra Bose, 'Epidemic Influenza in and around the City of Calcutta,' *IMG*, 55: 5 (1920), 169–74; E. S. Phipson, 'The Pandemic of Influenza in India in the Year 1918,' *IMG*, 58: 11 (1923), 509–24.

39. Edwin O. Jordan, *Epidemic Influenza: A Survey* (Chicago: American Medical Association, 1927), Bibliography.

40. Turner and Goldsmith, *Sanitation*, 597–619, 688–700.

41. Editorial, 'On the Seven Scourges of India', *IMG*, 59: 7 (1924), 351–5.

42. Seventh Congress of the Far Eastern Association of Tropical Medicine, *Souvenir: The Indian Empire* (Calcutta: FEATM, 1927).

43. Mike Davis, *The Monster at Our Door: The Global Threat of Avian Flu* (New York: New Press, 2005), 33.

44. Editorial, 'Influenza and Other Respiratory Infections,' *IMG*, 56: 7 (1921), 261–2.

45. James W. Best, *Forest Life in India* (London: John Murray, 1935), 251–3. Cf. Man Aman Singh Chhina, 'When Corpses of Influenza Victims Were Dumped in Narmada River in 1918,' *Indian Express*, 6 June 2021, https://indianexpress.com/article/explained/explained-when-corpse...f-influenza-victims-were-dumped-in-narmada-river-in-1918-7310909/.

46. 'Central Provinces Forest Administration Report, 1918–19,' *Indian Forester*, 47: 1 (1921), 36; *Report on the Administration of the Salt Department of the Bombay Presidency, 1918–19*, 6.

47. Jim Corbett, *The Man-Eaters of Kumaon* (London: Oxford University Press, 1952), xvi.

48. Alan R. Beals, 'Interplay among Factors of Change in a Mysore Village,' in *Village India*, ed. McKim Marriott (Chicago: University of Chicago Press, 1955), 90.

49. Corbett, *Man-Eaters*, xvi; *ARSC Central Provinces and Berar, 1918*, app. C, 2.

50. Best, *Forest*, 252.

51. For 'the complete helplessness of the people,' see *ARSC Central Provinces and Berar, 1918*, 8; and for 1918–19 as a tale of European initiative and philanthropy, Tallents, *Bihar and Orissa*, 13.

52. Best, *Forest*, 252–3.

53. David Arnold, 'Hunger in the Garden of Plenty: The Bengal Famine of 1770,' in *Dreadful Visitations: Confronting Natural Catastrophe in the Age of Enlightenment*, ed. Alessa Johns (New York: Routledge, 1999), 98–9.

54. F. Norman White, 'Retrospect,' *Transactions of the Royal Society of Tropical Medicine and Hygiene*, 47: 6 (1953), 442.

55. Best, *Forest*, 251, 253.

56. DeWitt C. Ellinwood, 'The Indian Soldier, the Indian Army, and Change, 1914–1918,' in *India and World War I*, ed. DeWitt C. Ellinwood and S. D. Pradhan (New Delhi: Manohar, 1978), 177–211.

57. See the concerns of Sir Walter Lawrence, special adviser on the Indian Army in France, Lawrence Papers, MSS Eur. F. 143/65, British Library.

58. M. S. Leigh, *The Punjab and the War* (Lahore: Government Printing, Punjab, 1922), 282–3.

59. *Neuve Chapelle: India's Memorial in France, 1914–1918* (London: Hodder and Stoughton, 1928); David A. Johnson, 'New Delhi's All-India War Memorial (India Gate): Death, Monumentality and the Lasting Legacy of Empire in India,' *Journal of Imperial and Commonwealth History*, 46: 2 (2018), 345–66; Samuel Hyson and Alan Lester, '"British India on Trial": Brighton Military Hospitals and the Politics of Empire in World War I,' *Journal of Historical Geography*, 38: 1 (2012), 18–34.

60. *ARSC Bombay, 1918*, 23.

61. David Arnold, *Burning the Dead: Hindu Nationhood and the Global Construction of Indian Tradition* (Oakland: University of California Press, 2021), chapter 7.

62. *ToI*, 15 July 1918, 8; 17 July 1918, 7.

63. Erik H. Erikson, *Gandhi's Truth: On the Origins of Militant Nonviolence* (London: Faber and Faber, 1970), 371–84.

64. Laura Spinney, *Pale Rider: The Spanish Flu of 1918 and How It Changed the World* (London: Jonathan Cape, 2017), 8, 254–60; Catharine Arnold, *Pandemic 1918: The Story of the Deadliest Influenza in History* (London: Michael O'Mara, 2018), 209–10.

65. Thomas Weber and Dennis Dalton, 'Gandhi and the Pandemic,' *Economic and Political Weekly*, 20 June 2020, https://www.epw.in/joiurnal/2020/25/perspectives/gandhi-and-pandemic.html.

66. Gandhi to Harilal, 23 November 1918, *Collected Works of Mahatma Gandhi* 17, online edition, 247.

67. Gandhi to Andrews, 10 January 1919, *Collected Works of Mahatma Gandhi* 17, online edition, 256.

68. Cited in Weber and Dalton, 'Gandhi.'

69. M. R. Jayakar, *The Story of My Life*, 2 vols. (Bombay: Asia Publishing House, 1958); Jawaharlal Nehru, *An Autobiography* (Bombay: Allied Publishers, 1962), 41.

70. E.g., Judith M. Brown, *Gandhi's Rise to Power: Indian Politics, 1915–1922* (Cambridge: Cambridge University Press, 1972), chapter 4.

71. *ABP*, 13 February 1919, 3.

72. E.g., D. W. Ferrell, 'The Rowlatt Satyagraha in Delhi,' in *Essays on Gandhian Politics: The Rowlatt Satyagraha of 1919*, ed. R. Kumar (Oxford: Clarendon Press, 1971), 198; C. A. Bayly, *The Local Roots of Indian Politics: Allahabad, 1880–1920* (Oxford: Oxford University Press 1975), 245–6.

73. See, for instance, the relatively small space given to Norman White's 'highly interesting preliminary report' and the figure of 6 million influenza deaths in *ABP*, 23 March 1919, 5, compared with the coverage in the same issue of the Rowlatt bills, Gandhi's forthcoming satyagraha, and the Paris peace conference.

74. Kim A. Wagner, *Amritsar 1919: An Empire of Fear and the Making of a Massacre* (New Haven: Yale University Press, 2019). Wagner makes passing reference to influenza, in ibid., 35.

75. Ida Milne, *Stacking the Coffins: Influenza, War and Revolution in Ireland, 1918–19* (Manchester: Manchester University Press, 2018).

76. Cited in Mridula Ramanna, 'Coping with the Influenza Pandemic: The Bombay Experience,' in *The Spanish Influenza Pandemic of 1918–19: New Perspectives*, ed. Howard Phillips and David Killingray (London: Routledge, 2003), 98. It has been doubted whether these were actually Gandhi's words or whether they appeared in *Young India* at all: Vinay Lal, *The Fury of COVID-19: The Politics, Histories, and Unrequited Love of the Coronavirus* (New Delhi: Macmillan, 2020), 243, n. 32.

77. Margrit Pernau, 'Introduction: Studying Emotions in South Asia,' *South Asian History and Culture* (2021), https://doi.org/10.1080/19472498.2021.1878 788.

78. David Omissi, *Indian Voices of the Great War: Soldiers' Letters, 1914–1918* (London: Macmillan, 1999); Santanu Das, *India, Empire, and First World War Culture: Writings, Images, and Songs* (Cambridge: Cambridge University Press, 2018).

79. *ToI*, 19 July 1918, 2.

80. 'Covid: India Launches Online Memorial to Commemorate Pandemic Victims,' BBC News, 2 February 2021, https://www.bbc.co.uk/news/world-asia-india-55884038.

81. *ToI*, 10 May 1919, 11.

82. Suryakant Tripathi Nirala, *A Life Misspent*, trans. Satti Khanna (New York: HarperCollins, 2016), 53–4.

83. Subhash Chandra Sarker, 'Sarat Chandra Chatterjee: The Great Humanist,' *Indian Literature*, 20: 1 (1977), 58.

84. In Christopher McKnight Nichols, Nancy Bristow, E. Thomas Ewing, Joseph M. Gabriel, Benjamin C. Montoya, and Elizabeth Outka, 'Reconsidering the 1918–19 Influenza Pandemic in the Age of Covid-19,' *Journal of the Gilded Age and Progressive Era*, 19: 4 (2020), 651.

85. Ahmed Ali, *Twilight in Delhi* (New York: New Directions, 1994), 169–72.

86. Prakash Tandon, *Punjabi Century, 1857–1947* (London: Chatto and Windus, 1961), 162.

87. Ibid.

88. *ToI*, 26 June 1918, 6.

89. *ToI*, 20 November 1919, 7.

90. *ToI*, 21 November 1919, 7.

91. D. E. Wacha, *Shells from the Sands of Bombay: Being My Recollections and Reminiscences, 1860–1875* (Bombay: Indian Newspaper Co., 1920), dedication.

92. Jadunath Sarkar, *House of Shivaji* (1955), 207–8, cited in Dipesh Chakrabarty, *The Calling of History: Sir Jadunath Sarkar and His Empire of Truth* (Chicago: University of Chicago Press, 2015), 240.

93. Kingsley Davis, *The Population of India and Pakistan* (Princeton: Princeton University Press, 1951); Mills, 'Influenza.'

94. Guy Beiner, 'Out in the Cold and Back: New-Found Interest in the Great Flu,' *Cultural and Social History*, 3: 4 (2006), 496–505.

95. Neil Ferguson, 'Poverty, Death, and a Future Influenza Pandemic,' *The Lancet*, 23 December 2006, 2187–8.

96. Siddharth Chandra and Julia Christensen, 'Preparing for Pandemic Influenza,' *Journal of World Historical Information*, 3–4: 1 (2016–17), 20, 24; Siddharth Chandra, Goran Kuljanin, and Jennifer Wray, 'Mortality from the Influenza Pandemic of 1918–19: The Case of India,' *Demography*, 49: 3 (2012), 857–65; Siddhartha Chandra and Eva Kassens-Noor, 'The Evolution of Pandemic Influenza: Evidence from India,' *BMC Infectious Diseases*, 14 (2014), https://bmcinfectdis.biomedcentral.com/articles/10.1186/1471-2334-14-510#citeas.

97. Lalit Kant and Randeep Guleria, 'Pandemic Flu 1918: After Hundred Years, India Is as Vulnerable,' *IJMR*, 147: 3 (2018), 221–4. Also, Christopher J. Murray, Alan D. Lopez, Brian Chin, Dennis Feehan, and Kenneth H. Hill, 'Estimation of Global Pandemic Influenza Mortality on the Basis of Vital Registration Data from the 1918–20 Pandemic: A Quantitative Analysis,' *The Lancet*, 23 December 2006, 2211–18.

98. Kant and Guleria, 'Pandemic,' 221; Robert J. Barro, José F. Ursúa, and Joanna Weng, 'The Coronavirus and the Great Influenza Pandemic: Lessons from the "Spanish Flu" for the Coronavirus's Potential Effects on Mortality and Economic Activity,' working paper 26866, National Bureau of Economic Research, Cambridge, MA, 2020, https://doi.org/10.3386/w26866.

6. IN THE TIME OF THE NATION

1. Raymond Williams, *Keywords: A Vocabulary of Culture and Society* (London: Fontana, 1975).
2. Jawaharlal Nehru, 'A Tryst with Destiny,' 14 August 1947, https://www.files.ethz.ch/isn/125396/1154_trystnehru.pdf.
3. Vikram Patel, 'India's Tryst with Covid-19,' https://www.theindiaforum.in/article/indi-s-tryst-covid-19.
4. 'Delhi's Tryst with the Third Wave of Covid-19 Infections,' *The Week*, 22 November 2020, https://www.theweek.in/news/india/2020/11/22/delhi-tryst-with-the-third-wave-of-covid-19-infections-what-numbers-tell-us.html; Anilkumar Kamat, 'My Tryst with Coronavirus and Home Quarantine,' *ToI*, 11 February 2021, https://timesofindia.indiatimes.com/readersblog/kamatsense/my-tryst-with-coronavirus-home-quarantine-29683/; Bibek Debray, 'Lessons from India's Tryst with Lockdown,' *The Mint*, 25 March 2021, https://www.livemint.com/news/india/lessons-from-india-s-tryst-with-lockdown-11616599176632.html.
5. For 'the unexpected vulnerability of modern society' to new or returning pandemic diseases, see Frank M. Snowden, *Epidemics and Society: From the Black Death to the Present* (New Haven: Yale University Press, 2019), 1.
6. Roald Dahl, *Tales of the Unexpected* (London: Michael Joseph, 1979).
7. I. J. Catanach, 'The "Globalization" of Disease? India and the Plague,' *Journal of World History*, 12: 1 (2001), 131.
8. F. M. Burnet, *Natural History of Infectious Disease* (2nd ed., Cambridge: Cambridge University Press, 1953), 3.
9. Quoted in Prema-Chandra Athukorala and Chaturica Athukorala, 'The Great Influenza Pandemic of 1918–20: An Interpretive Survey at the Time of Covid-19,' discussion paper, Australian National University, Canberra, 2020, 3.
10. Quoted in Larry Brilliant, 'The Age of Pandemics,' *Wall Street Journal*, 2 May 2009, https://www.wsj.com/articles/SB124121965740478983.
11. D. Mahalanabis, A. B. Choudhuri, N. G. Bagchi, A. K. Bhattacharya, and T. W. Simpson, 'Oral Fluid Therapy of Cholera among Bangladesh Refugees,' *WHO South-East Asia Journal of Public Health*, 1: 1 (2012), 105–12.
12. I. G. K. Menon, 'The 1957 Pandemic of Influenza in India,' *Bulletin of the World Health Organization*, 20: 2–3 (1959), 199–224; Sumi Krishna, 'I Survived a Pandemic in the Last Century. Now, I Fight One More,' *The Wire*, 3 April 2020, https://science.thewire.in/health/coronavirus-asian-flu-igk-menon-coonoor-epidemic/.
13. Kavita Sivaramakrishnan, '"Endemic Risks": Influenza Pandemics, Public Health, and Making Self-reliant Indian Citizens,' *Journal of Global History*, 15: 3 (2020), 459–77.
14. Jean Drèze, 'Famine Prevention in India,' in *The Political Economy of Hunger*, vol. 2: *Famine Prevention*, ed. Jean Drèze and Amartya Sen (Oxford: Clarendon Press, 1991), 13–122.

15. Benjamin Robert Siegal, *Hungry Nation: Food, Famine, and the Making of Modern India* (Cambridge: Cambridge University Press, 2018).

16. A. K. Sen, 'Famine Mortality: A Study of the Bengal Famine of 1943,' in *Peasants in History: Essays in Memory of Daniel Thorner*, ed. Eric J. Hobsbawm, Witold Kula, Ashok Mitra, K. N. Raj, and Ignacy Sachs (Calcutta: Oxford University Press, 1980), 194–220.

17. Ira Klein, 'Population Growth and Mortality, Part 1: The Climacteric of Death,' *Indian Economic and Social History Review*, 26: 4 (1989), 387–403; Kingsley Davis, *The Population of India and Pakistan* (Princeton: Princeton University Press, 1951), chapter 6.

18. Sumit Guha, *Health and Population in South Asia: From the Earliest Times to the Present Day* (London: Hurst, 2001), 26.

19. Sumit Guha, 'India in the Pandemic Age,' *Indian Economic Review*, 55: 1 (2020), 28.

20. Tirthankar Roy, 'Water, Climate, and Economy in India from 1880 to the Present,' *Journal of Interdisciplinary History*, 51: 4 (2021), 565–94. Davis, *Population*, 41, argued that from about 1900 onward, irrigation had 'probably done more than any other technological factor to eliminate famines from the Indian subcontinent.'

21. Gyanshyam Shah, *Public Health and Urban Development: The Plague in Surat* (New Delhi: Sage, 1997).

22. Ashok K. Dutt, Rais Akhtar, and Melinda McVeigh, 'Surat Plague of 1994 Re-examined,' *Southeast Asian Journal of Tropical Medicine and Public Health*, 37: 4 (2006), 755–60.

23. J. C. Suri and M. K. Sen, 'Pandemic Influenza: Indian Experience,' *Lung India*, 28: 1 (2011), 2–4.

24. Chinmay Tumbe, *The Age of Pandemics, 1817–1920: How They Shaped India and the World* (Noida: HarperCollins, 2020), 182.

25. Robert Peckham, *Epidemics in Modern Asia* (Cambridge: Cambridge University Press, 2016), 252.

26. Susan Sontag, 'AIDS and Its Metaphors,' *New York Review of Books*, 27 October 1988, https://www.nybooks.com/articles/1988/10/27/aids-and-its-metaphors/; Charles E. Rosenberg, *Explaining Epidemics and Other Studies in the History of Medicine* (Cambridge: Cambridge University Press, 1992); Dorothy Nelkin and Sander L. Gilman, 'Placing Blame for Devastating Disease,' *Social Research*, 55: 2 (1988), 361–78.

27. 'HIV/AIDS in India,' https://en.wikipedia.org/wiki/HIV/AIDS_in_india; 'HIV and AIDS in India,' https://www.avert.org/printpdf/node/417.

28. Mark Honigsbaum, *The Pandemic Century: A History of Global Contagion from the Spanish Flu to Covid-19* (London: Penguin, 2020), chapter 6.

29. Sreejith Radhakrishnan, Abi Tamim Vanak, Pierre Nouvellet, and Christl A. Donnelly, 'Rabies as a Public Health Concern in India: A Statistical Perspective,' *Tropical Medicine and Infectious Disease*, 5: 4 (2020), doi: 10.3390/tropicalmed5040162.

30. Sheetal Chhabria, 'Manufacturing Epidemics: Pathogens, Poverty, and Public Health Crises in India,' *India Forum*, 5 June 2020, www.TheIndiaForum.in.

31. Prachi Singh, Shamika Ravi, and Sikim Chakraborty, 'COVID-19: Is India's Health Infrastructure Equipped to Handle an Epidemic?', *Brookings*, 24 March 2020, https://www.brookings.edu/blog/up-front/2020/03/24/is-indias-health-infrastructure-equipped-to-handle-an-epidemic/.

32. Roger Jeffery, *The Politics of Health in India* (Berkeley: University of California Press, 1988), 112–14, 236–44.

33. Meera Chatterjee, *Implementing Health Policy* (New Delhi: Manohar, 1988), 1.

34. Sumit Ganguly, 'Mangling the COVID Crisis: India's Response to the Pandemic,' *Washington Quarterly*, 43: 4 (2021), 113.

35. Jean Drèze and Amartya Sen, *An Uncertain Glory: India and Its Contradictions* (London: Allen Lane, 2013), 149.

36. Banu Subramaniam, *Holy Science: The Biopolitics of Hindu Nationalism* (Seattle: University of Washington Press, 2019), 167–70.

37. Drèze and Sen, *Uncertain*, 143; V. Sujatha, 'COVID-19 Pandemic and the Politics of Risk: Perspectives on Science, State and Society in India,' *Contributions to Indian Sociology*, 55: 2 (2021), 267.

38. In the resulting international blame game, Chinese researchers claimed that India had been the original source: 'Now Chinese Scientists Claim Coronavirus Originated in India,' https://www.dailymail.co.uk/news/article-8993667/Now-Chinese-scientists-claim-coronavirus-originated-INDIA-summer-2019.html.

39. 'WHO Director-General's Opening Remarks at the Media Briefing on COVID-19 – 11 March 2020,' https://www.who.int/director-general/speeches/detail/who-director-general-s-opening-remarks-at-the-media-briefing-on-covid-19---11-march-2020.

40. T. Sundararaman and Alok Ranjan, 'Challenges to India's Rural Healthcare System in the Context of Covid-19,' *Review of Agrarian Studies* 10: 1 (2020), http://ras.org.in/79332f54f12620b88534aa93a142dc1f.

41. Ganguly, 'Mangling,' 105; Prabash K. Dutta, 'SARS: How India Tackled Previous Coronavirus Outbreak,' *India Today*, 29 May 2020, https://www.indiatoday.in/india/story/sars-2002-03-india-coronavirus-outbreak-1683404-2020-05-29.

42. Soutik Biswas, 'India's Frightful Pandemic Projections,' *BBC News*, 25 March 2020, https://www.bbc.co.uk/news/live/world-52026908.

43. Anup Malani, Arpit Gupta, and Reuben Abraham, 'Why Does India Have So Few Covid-19 Cases and Deaths?,' *Quartz India*, 16 April 2020, https://qz.com/india/1839018/why-does-india-have-so-few-coronavirus-covid-19-cases-and-deaths/.

44. 'I Don't Expect That Fatalities from Covid-19 Will Be Comparable to Those from the 1918 Influenza: Prof. Siddharth Chandra,' *Indian Express*, 23 March 2020, https://indianexpress.com/article/coronavirus/coronavirus-pandemic-covid-19-siddharth-chandra-interview-6327127/.

45. 'India Covid-19: PM Modi "Did Not Consult" before Lockdown,' BBC News, 29 March 2021, https://www.bbc.co.uk/news/world-asia-india-56561095.

46. 'Coronavirus: India Enters "Total Lockdown" after Spike in Cases,' BBC News, 25 March 2020, https://www.bbc.co.uk/news/world-asia-india-52024239.

47. 'Coronavirus: India's PM Modi Seeks "Forgiveness" over Lockdown,' BBC News, 29 March 2020, https://www.bbc.co.uk/news/world-asia-india-52081396.

48. Catherine Connolly, 'War and the Coronavirus Pandemic,' *Third World Approaches to International Law Review* (2020), https://twailr.com/war-and-the-coronavirus-pandemic/.

49. Sujatha, 'COVID-19,' 255.

50. Pushpa Arabindoo, 'Pandemic Cities: Between Mimicry and Trickery,' *City and Society*, 32 (2020), https://doi.org/10.1111/ciso.12263.

51. Ravinder Kaur and Sumathi Ramaswamy, 'The Goddess and the Virus,' in *The Pandemic: Perspectives on Asia*, ed. Vinayak Chaturvedi (Ann Arbor: Association for Asian Studies, 2020), 75–94; 'Art of the Pandemic: COVID-Inspired Street Graffiti,' https://www.reuters.com/news/picture/art-of-the-pandemic-covid-inspired-stree-idUSRTXA3GSN.

52. Ramanan Laxminarayan, Shahid Jameel, and Swarup Sarkar, 'India's Battle against COVID-19: Progress and Challenges,' *American Journal of Tropical Medicine and Hygiene*, 103: 4 (2020), 1346.

53. Pranav Tanwar and Saurabh Pandey, 'Epidemic Diseases Act, 1897: 123 Year Old Weapon against Coronavirus,' https://ijlpp.com/epidemic-disease-act-1897-123-year-old-weapon-against-corona/.

54. P. S. Rakesh, 'The Epidemic Diseases Act of 1897: Public Health Relevance in the Current Scenario,' *Indian Journal of Medical Ethics*, 1: 3 (2016), 156.

55. Dilip M. Menon, 'Viral Histories: Will Covid-19 Help Us Generate New Thinking?,' *Scroll.in*, 7 August 2020, https://scroll.in/article/969649/viral-histories-will-covid-19-help-us-to-generate-new-thinking.

56. Antonia Noori Farzan, 'Amid "Heartbreaking" Coronavirus Surge in India, Government Orders Twitter to Remove Posts Critical of Response,' *Washington Post*, 26 April 2021, https://www.washingtonpost.com.world/2021/04/26/twitter-india-coronavirus/.

57. 'Statement Condemning Crackdown on Women Activists in Delhi,' *Focus on the Global South*, 7 May 2020, https://focusweb.org/statement-condemning-crackdown-on-women-activists-in-delhi/23; Soutik Biswas, 'Why Journalists in India Are under Attack,' BBC News, 4 February 2021, https://www.bbc.co.uk/news/world-asia-india-55906345; Shruti Menon, 'Farmer Protests: India's Sedition Law Used to Muffle Dissent,' BBC News, 24 February 2021, https://www.bbc.co.uk/news/world-asia-india-56111289. On the increasingly autocratic style of Narendra Modi and the BJP, see Ramachandra Guha, 'Supreme Court Must Reflect on Its Calling

as Defined by the Constitution,' *Indian Express*, 13 August 2020, https://indianexpress.com/article/opinion/columns/supreme-court-democracy-politicisation-judiciary-kashmir-covid-6552287/.

58. 'India Is Now Only "Partly Free" under Modi, Says Report,' BBC News, 3 March 2021, https://www.bbc.co.uk/news/world-asia-india-56249596.

59. Soutik Biswas, 'Manmohan Singh's "Three Steps" to Stem India's Economic Crisis,' BBC News, 9 August 2020, https://www.bbc.co.uk/news/world-asia-india-53675858.

60. Ganguly, 'Mangling,' 105.

61. John Harriss, '"Responding to an Epidemic Requires a Compassionate State": How Has the Indian State Been Doing in the Time of COVID-19?,' *Journal of Asian Studies*, 79: 3 (2020), 619.

62. Nikhil Inamdar and Aparna Alluri, 'India Economy: Seven Years of Modi in Seven Charts,' BBC News, 22 June 2021, https://www.bbc.co.uk/news/world-asia-india-57437944.

63. 'India Covid Map and Case Count,' *New York Times*, 20 October 2020, https://www.nytimes.com/interactive/2020/world/asia/india-coronavirus-cases-html.

64. Ganguly, 'Mangling,' 112.

65. Amy Kazmin, 'India Unveils $10bn Plan to Boost Growth,' *Financial Times*, 13 October 2020, 8.

66. Nikhil Inamdar, 'Three Takeaways from India's "Pandemic Budget"', BBC News, 1 February 2021, https://www.bbc.co.uk/news/world-asia-india-55884215.

67. Ganguly, 'Mangling,' 107.

68. Soutik Biswas, 'Coronavirus: India's Pandemic Lockdown Turns into a Human Tragedy,' BBC News, 30 March 2020, www.bbc.com/news/world-asia-india-52086274.

69. Maria K. Johns, 'The Violence of Abandonment: Urban Indigenous Health and the Settler-Colonial Politics of Nonrecognition in the United States and Australia,' *Native American and Indigenous Studies*, 7: 1 (2020), 87–120.

70. Ramachandra Guha, 'Repeating the Past,' *Telegraph*, 24 April 2020, https://www.telegraphindia.com/opinion/coronavirus-india-the-gover...ious-minorities-during-covid-19-lockdown-and-pandemic/cid/1767769.

71. Ranjini Basu, 'Migrant Agricultural Workers in India and the COVID-19 Lockdown,' *Focus on the Global South*, 29 April 2020, https://focusweb.org/migrant-agricultural-workers-in-india-and-the-covid-19-lockdown/.

72. Samata Biswas, 'Bringing the Border Home: Indian Partition 2020,' in *Borders of an Epidemic: COVID-19 and Migrant Workers*, ed. Ranabir Samaddar (Kolkata: Calcutta Research Group, 2020), 104–14; Menon, 'Viral Histories.'

73. Mohammad Tareq Hasan, 'Homecoming from the City: Covid-19 and Dhaka,' *Medical Anthropology at UCL*, 15 April 2020, https://medanthucl.com/2020/04/15/homecoming-from-the-city-covid-19-dhaka/.

74. Arabindoo, 'Pandemic.'

75. William Digby, *The Famine Campaign in Southern India, 1876–78*, 2 vols. (London: Longmans, Green 1878).

76. Tanushree Ghosh, 'Witnessing Famine: The Testimonial Work of Famine Photographs and Anti-colonial Spectatorship,' *Journal of Visual Culture*, 18: 3 (2019), 327–57.

77. '12-Year-Old Dies after Walking for 3 Days from Telangana to Reach Her Home in Chhattisgarh,' *Times of India*, 21 April 2020, https://timesofindia. indiatimes.com/india/12-year-old-dies-after-w...langana-to-reach-her-home-in-chhattisgarh/articleshow/75278563.cms; Harsh Mander, *Locking Down the Poor: The Pandemic and India's Moral Centre* (New Delhi: Speaking Tiger, 2020).

78. E.g., Samuel K. Cohn, *Epidemics: Hate and Compassion from the Plague of Athens to AIDS* (Oxford: Oxford University Press, 2018).

79. Data here and in subsequent paragraphs were taken online from the Johns Hopkins University Corona Virus Resources Center.

80. Amitabh Sinha, 'India Coronavirus Numbers Explained: A Scary Runaway Phase Begins,' *Indian Express*, 15 September 2020, https://indianexpress. com/article/explained/september-7-india-coronavirus-covid-19-cases-deaths-numbers-explained-6586353/.

81. Soutik Biswas, 'Coronavirus: Is the Epidemic Finally Coming to an End in India?,' BBC News, 15 February 2021, https://www.bbc.co.uk/news/world-asia-india-56037565.

82. Soutik Biswas, 'Coronavirus: Is the Pandemic Slowing Down in India?,' BBC News, 6 October 2020, https://www.bbc.co.uk/news/world-asia-india-54419959; Amy Kazmin, 'India Has Reached Coronavirus Peak, Says Government Panel,' *Financial Times*, 19 October 2020, https://app.ft.com/content/734102c3-b5f8-486a-bb65-a2ab85bffe3f.

83. P. K. Yasser Arafath, 'Success of the Kerala Model,' *Telegraph*, 23 April 2020, https://www.telegraphindia.com/opinion/coronavirus-kerala-success-with...-by -its-high-level-of-literacy-and-secular-sensibilities/cid/1767508.

84. Jyotsna Jalan and Arijit Sen, 'Controlling a Pandemic with Public Actions and Public Trust: The Kerala Story,' *Indian Economic Review*, 55: 1 (2020), 105–24.

85. Soutik Biswas, 'India Coronavirus: How a Group of Volunteers "Exposed" Hidden Covid-19 Deaths,' BBC News, 20 November 2020, https://www. bbc.co.uk/news/world-asia-india-54985981.

86. 'Maharashtra: Nagpur Becomes First Major Indian City to Return to Lockdown,' BBC News, 12 March 2021, https://www.bbc.co.uk/news/world-asia-india-56369590.

87. 'India Coronavirus: Patients Stranded as Delhi Struggles with Covid,' BBC News, 8 June 2020, https://www.bbc.co.uk/news/world-asia-india-52961589.

88. Ganguly, 'Mangling,' 114–15; Madhuparna Das, '"Never Seen Such Devastation Before,"' *ThePrint*, 21 May 2020, https://theprint.in/india/

never-seen-such-devastation-before-shocked-cm-mamata-says-as-cyclone-amphan-ravages-bengal/426168/.

89. Malani, 'Why Does India?'; Soutik Biswas, 'India Coronavirus: The "Mystery" of Low Covid-19 Death Rates,' BBC News, 27 April 2020, https://www.bbc.co.uk/news/world-asia-india-52435463.

90. Chris Pleasance and Rachel Bunyan, 'Why Did COVID Fail to Take Off in India and Has Now Collapsed?,' Mail Online, 17 February 2021, https://www.dailymail.co.uk/news/article-9265495/Mystery-plunge-coronavirus-cases-India-baffles-experts-country-recorded-11m-infections.html?ito=social-twitter_mailonline.

91. Soutik Biswas, 'Coronavirus: Are Indians More Immune to Covid-19?,' BBC News, 2 November 2020, https://www.bbc.co.uk/news/world-asia-india-54730290.

92. Laxminarayan, 'India's Battle,' 1343–5.

93. 'India Coronavirus: Four Modi Claims Fact-Checked,' BBC News, 21 October 2020, https://www.bbc.co.uk/news/world-asia-india-54615353.

94. Naorem Pushparani Chanu and Gorky Chakraborty, 'A Novel Virus, A New Racial Slur,' India Forum, 3 July 2020, https://www.theindiaforum.in/article/novel-virus-new-racial-slur.

95. Niraja Gopal Jayal, 'Faith-Based Citizenship,' India Forum, 1 November 2019, https://www.theindiaforum.in/article/faith-criterion-citizenship.

96. Hannah Ellis-Petersen and Shaikh Azizur Rahman, 'Delhi Muslims Fear They Will Never See Justice for Religious Riot Atrocities,' The Observer, 28 March 2020, 24–5.

97. William Gould, Hindu Nationalism and the Language of Politics in Late Colonial India (Cambridge: Cambridge University Press, 2004).

98. Christophe Jaffrelot, Modi's India: Hindu Nationalism and the Rise of Ethnic Democracy, trans. Cynthia Schoch (Princeton: Princeton University Press, 2021).

99. Quoted in Billy Perrigo, 'It Was Already Dangerous to Be Muslim in India. Then Came the Coronavirus,' Time, 3 April 2020, https://time.com/5815264/coronavirus-india-islamophobia-coronajihad/.

100. 'Coronavirus: Search for Hundreds of People after Delhi Prayer Meeting,' BBC News, 31 March 2020, https://www.bbc.co.uk/news/world-asia-india-52104753; 'Islamophobia Concerns after India Mosque Outbreak,' BBC News, 3 April 2020, https://www.bbc.co.uk/news/world-asia-india-52147260.

101. Cited in Shweta Desai and Amarnath Amarasingam, 'Corona Jihad: COVID-19, Misinformation, and Anti-Muslim Violence in India,' https://strongcitiesnetwork.org/en/coronajihad-covid-19-misinformation-and-anti-muslim-violence-in-india/.

102. Hannah Ellis-Petersen and Shaik Azizur Rahman, 'Coronavirus Conspiracy Theories Targeting Muslims Spread in India,' The Guardian, 13 April 2020, https://www.theguardian.com/world/2020/apr/13/coronavirus-

conspiracy-theories-targeting-muslims-spread-in-india; Apoorvanand, 'How the Coronavirus Outbreak in India Was Blamed on Muslims,' *Al Jazeera*, 18 April 2020, https://www.aljazeera.com/indepth/opinion/coronavirus-outbreak-india-blamed-muslims-200418143252362.html.

103. Cited in Desai and Amarasingam, 'Corona,' 17.

104. Ian McDonald, '"Physiological Patriots"? The Politics of Physical Culture and Hindu Nationalism in India,' *International Review for the Sociology of Sport*, 34: 4 (1999), 343–58.

105. For the Hindu 'vulnerability syndrome,' see Christophe Jaffrelot, 'Hindu Nationalism and the (Not So Easy) Art of Being Outraged: The *Ram Setu* Controversy,' *South Asia Multidisciplinary Academic Journal*, 2 (2008), https://journals.openedition.org/samaj/1372.

106. Kaveree Bamzai, 'Between Sanitiser and Gaumutra for Covid-19,' *ThePrint*, 21 March 2020, https://theprint.in/opinion/gaumutra-for-covid-19-modis-india-made-historical-choice.

107. 'Cow Urine, Cow Dung, Can Cure Coronavirus,' *Outlook*, 2 March 2020, https://www.outlookindia.com/website/story/india-news-cow-urine-cow-dung-can-cure-coronavirus-assam-bjp-mla-suman-haripriya/348159.

108. 'Don't Eat Non-veg Which Creates Viruses,' *India Today*, 14 March 2020, https://www.indiatoday.in/india/story/haryana-health-minister-anil-vij-coronavirus-non-vegetarian-food-1655591-2020-03-14.

109. 'Coronavirus: Group Hosts "Cow Urine Party", Says COVID-19 Due to Meat-Eaters,' *The Hindu*, 14 March 2020, https://www.thehindu.com/news/national/coronavirus-group-hosts-cow-urine-party-says-covid-19-due-to-meat-eaters/article31070516.ece.

110. Subramaniam, *Holy Science*, Introduction.

111. Quoted in Shreekant Gupta, 'Pandemics, COVID-19 and India,' *Indian Economic Review*, 55: 1 (2020), 1, n. 2.

112. Karishma Patel, 'Covid-19: Fake "Immunity Booster" Found on Sale in London Shops,' BBC News, 19 December 2020, https://www.bbc.co.uk/news/uk-england-london-55318095. On Ramdev, see Venera Khailkova, 'The Ayurveda of Baba Ramdev: Biomoral Consumerism, National Duty and the Politics of "Homegrown" Medicine in India,' *South Asia*, 40: 1 (2017), 105–22.

113. Unnikrishnan Payyappallimana, 'Doctors at the Borders: Ayurveda's Encounter with Public Health and Epidemics,' https://culanth.org/fieldsights/doctors-at-the-borders-ayurvedas-encounter-with-public-health-and-epidemics.

114. Konya Tomar, 'Ayurveda in the (Mis)Information Age,' *Society for Cultural Anthropology*, 23 June 2020, https://culanth.org/fieldsights/ayurveda-in-the-misinformation-age.

115. 'PM Narendra Modi Gets Covid Jab as India Scales Up Vaccination,' BBC News, 1 March 2021, https://www.bbc.co.uk/news/world-asia-india-56237436.

116. 'India PM Modi Lays Foundation for Ayodhya Ram Temple amid Covid Surge,' BBC News, 5 August 2020, https://www.bbc.co.uk/news/world-asia-india-53577942.

117. Shruti Menon and Jack Goodman, 'India Covid Crisis: Did Election Rallies Help Spread Virus?,' BBC News, 24 April 2021, https://www.bbc.co.uk/news/56858980; Chetan Chauhan, 'Half of All Covid Deaths in India Took Place in April–May,' https://www.hindustantimes.com/india-news/half-of-all-covid-deaths-in-india-took-place-in-april-may-shows-government-data-101627204345380.html.

118. Geeta Pandey, 'India Covid: Kumbh Mela Pilgrims Turn into Super-spreaders,' BBC News, 10 May 2021, https://www.bbc.co.uk/news/world-asia-india-57005563; Shuddhabrata Sengupta, 'Kumbh 2021: Astrology, Mortality and the Indifference to Life of Leaders and Stars,' *TheWire*, 20 April 2021, https://thewire.in/government/kumbh-2021-astrology-mortality-and-the-indifference-to-life-of-leaders-and-stars.

119. Quoted in Benjamin Parkin, Jyotsna Singh, Stephanie Findlay, and John Burn-Murdoch, '"It Is Much Worse This Time": India's Devastating Second Wave,' *Financial Times*, 21 April 2021, https://www.ft.com/content/683914a3-134f-40b6-989b-21e0ba1dc403.

120. 'India in "Endgame of Pandemic", Says Health Minister,' NDTV, 8 March 2021, https://www.ndtv.com/india-news/coronavirus-india-in-endgame-of-pandemic-says-health-minister-2385882.

121. Quoted in Arundhati Roy, 'We Are Witnessing a Crime against Humanity,' *The Guardian*, 29 April 2021, https://www.theguardian.com/news/2021/apr/28/crime-against-humanity-arundhati-roy-india-covid-catastrophe.

122. Parkin, 'Much Worse.'

123. Joe Wallen, 'India's Covid Excess Death Toll Nearly 10 Times Higher Than Official Estimates,' *The Telegraph*, 20 July 2021, https://www.telegraph.co.uk/global-health/science-and-disease/indias-covid-excess-death-toll-nearly-10-times-higher-official/.

124. Hannah Ellis-Petersen, 'The System Has Collapsed: India's Descent into Covid Hell,' *The Guardian*, 21 April 2021, https://www.theguardian.com/world/2021/apr/21/system-has-collapsed-india-descent-into-covid-hell.

125. Barkha Dutt, 'India: A Broken Country, a Country in Torment,' BBC News, 23 April 2021, https://www.bbc.co.uk/news/world-asia-india; 'India Covid-19: Delhi Adds Makeshift Crematoriums as Deaths Climb,' BBC News, 27 April 2021, https://www.bbc.co.uk/news/world-asia-india-56897970.

126. Parkin, 'Much Worse.'

127. Rebecca Morelle, 'Why India's Covid Crisis Matters to the Whole World,' BBC News, 28 April 2021, https://www.bbc.co.uk/news/world-asia-india-56907007.

128. Geeta Pandey, 'India's Holiest River Is Swollen with Covid Victims,' BBC News, 19 May 2021, https://www.bbc.co.uk/news/world-asia-india-57154564; Hannah Ellis-Petersen and Saurabh Sharma, 'Stench

of Death Pervades Rural India as Ganges Swells with Covid Victims,' *The Guardian*, 20 May 2021, https://www.theguardian.com/world/2021/may/20/stench-death-pervades-rural-india-ganges-swells-covid-victims.

129. Parkin, 'Much Worse.'

130. Channel 4 News, 4 May 2021.

131. Shareen Joshi, 'Funeral Pyres Should Not Be the Symbol of India's Covid Crisis,' CNN Opinion, 2 June 2021, https://edition.cnn.com/2021/06/02/opinions/india-funeral-pyres-should-not-be-covid-symbol-joshi/index.html.

132. Nandagopal R. Menon, 'Like Modi's Government, India's Colonial Rulers Also Knew That Sight of Pyres Could Be Contentious,' *Scroll.in*, 16 May 2021, https://scroll.in/article/994599/like-modi-government-indias-colonial-rulers-also-knew-that-sight-of.

133. Tavleen Singh, 'India Feels like a Ship That Is Totally Adrift,' *Indian Express*, 25 April 2021, https://indianexpress.com/article/opinion/columns/india-covid-19-crisis-oxygen-election.

134. Dutt, 'India.'

135. 'India Surpasses 200,000 Covid Deaths amid Surge,' BBC News, 28 April 2021, https://www.bbc.co.uk/news/live/world-56890174.

136. Editorial, *The Guardian*, 24 April 2021, 2.

137. Aparna Alluri, 'India's Covid Crisis Delivers a Blow to Brand Modi,' BBC News, 8 May 2021, https://www.bbc.co.uk/news/world-asia-india-56970569.

7. CORONAVIRUS AND THE USES OF HISTORY

1. R. P. Karkaria, '1837 and 1897: Two Years of Calamities,' *Calcutta Review*, 106 (1898), 1.

2. Ibid., 20.

3. *ToI*, 6 May 1919, 7.

4. *ToI*, 22 May 1957, 6.

5. *ToI*, 14 July 1957, 5.

6. Ibid.

7. Mohammad Sajjad, 'When Will We Learn Our Lessons from Previous Pandemics?,' *Sabrangindia*, 1 June 2020, https://sabrangindia.in/article/when-will-we-learn-our-lessons-previous-pandemics.

8. Suhail-ul-Rehman Lone, 'What Epidemics from the Colonial Era Can Teach Us about Society's Response,' *The Wire*, 8 April 2020, https://thewire.in/history/colonial-era-epidemics-india.

9. Tarangini Sriraman, 'Plague Passport to Detention: Epidemic Act Was a Surveillance Tool in British India,' *ThePrint*, 22 March 2020, https://theprint.in/opinion/plague-passport-to-detention-epidemic-act-was-a-medical-surveillance-tool-in-british-india/385121/; Prerna Agarwal, 'The Government Will Come to Its Senses,' *India Forum*, 2 May 2020, www.TheIndiaForum.in.

10. Sagaree Jain, 'Anti-Asian Racism in the 1817 Cholera Pandemic,' 20 April 2020, https://daily.jstor.org/anti-asian-racism-in-the-1817-cholera-pandemic/.

11. Sheetal Chhabria, 'Pathogens Need Poverty: Manufacturing Epidemics in India,' https://www.platformspace.net/home/pathogens-need-poverty-manufacturing-epidemics-in-india.

12. Anirban Chanda and Sahil Bansal, 'The 1896 Bombay Plague: Lessons in What Not to Do,' *Outlook*, 9 April 2020, https://www.outlookindia.com/website/story/opinion-colonial-experiences-from-the-bombay-plague-of-1896-no-lessons-learned/350389.

13. Dwaipayan Banerjee, 'Fantasies of Control,' *The Caravan*, July 2020, https://www.magzter.com/article/News/The-Caravan/Fantasies-Of-Control.

14. Maura Chhun, '1918 Flu Pandemic Killed 12 Million Indians,' *The Conversation*, 17 April 2020, https://theconversation.com/1918-flu-pandemic-killed-12-million-in..rlords-indifference-strengthened-the-anti-colonial-movement-133605.

15. Hardeep Dhillon, 'The Deadly Fever,' *India Forum*, 3 September 2021, www.TheIndiaForum.in.

16. Ramachandra Guha, 'Repeating the Past,' *The Telegraph*, 24 April 2020, https://www.telegraphindia.com/opinion/cornavirus-india-the-gover...ious-minorities-during-covid-19-lockdown-and-pandemic/cid/1767769.

17. Yaqoob Khan Bangash, 'Epidemics in South Asia-I,' *News on Sunday*, 3 May 2020, https://www.thenews.com.pk/tns/detail/652672-epidemics-in-south-asia-i.

18. Yaqoob Khan Bangash, 'Epidemics in South Asia,' *News on Sunday*, 6 September 2020, https://www.thenews.com.pk/tns/detail/710480-epidemiic-in-soouth-asia.

19. Shuddhabrata Sengupta, 'Kumbh 2021: Astrology, Mortality and the Indifference to Life of Leaders and Stars,' *The Wire*, 20 April 2021, https://thewire.in/government/kumbh-2021-astrology-mortality-and-the-indifference-to-life-of-leaders-and-stars.

20. E.g., Md Toriqul Islam, 'Pandemic and Politics in Colonial Bengal: Lessons from History,' *Prothom Alo*, 15 April 2020, https://en.prothomalo.com/opinion/op-ed/pandemic-politics-in-colonial-bengal-lessons-for-history.

21. Guillaume Lachenal and Gaëtan Thomas, 'COVID-19: When History Has No Lessons,' 30 March 2020, https://www.historyworkshop.org.uk/covid-19-when-history-has-no-lessons/.

22. Robert Peckham, 'COVID-19 and the Anti-lessons of History,' *The Lancet*, 14 March 2020, 10.1016/S0140-6736(20)30468-2.

23. Dhillon, 'Deadly Fever,' quoting the Punjab sanitary commissioner's 1918 report. The same passage is quoted in Praveen Swami, 'Covid-19 in India: Leaders Are Accountable for Near-Collapse of the State,' *Firstpost*, 4 May 2021, https://www.firstpost.com/india/covid-19-in-india-leaders-are-accou...for-near-collapse-of-the-state-apocalypse-must-matter-9589821.html.

24. Sajjad, 'Lessons?'

25. Basant Kumar Mohanty, 'UGC Asks Colleges to Go Back 100 Years to Rate Covid-19 Handling,' *The Telegraph*, 13 June 2020, https://www. telegraphindia.com/india/ugc-asks-colleges-to-go-back-100-years-to-rate-coronavirus-handling/cid/1780467.

26. Chinmay Tumbe, *The Age of Pandemics: How They Shaped India and the World* (Noida: HarperCollins, 2020), 1.

27. Mike Davis, *The Monster at Our Door: The Global Threat of Avian Flu* (New York: New Press, 2005), 25; idem, *Late Victorian Holocausts: El Niño Famines and the Making of the Third World* (London: Verso, 2001).

28. Sathnam Sanghera, *Empireland: How Imperialism Has Shaped Modern Britain* (London: Viking, 2021).

29. Manjari Chatterjee Miller, *Wronged by Empire: Post-imperial Ideology and Foreign Policy in India and China* (Stanford: Stanford University Press, 2013), 17, citing Jeffrey C. Alexander, 'Toward a Theory of Cultural Trauma,' in *Cultural Trauma and Collective Identity*, ed. Jeffrey C. Alexander at al. (2004).

30. Miller, *Wronged*, 15.

31. Sunil S. Amrith, *Unruly Waters: How Mountain Rivers and Monsoons Have Shaped South Asia's History* (London: Penguin, 2018), 12.

32. Ashis Nandy, *The Intimate Enemy: Loss and Recovery of Self under Colonialism* (New Delhi: Oxford University Press, 1983); Shashi Tharoor, *Inglorious Empire: What the British Did to India* (London: Penguin, 2017).

33. Islam, 'Pandemics.'

34. Banu Subramaniam, *Holy Science: The Biopolitics of Hindu Nationalism* (Seattle: University of Washington Press, 2019), 15.

35. Richard J. Evans, *In Defence of History* (London: Granta, 1997), 59.

36. Adam Kucharski, *The Rules of Contagion: Why Things Spread—and Why They Stop* (London: Profile Books, 2020), 3.

37. Peckham, 'Covid-19.'

38. Simon Tisdall, 'Amnesty Specialises in Hard Truths: No Wonder India's Modi Froze It Out,' *The Observer*, 4 October 2020, 25.

39. For India's role in international health in the mid-twentieth century, see Sunil S. Amrith, *Decolonizing International Health: India and Southeast Asia, 1930–65* (Cambridge: Cambridge University Press, 2006); for the immunization campaign against polio: Patralekha Chatterjee, 'How India Managed to Defeat Polio,' BBC News, 13 January 2014, https://www.bbc.co.uk/news/world-asia-india-25709362.

40. Geeta Pandey, 'Narendra Modi: "Why Is the Indian PM's Photo on My Covid Vaccine Certificate?",' BBC News, 19 October 2021, https://www.bbc.co.uk/news/world-asia-india-58944475.

41. For India's antituberculosis campaign and resistance to it, see Niels Brimnes, 'Fallacy, Sacrilege, Betrayal and Conspiracy: The Cultural Construction of Opposition to Immunisation in India,' in *The Politics of Vaccination: A Global*

History, ed. Christine Holmberg, Stuart Blume, and Paul Greenough (Manchester: Manchester University Press, 2017), 51–76.

42. T. V. Padma, 'India: The Fight to Become a Science Superpower,' *Nature*, 521 (2015), https://www.nature.com/news/india-the-fight-to-become-a-science-superpowert-1.17518.

43. 'Hydroxychloroquine: India Agrees to Release Drug after Trump Retaliation Threat,' BBC News, 7 April 2020, https://www.bbc.co.uk/news/world-asia-india-52196730.

44. Jeffrey Gentleman, 'Indian Billionaires Bet Big on Head Start in Coronavirus Vaccine Race,' *New York Times*, 1 August 2020, https://www.nytimes.com/2020/08/01/world/asia/coronavirus-vaccine-india-html.

45. 'Covaxin: Concern over "Rushed" Approval for India Covid Jab,' BBC News, 4 January 2021, www.bbc.co.uk/news/world-asia-india-55526123; Soutik Biswas, 'Covaxin: What Was the Rush to Approve Homegrown Vaccine?,' BBC News, 5 January 2021, www.bbc.co.uk/news/world-asia-india-55534902.

46. Soutik Biswas, 'Covid Vaccine: India Expects to "Begin Vaccination in January,"' BBC News, 18 December 2020, https://www.bbc.co.uk/news/world-asia-india-55314709; Michael Safi, 'Vaccine Tensions Looming in Asia,' *The Observer*, 21 March 2021, 37.

47. 'COVID-19 Vaccination in India,' https://en.wikipedia.org/wiki/COVID-19_vaccination_in_India.

48. Chinki Sinha, 'Covid India: Women in Rural Bihar Hesitant to Take Vaccines,' BBC News, 1 July 2021, https://www.bbc.co.uk/news/world-asia-india-57551345.

49. *The Guardian*, 24 April 2021, 15.

50. 'Coronavirus: India Temporarily Halts Oxford-AstraZeneca Vaccine Exports,' BBC News, 24 March 2021, https://www.bbc.co.uk/news/world-asia-india-56513371.

51. Nikhil Inamdar and Aparna Alluri, 'How India's Vaccine Drive Went Horribly Wrong,' BBC News, 14 May 2021, https://www.bbc.co.uk/news/world-asia-india-57007004.

52. Aparna Alluri, 'India's Covid Vaccine Shortage: The Desperate Wait Gets Longer,' BBC News, 1 May 2021, https://www.bbc.co.uk/news/world-asia-india-56912977.

53. 'COVID-19 Vaccination.'

54. Roberts, 'Pandemics,' 8.

55. Mark Honigsbaum, *The Pandemic Century: A History of Global Contagion from the Spanish Flu to Covid-19* (London: Penguin, 2020).

56. Navin Singh Khadka, 'Why India and Nepal's Forest Fires Are Worrying Scientists,' BBC News, 12 April 2021, https://www.bbc.co.uk/news/world-asia-india-56671148.

57. Matt McGrath, 'Climate Change: Net Zero Targets Are "Pie in the Sky,"' BBC News, 1 April 2021, https://www.bbc.co.uk/news/science-environment-56596200; 'India and China Weaken Pledge to Phase Out Coal

as COP26 Ends,' *Financial Times*, 13 November 2021, https://www.ft.com/content/471c7db9-925f-479e-ad57-09162310a21a. For a defense of India's position, see David Parsons and Martin Taylor, 'Coal: Why China and India Aren't the Climate Villains of COP26,' *The Conversation*, 17 November 2021, https://theconversation.com/coal-why-china-and-india-arent-the-climate-villains-of-cop26-171879.

58. David Wallace-Wells, *The Uninhabitable Earth: A Story of the Future* (London: Penguin, 2019); Amrith, *Unruly Waters*.

59. Amitav Ghosh, *The Great Derangement: Climate Change and the Unthinkable* (Chicago: University of Chicago Press, 2016).

60. Vikas Pandey, 'Covid 19 and Pollution: "Delhi Staring at Coronavirus Disaster,"' BBC News, 20 October 2020, https://www.bbc.co.uk/news/world-asia-india-54596245; 'Air Quality Index: Delhi Air Turns Toxic after Diwali Fireworks,' BBC News, 5 November 2021, https://www.bbc.co.uk/news/world-asia-india-59172888.

CONCLUSION

1. Alex de Waal, *Famine that Kills: Darfur, Sudan, 1984–85* (Oxford: Oxford University Press, 1989), 6.

BIBLIOGRAPHY

Archival Sources

India Office Records, British Library, London
Board's Collections, F/4
India Education (Sanitary), Home (Judicial), Home (Public), Revenue and
Agriculture (Famine)
Bengal Judicial, Municipal (Sanitation)
Bombay Revenue (Famine)
Madras Board of Revenue
Lawrence Papers, MSS Eur. F. 143/65
Willingdon Papers, MSS Eur. F. 93/1

National Archives of India, New Delhi

India Home (Judicial), Home (Legislative), Home (Medical), Home (Public),
Home (Sanitary)

Official Reports and Publications

The Etiology and Epidemiology of Plague: A Summary of the Work of the Plague Commission,
Calcutta: Superintendent of Government Printing, 1908.
*Proceedings of the International Sanitary Conference Opened at Constantinople on the 13th
February 1866*, Calcutta: Superintendent of Government Printing, 1868.
Punjab Plague Manual, Lahore: Punjab Government Press, 1909.
Report of the Cholera Committee, Madras: Gantz, 1868.
*Report of the Commissioners Appointed to Inquire into the Cholera Epidemic of 1861 in
Northern India*, Calcutta: Cutter, 1864.
Report of the Pilgrim Committee: Bihar and Orissa, 1913, Simla: Government Central
Branch Press 1915.

Report Regarding the Control of Pilgrimages in the Madras Presidency, Madras: Gantz, 1868.

Rules Regarding the Measures to Be Adopted on the Outbreak of Cholera or the Appearance of Small-Pox, Calcutta: Office of Superintendent of Government Printing, 1870.

Blunt, E. A. H., *Census of India, 1911, XV: 1, United Provinces, Report*, Allahabad: Government Press, United Provinces, 1912.

Boag, G. T., *Census of India, 1921, XIII: 1, Madras, Report*, Madras: Government Press, 1923.

Edye, E. H. H., *Census of India, 1921, XVI: 1, United Provinces, Report*, Allahabad: Government Press, United Provinces, 1923.

Gopalaswami, R. A., *Census of India, 1951, 1: 1A, Report*, Delhi: Government of India, Manager of Publications, 1957.

Lloyd, G. T., *Census of India, 1921, III: 1, Assam, Report*, Shillong: Government Press, 1923.

Middleton, L., and S. M. Jacob, *Census of India, 1921, XV: 1, Punjab, Report*, Lahore: Civil and Military Gazette, 1923.

Sedgwick, L. J., *Census of India, 1921, VIII, 1: Bombay, Report*, Bombay: Government Central Press, 1922.

Tallents, P. C., *Census of India, 1921, VII: 1, Bihar and Orissa, Report*, Patna: Superintendent of Government Printing, Bihar and Orissa, 1923.

Official Series

Annual Report of the Director of Public Health (various provinces).
Annual Report on the Municipal Administration of Calcutta.
Annual Report of the Municipal Commissioner for the City of Bombay.
Annual Report of the Sanitary Commissioner (India and provinces).
Reports on the Native Press (various provinces).

Printed Sources

Ackerknecht, Erwin H., *History and Geography of the Most Important Diseases*, New York: Hafner Publishing, 1965.

Ali, Ahmed, *Twilight in Delhi*, New York: New Directions, 1994.

Amrith, Sunil S., *Decolonizing International Health: India and Southeast Asia, 1930–65*, Cambridge: Cambridge University Press, 2006.

———, *Unruly Waters: How Mountain Rivers and Monsoons Have Shaped South Asia's History*, London: Penguin, 2018.

Annesley, James, *Sketches of the Most Prevalent Diseases of India*, London: Underwood, 1829.

Anon., 'The Asiatic Cholera,' *Fraser's Magazine*, December 1831, 613–25.

Antrobus, H. A., *A History of the Assam Company, 1839–1953*, Edinburgh: T. and A. Constable, 1957. *The Army in India and Its Evolution*, Calcutta: Superintendent, Government Printing, 1924.

Arnold, Catharine, *Pandemic 1918: The Story of the Deadliest Influenza in History*, London: Michael O'Mara, 2018.

Arnold, David, *Burning the Dead: Hindu Nationhood and the Global Construction of Indian Tradition*, Oakland: University of California Press, 2021.

———, 'Cholera and Colonialism in British India,' *Past and Present*, no. 113 (1986), 118–51.

———, *Colonizing the Body: State Medicine and Epidemic Disease in Nineteenth-Century India*, Berkeley: University of California Press, 1993.

———, 'Hunger in the Garden of Plenty: The Bengal Famine of 1770,' in *Dreadful Visitations: Confronting Natural Catastrophe in the Age of Enlightenment*, ed. Alessa Johns, New York: Routledge, 1999, 81–111.

———, 'Looting, Grain Riots and Government Policy in South India, 1918,' *Past and Present*, 84 (1979), 111–45.

———, 'Picturing Plague: Photography, Pestilence and Cremation in Late Nineteenth- and Early Twentieth-Century India,' in *Plague Image and Imagination from Medieval to Modern Times*, ed. Christos Lynteris, London: Palgrave Macmillan, 2021, 111–39.

———, 'Touching the Body: Perspectives on the Indian Plague, 1896–1900,' *Subaltern Studies V*, ed. Ranajit Guha, New Delhi: Oxford University Press, 1987, 55–90.

Arnold, David, ed., *Warm Climates and Western Medicine: The Emergence of Tropical Medicine, 1500–1900*, Amsterdam: Rodopi, 1996.

Athukorala, Prema-Chandra, and Chaturica Athukorala, 'The Great Influenza Pandemic of 1918–20: An Interpretive Survey at the Time of Covid-19,' discussion paper, Centre for Economic History, Australian National University, Canberra, 2020.

Attewell, Guy N. A., *Refiguring Unani Tibb: Plural Healing in Late Colonial India*, Hyderabad: Orient Longman, 2007.

Bala, Ruby, 'The Spread of Influenza Epidemic in the Punjab (1918–1919),' *Proceedings of the Indian History Congress*, 72 (2011), 986–96.

Banerjea, A. C., 'Note on Cholera in the United Provinces,' *Indian Journal of Medical Research*, 39: 1 (1951), 17–40.

Bannerman, W. B., *The Plague Prophylactic: What It Is, How It Is Prepared, and What Its Uses Are*, Bombay: Government Central Press, 1905.

———, *Statistics of Inoculations with Haffkine's Anti-plague Vaccine, 1897–1900*, Bombay: Government Central Press, 1900.

Barry, John M., *The Great Influenza: The Story of the Greatest Pandemic in History*, London: Penguin, 2004.

Bayly, C. A., *The Local Roots of Indian Politics: Allahabad, 1880–1920*, Oxford: Oxford University Press, 1975.

Beals, Alan R., 'Interplay among Factors of Change in a Mysore Village,' in *Village India*, ed. McKim Marriott, Chicago: University of Chicago Press, 1955, 78–101.

Beiner, Guy, 'Out in the Cold and Back: New-Found Interest in the Great Flu,' *Cultural and Social History*, 3: 4 (2006), 496–505.

Bellew, H. W., *The History of Cholera in India from 1862 to 1881*, London: Trübner, 1885.

Berger, Rachel, 'From the Biomoral to the Biopolitical: Ayurveda's Political Histories,' *South Asian History and Culture*, 4: 1 (2013), 48–64.

Best, James W., *Forest Life in India*, London: John Murray, 1935.

Bewell, Alan, *Romanticism and Colonial Disease*, Baltimore: Johns Hopkins University Press, 1999.

Bhattacharyya, Debjani, *Empire and Ecology in the Bengal Delta: The Making of Calcutta*, Cambridge: Cambridge University Press, 2018.

Biswas, Samata, 'Bringing the Border Home: Indian Partition 2020,' in *Borders of an Epidemic: COVID-19 and Migrant Workers*, ed. Ranabir Samaddar, Kolkata: Calcutta Research Group, 2020, 104–14.

Bloch, Marc, *The Royal Touch: Sacred Monarchy and Scrofula in England and France*, trans. J. E. Anderson [originally published as *Les rois thaumaturges*], London: Routledge and Kegan Paul, 1973.

Bose, Koilas Chandra, 'Epidemic Influenza in and around the City of Calcutta,' *Indian Medical Gazette*, 55: 5 (1920), 169–74.

Brahmachari, U. N., and S. N. Ghosh, 'The Bacteriology of the Blood and Treatment of Influenza Occurring Epidemically in Calcutta,' *Indian Medical Gazette*, 54: 3 (1919), 90–2.

Brewis, Georgina, '"Fill Full the Mouth of Famine": Voluntary Action in Famine Relief in India, 1896–1901,' *Modern Asian Studies*, 44: 4 (2010), 887–918.

Brimnes, Niels, 'Fallacy, Sacrilege, Betrayal and Conspiracy: The Cultural Construction of Opposition to Immunisation in India,' in *The Politics of Vaccination: A Global History*, ed. Christine Holmberg, Stuart Blume, and Paul Greenough, Manchester: Manchester University Press, 2017, 51–76.

Bristow, Nancy K., *American Pandemic: The Lost Worlds of the 1918 Influenza Epidemic*, Oxford: Oxford University Press, 2012.

British Medical Journal, Editorial, 'The Teachings of the Late Epidemic of Cholera,' 9 May 1868, 456.

Brown, Judith M., *Gandhi's Rise to Power: Indian Politics, 1915–1922*, Cambridge: Cambridge University Press, 1972.

Bryden, James L., *Epidemic Cholera in the Bengal Presidency*, Calcutta: Superintendent of Government Printing, 1869.

Burnet, F. M., *Natural History of Infectious Disease*, 2nd ed., Cambridge: Cambridge University Press, 1953.

Bynum, W. F., 'Policing Hearts of Darkness: Aspects of the International Sanitary Conferences,' *History and Philosophy of the Life Sciences*, 15: 3 (1993), 421–34.

Campbell, J. M., *Report of the Bombay Plague Committee on the Plague in Bombay, 1st July 1897 to the 30th April 1898*, Bombay: Times of India, 1898.

Cantlie, James, 'Plague and Its Spread,' *Journal of the Royal Society of Arts*, 59: 3042 (1911), 434–41.

Carpenter, Charles C. J., William B. Greenough, and Robert S. Gordon, 'Pathogenesis and Pathophysiology of Cholera,' in *Cholera*, ed. Dhiman Barua and William Burrows, Philadelphia: Saunders, 1974, 129–31.

Catanach, I. J., '"Fatalism"? Indian Responses to Plague and Other Crises,' *Asian Profile*, 12: 2 (1984), 183–92.

———, 'The "Globalization" of Disease? India and the Plague,' *Journal of World History*, 12: 1 (2001), 131–53.

———, 'Plague and the Tensions of Empire, 1896–1918,' in *Imperial Medicine and Indigenous Societies*, ed. David Arnold, Manchester: Manchester University Press, 1988, 149–71.

———, 'Poona Politicians and the Plague,' *South Asia*, 7: 2 (1984), 1–18.

Cell, John W., *Hailey: A Study in British Imperialism, 1872–1969*, Cambridge: Cambridge University Press, 1992.

Chakrabarti, Pratik, *Bacteriology in British India: Laboratory Medicine and the Tropics*, Rochester, NY: Rochester University Press, 2012.

Chakrabarty, Dipesh, *Provincializing Europe: Postcolonial Thought and Historical Difference*, Princeton: Princeton University Press, 2000.

Chandavarkar, Rajnarayan, *The Origins of Industrial Capitalism in India: Business Strategies and the Working Classes in Bombay, 1900–1940*, Cambridge: Cambridge University Press, 1994.

———, 'Plague Panic and Epidemic Politics in India, 1896–1914,' in *Epidemics and Ideas: Essays on the Historical Perception of Pestilence*, ed. Terence Ranger and Paul Slack, Cambridge: Cambridge University Press, 1992, 203–40.

Chandra, Siddharth, and Julia Christensen, 'Preparing for Pandemic Influenza,' *Journal of World Historical Information*, 3–4: 1 (2016–17), 19–30.

Chandra, Siddharth, Goran Kuljanin, and Jennifer Wray, 'Mortality from the Influenza Pandemic of 1918–19: The Case of India,' *Demography*, 49: 3 (2012), 857–65.

Charters, Erica, and Richard A. McKay, 'The History of Science and Medicine in the Context of COVID-19,' *Centaurus*, 62: 2 (2020), 223–33.

Chatterjee, Meera, *Implementing Health Policy*, New Delhi: Manohar, 1988.

Christie, A. T., *Observations on the Nature and Treatment of Cholera*, Edinburgh: Maclachlan and Stewart, 1828.

Clemow, Frank G., *The Geography of Disease*, Cambridge: Cambridge University Press, 1903.

Clutterbuck, George W., *In India, the Land of Famine and of Plague*, London: Ideal Publishing Union, 1897.

Cohn, Samuel K., *Epidemics: Hate and Compassion from the Plague of Athens to AIDS*, Oxford: Oxford University Press, 2018.

Condon, J. K., *The Bombay Plague: Being a History of the Progress of Plague in the Bombay Presidency from September 1896 to June 1899*, Bombay: Education Society, 1900.

Cook, J. Neild, *Report of the Epidemics of Plague in Calcutta during the Years 1898–99, 1899–1900 and up to 30th June 1900-01*, Calcutta: Municipal Press, 1900.

Corbett, Jim, *The Man-Eaters of Kumaon*, London: Oxford University Press, 1952.

Couchman, M. E., *Account of the Plague Administration in the Bombay Presidency, from September 1896 till May 1897*, Bombay: Government Central Press, 1897.

Cowell, Rita R., 'Global Climate and Infectious Disease: The Cholera Paradigm,' *Science*, 274: 5295 (1996), 2025–31.

Crawford, Arthur, *Our Troubles in Poona and the Deccan*, Westminster: Constable, 1897.

Crooke, William, *Religion and Folklore of Northern India*, 3rd ed., London: Oxford University Press, 1926.

Crosby, Alfred W., *America's Forgotten Pandemic: The Influenza of 1918*, 2nd ed., Cambridge: Cambridge University Press, 1989.

Cueto, Marcos, Theodore M. Brown, and Elizabeth Fee, *The World Health Organization: A History*, Cambridge: Cambridge University Press, 2019.

Das, Santanu, *India, Empire, and First World War Culture: Writings, Images, and Songs*, Cambridge: Cambridge University Press, 2018.

Davis, Kingsley, *The Population of India and Pakistan*, Princeton: Princeton University Press, 1951.

Davis, Mike, *Late Victorian Holocausts: El Niño Famines and the Making of the Third World*, London: Verso, 2001.

————, *The Monster at Our Door: The Global Threat of Avian Flu*, New York: New Press, 2005.

De Waal, Alex, *Famine That Kills: Darfur, Sudan, 1984–85*, Oxford: Oxford University Press, 1989.

Digby, William, *The Famine Campaign in Southern India, 1876–78*, 2 vols., London: Longmans, Green, 1878.

Doniger, Wendy, *The Hindus: An Alternative History*, New York: Penguin, 2009.

Drèze, Jean, 'Famine Prevention in India,' in *The Political Economy of Hunger*, vol. 2: *Famine Prevention*, ed. Jean Drèze and Amartya Sen, Oxford: Clarendon Press, 1991, 13–122.

Drèze, Jean, and Amartya Sen, *An Uncertain Glory: India and Its Contradictions*, London: Allen Lane, 2013.

Dutt, Ashok K., Rais Akhtar, and Melinda McVeigh, 'Surat Plague of 1994 Reexamined,' *Southeast Asian Journal of Tropical Medicine and Public Health*, 37: 4 (2006), 755–60.

Dutton, H. R., 'Note on a Recent Outbreak of Influenza,' *Indian Medical Gazette*, 56: 2 (1921), 56.

Echenberg, Myron, *Plague Ports: The Global Urban Impact of Bubonic Plague, 1894–1901*, New York: New York University Press, 2007.

Eisenberg, Merle, and Lee Mordechai, 'The Justinianic Plague and Global Pandemics: The Making of the Plague Concept,' *American Historical Review*, 125: 5 (2020), 1632–67.

Eliade, Mircea, *Patterns in Comparative Religion*, London: Sheed and Ward, 1958.

Ellinwood, DeWitt C., 'The Indian Soldier, the Indian Army, and Change, 1914–1918,' in *India and World War I*, ed. DeWitt C. Ellinwood and S. D. Pradhan, New Delhi: Manohar, 1978, 177–211.

Enthoven, R. E., *The Folklore of Bombay*, Oxford: Clarendon Press, 1924.

Erikson, Erik H., *Gandhi's Truth: On the Origins of Militant Nonviolence*, London: Faber and Faber, 1970.

Evans, Nicholas H. A., 'Blaming the Rat? Accounting for Plague in Colonial Indian Medicine,' *Medicine, Anthropology, Theory*, 5: 3 (2018), 15–42.

Evans, Richard J., *In Defence of History*, London: Granta, 1997.

——, *The Pursuit of Power: Europe, 1815–1914*, London: Penguin, 2017.

Ewart, Joseph, *A Digest of the Vital Statistics of the European and Native Armies in India*, London: Smith, Elder, 1859.

Fenske, James, Bishnupriya Gupta, and Song Yuan, 'Demographic Shocks and Women's Labor Market Participation: Evidence from the 1918 Influenza Pandemic in India,' discussion paper 15077, Centre for Economic Policy Research, London, 2020.

Ferguson, Neil, 'Poverty, Death, and a Future Influenza Pandemic,' *The Lancet*, 23 December 2006, 2187–8.

Ferrell, D. W., 'The Rowlatt Satyagraha in Delhi,' in *Essays on Gandhian Politics: The Rowlatt Satyagraha of 1919*, ed. R. Kumar, Oxford: Clarendon Press, 1971, 189–235.

Fischer-Tiné, Harald, *Shyamji Krishnavarma: Sanskrit, Sociology and Anti-imperialism*, London: Routledge, 2014.

Forbes, Geraldine, *Women in India*, Cambridge: Cambridge University Press, 1996.

Forth, Aidan, *Barbed Wire Imperialism: Britain's Empire of Camps, 1873–1903*, Oakland: University of California Press, 2017.

Foucault, Michel, *The Order of Things: An Archaeology of the Human Sciences*, trans. Alan Sheridan, London: Tavistock Publications, 1970.

——, *The Archaeology of Knowledge*, trans. Alan Sheridan, London: Tavistock Publications, 1972.

Furnell, M. C., *Cholera and Water in India*, London: J. and A. Churchill, 1887.

Ganguly, Sumit, 'Mangling the COVID Crisis: India's Response to the Pandemic,' *Washington Quarterly*, 43: 4 (2021), 105–20.

Ghosh, Amitav, *The Great Derangement: Climate Change and the Unthinkable*, Chicago: University of Chicago Press, 2016.

Ghosh, Tanushree, 'Witnessing Famine: The Testimonial Work of Famine Photographs and Anti-colonial Spectatorship,' *Journal of Visual Culture*, 18: 3 (2019), 327–57.

Gill, Clifford Allchin, 'The Epidemiology of Plague,' *The Lancet*, 25 January 1908, 213–16.

——, *The Genesis of Epidemics and the Natural History of Disease*, London: Ballière, Tindall, and Cox, 1928.

Gould, William, *Hindu Nationalism and the Language of Politics in Late Colonial India*, Cambridge: Cambridge University Press, 2004.

Guha, Sumit, *Health and Population in South Asia: From the Earliest Times to the Present Day*, London: Hurst, 2001.

——, 'India in the Pandemic Age,' *Indian Economic Review*, 55: 1 (2020), 13–30.

Gupta, Shreekant, 'Pandemics, COVID-19 and India,' *Indian Economic Review*, 55: 1 (2020), 1–12.

Haffkine, W. M., *Anti-cholera Inoculation*, Calcutta: Thacker, Spink, 1895.

Hamlin, Christopher, *Cholera: The Biography*, Oxford: Oxford University Press, 2009.

Hardiman, David, 'The Influenza Epidemic of 1918 and the *Adivasis* of Western India,' *Social History of Medicine*, 25: 3 (2012), 644–64.

Harnetty, Peter, 'The Famine That Never Was: Christian Missionaries in India, 1918–1919,' *Historian*, 63: 3 (2001), 555–75.

Harrison, Mark, *Climates and Constitutions: Health, Race, Environment and British Imperialism in India, 1600–1850*, New Delhi: Oxford University Press, 1999.

———, *Contagion: How Commerce Has Spread Disease*, New Haven: Yale University Press, 2012.

———, 'A Dreadful Scourge: Cholera in Early Nineteenth-Century India,' *Modern Asian Studies*, 54: 2 (2020), 502–53.

———, *Medicine in an Age of Commerce and Empire: Britain and Its Tropical Colonies*, Oxford: Oxford University Press, 2010.

———, 'Pandemics,' in *The Routledge History of Disease*, ed. Mark Jackson, London: Routledge, 2016, 129–46.

———, 'A Question of Locality: The Identity of Cholera in British India, 1860–1890,' in *Warm Climates and Western Medicine: The Emergence of Tropical Medicine, 1500–1900*, ed. David Arnold, Amsterdam: Rodopi, 1996, 133–59.

Harriss, John, '"Responding to an Epidemic Requires a Compassionate State": How Has the Indian State Been Doing in the Time of COVID-19?,' *Journal of Asian Studies*, 79: 3 (2020), 609–20.

Hecker, J. F. C., *The Epidemics of the Middle Ages*, 2nd ed., trans. B. G. Babington, London: George Woodfall and Son, 1835.

Heiser, Victor, *An American Doctor's Odyssey: Adventures in Forty-Five Countries*, New York: W. W. Norton, 1936.

[Higginbottom, Sam], *Sam Higginbottom, Farmer: An Autobiography*, New York: Charles Scribner's Sons, 1949.

Hill, Kenneth, 'Influenza in India in 1918: Excess Mortality Reassessed,' *Genus*, 67: 2 (2011), 9–29.

Hirsch, August, *Handbook of Geographical and Historical Pathology*, vol. I: *Acute Infective Diseases*, trans. Charles Creighton, London: New Sydenham Society, 1883.

———, *Handbuch der Historisch-Geographischen Pathologie*, 2 vols., Erlangen: Verlag von Ferdinand Enke, 1859.

Hirst, L. Fabian, *The Conquest of Plague: A Study of the Evolution of Epidemiology*, Oxford: Clarendon Press, 1953.

Honigsbaum, Mark, *The Pandemic Century: A History of Global Contagion from the Spanish Flu to Covid-19*, London: Penguin, 2020.

Hora, Sunder Lal, 'Worship of the Deities Ola, Jhola and Bon Bibi in Lower Bengal,' *Journal of the Asiatic Society of Bengal*, 29: 1 (1933), 1–4.

Hornabrook, R. W., *Report on the Dharwar Plague Hospital, August 28th – December 18th 1898*, Dharwar: Dharwar Plague Hospital, 1899.

Howard-Jones, Norman, *The Scientific Background of the International Sanitary Conferences, 1851–1938*, Geneva: WHO, 1975.

Huber, Valeska, 'The Unification of the Globe by Disease? The International Sanitary Conferences on Cholera, 1851–1894,' *Historical Journal*, 49: 2 (2006), 453–76.

Hume, John C., 'Rival Traditions: Western Medicine and Yunan-i Tibb in the Punjab, 1849–1889,' *Bulletin of the History of Medicine*, 51: 2 (1977), 214–31.

Hunter, W. W., *Orissa*, 2 vols., London: Smith, Elder, 1872.

Hyson, Samuel, and Alan Lester, '"British India on Trial": Brighton Military Hospitals and the Politics of Empire in World War I,' *Journal of Historical Geography*, 38: 1 (2012), 18–34.

Indian Medical Gazette, Editorial, 'Influenza,' 25: 4 (1890), 112–13.

Indian Medical Gazette, Editorial, 'Influenza and Other Respiratory Infections,' 56: 7 (1921), 261–2.

Indian Medical Gazette, Editorial, 'On the Seven Scourges of India', 59: 7 (1924), 351–5.

Jaffrelot, Christophe, *Modi's India: Hindu Nationalism and the Rise of Ethnic Democracy*, trans. Cynthia Schoch, Princeton: Princeton University Press, 2021.

Jalan, Jyotsna, and Arijit Sen, 'Controlling a Pandemic with Public Actions and Public Trust: The Kerala Story,' *Indian Economic Review*, 55: 1 (2020), 105–24.

Jameel, Shahid, 'On Ecology and Environment as Drivers of Human Disease and Pandemics,' *ORF Issue Brief*, no. 388, July 2020.

James, C. H., *Report on the Outbreak of Plague in the Jullundur and Hoshiapur Districts of the Punjab during the Year 1898–99*, Lahore: Punjab Government Press, 1902.

James, Paul, and Manfred Steger, 'A Genealogy of "Globalization": The Career of a Concept,' *Globalizations*, 11: 4 (2014), 417–34.

Jameson, James, *Report on the Epidemick Cholera Morbus, as It Visited the Territories Subject to the Presidency of Bengal in the Years 1817, 1818 and 1819*, Calcutta: Government Gazette Press, 1820.

Jayakar, M. R., *The Story of My Life*, 2 vols., Bombay: Asia Publishing House, 1958.

Jeffery, Roger, *The Politics of Health in India*, Berkeley: University of California Press, 1988.

Johns, Maria K., 'The Violence of Abandonment: Urban Indigenous Health and the Settler-Colonial Politics of Nonrecognition in the United States and Australia,' *Native American and Indigenous Studies*, 7: 1 (2020), 87–120.

Johnson, David A., 'New Delhi's All-India War Memorial (India Gate): Death, Monumentality and the Lasting Legacy of Empire in India,' *Journal of Imperial and Commonwealth History*, 46: 2 (2018), 345–66.

Johnson, Niall, *Britain and the 1918–19 Influenza Pandemic: A Dark Epilogue*, Abingdon: Routledge, 2006.

Johnson, Niall, and Juergen Mueller, 'Updating the Accounts: Global Mortality of the 1918–20 "Spanish" Influenza Pandemic,' *Bulletin of the History of Medicine*, 76: 1 (2002), 105–15.

Jordan, Edwin O., *Epidemic Influenza: A Survey*, Chicago: American Medical Association, 1927.

Kant, Lalit, and Randeep Guleria, 'Pandemic Flu 1918: After Hundred Years, India Is as Vulnerable,' *Indian Journal of Medical Research*, 147: 3 (2018), 221–4.

Kanungo, S., et al., 'Cholera in India: An Analysis of Reports, 1997–2006,' *Bulletin of the World Health Organization*, 88: 3 (2010), 185–91.

Karkaria, R. P., '1837 and 1897: Two Years of Calamities,' *Calcutta Review*, 106 (1898), 1–20.

Kaur, Ravinder, and Sumathi Ramaswamy, 'The Goddess and the Virus,' in *The Pandemic: Perspectives on Asia*, ed. Vinayak Chaturvedi, Ann Arbor: Association for Asian Studies, 2020, 75–94.

Kennedy, Margaret F., *Flame of the Forest: Canadian Presbyterians in India*, Ontario: Board of World Missions, c.1980.

Kennedy, R. H., *Notes on the Epidemic Cholera*, Calcutta: Baptist Mission Press, 1827.

Kerr, Ian J., *Building the Railways of the Raj, 1850–1900*, Delhi: Oxford University Press, 1995.

Khailkova, Venera, 'The Ayurveda of Baba Ramdev: Biomoral Consumerism, National Duty and the Politics of "Homegrown" Medicine in India,' *South Asia*, 40: 1 (2017), 105–22.

Khan, Enayattulah, 'Visitations of Plague in Mughal India,' *Proceedings of the Indian History Congress*, 74 (2013), 305–12.

King, H. H., and C. G. Pandit, 'A Summary of the Rat-Flea Survey of the Madras Presidency,' *Indian Journal of Medical Research*, 19: 2 (1931), 357–92.

Kingsbury, Benjamin, *An Imperial Disaster: The Bengal Cyclone of 1876*, London: Hurst, 2018.

Klein, Ira, 'Cholera Therapy and Treatment in Nineteenth Century India,' *Journal of Indian History*, 58 (1980), 35–51.

———, 'Death in India, 1871–1921,' *Journal of Asian Studies*, 32: 4 (1973), 639–59.

———, 'Plague, Policy and Popular Unrest in British India,' *Modern Asian Studies*, 22: 4 (1988), 723–55.

———, 'Population Growth and Mortality in British India, Part 1: The Climacteric of Death,' *Indian Economic and Social History Review*, 26: 4 (1989), 387–403.

———, 'Population Growth and Mortality in British India, Part 2: The Demographic Revolution,' *Indian Economic and Social History Review*, 27: 1 (1990), 33–63.

———, 'When the Rains Failed: Famine, Relief, and Mortality,' *Indian Economic and Social History Review*, 21: 2 (1984), 185–214.

Kucharski, Adam, *The Rules of Contagion: Why Things Spread—and Why They Stop*, London: Profile Books, 2020.

Ladurie, Emmanuel Le Roy, *The Mind and Method of the Historian*, trans. Sian Reynolds, Brighton: Harvester Press, 1981.

Lal, Vinay, *The Fury of COVID-19: The Politics, Histories, and Unrequited Love of the Coronavirus*, New Delhi: Macmillan, 2020.

The Lancet, Editorial, 'Cholera: A Forecast and Forewarning,' 25 May 1867, 632.

Langford, Christopher, 'Did the 1918–19 Influenza Pandemic Originate in China?,' *Population and Development Review*, 31: 3 (2005), 473–505.

Laxminarayan, Ramanan, Shahid Jameel, and Swarup Sarkar, 'India's Battle against COVID-19: Progress and Challenges,' *American Journal of Tropical Medicine and Hygiene* 103: 4 (2020), 1343–7.

Lee, Kelley, and Richard Dodgson, 'Globalization and Cholera: Implications for Global Governance,' *Global Governance*, 6: 2 (2000), 213–36.

Leigh, M. S., *The Punjab and the War*, Lahore: Government Printing, Punjab, 1922.

Liston, W. Glen, *The Cause and Prevention of the Spread of Plague in India*, Bombay: Times Press, 1908.

Lombardo, Nick, 'Controlling Mobility and Regulation in Urban Space: Muslim Pilgrims to Mecca in Colonial Bombay, 1880–1914,' *International Journal of Urban and Regional Research*, 40: 5 (2016), 983–99.

Longrigg, James, 'Epidemic, Ideas and Classical Athenian Society,' in *Epidemics and Ideas: Essays on the Historical Perception of Pestilence*, ed. Terence Ranger and Paul Slack, Cambridge: Cambridge University Press, 1992, 21–44.

Lukis, C. P., and R. J. Blackham, *Tropical Hygiene for Anglo-Indians and Indians*, Calcutta: Thacker, Spink, 1911.

McDonald, Ian, '"Physiological Patriots?" The Politics of Physical Culture and Hindu Nationalism in India,' *International Review for the Sociology of Sport*, 34: 4 (1999), 343–58.

M'Gregor, James, *Medical Sketches of the Expedition to Egypt from India*, London: J. Murray, 1804.

Maclean, Kama, *Pilgrimage and Power: The Kumbh Mela in Allahabad, 1765–1954*, Oxford: Oxford University Press, 2008.

Maclean, William Campbell, *Diseases of Tropical Climates*, London: Macmillan, 1886.

McMillen, Christian W., *Pandemics: A Very Short Introduction*, Oxford: Oxford University Press, 2016.

McNeill, J. R., and William H. McNeill, *The Human Web: A Bird's-Eye View of World History*, New York: W. W. Norton, 2003.

McNeill, William H., *Plagues and Peoples*, Harmondsworth: Penguin, 1979.

Macpherson, John, *Annals of Cholera from the Earliest Periods to the Year 1817*, London: Ranken, 1872.

MacWatt, R. C., *Report on Malaria in the Punjab during the Year 1918*, Lahore: Superintendent of Government Printing, Punjab, 1919.

Mahalanabis, D., A. B. Choudhuri, N. G. Bagchi, A. K. Bhattacharya, and T. W. Simpson, 'Oral Fluid Therapy of Cholera among Bangladesh Refugees,' *WHO South-East Asia Journal of Public Health*, 1: 1 (2012), 105–12.

Mahammadh, Vempalli Raj, 'Plague Mortality and Control Policies in Colonial South India, 1900–47,' *South Asia Research*, 40: 3 (2020), 323–43.

[Maitland, Julia], *Letters from Madras, during the Years 1836–1839, by a Lady*, London: John Murray, 1846.

Malone, R. H., 'A Bacteriological Investigation of Influenza Carried Out under the Indian Research Fund Association,' *Indian Journal of Medical Research*, 7: 3 (1919–20), 495–518.

Mander, Harsh, *Locking Down the Poor: The Pandemic and India's Moral Centre*, New Delhi: Speaking Tiger, 2020.

Márquez, Gabriel García, *Love in the Time of Cholera*, trans. Edith Grossman, London: Penguin, 1989.

Marten, J. T., 'The Census of India of 1921,' *Journal of the Royal Society of Arts*, 71: 3672 (1923), 355–71.

Martin, James Ranald, *The Influence of Tropical Climates on European Constitutions*, London: Churchill, 1856.

Menon, I. G. K., 'The 1957 Pandemic of Influenza in India,' *Bulletin of the World Health Organization*, 20: 2–3 (1959), 199–224.

Miller, Manjari Chatterjee, *Wronged by Empire: Post-imperial Ideology and Foreign Policy in India and China*, Stanford: Stanford University Press, 2013.

Mills, I. D., 'The 1918–1919 Influenza Pandemic: The Indian Experience,' *Indian Economic and Social History Review*, 23: 1 (1986), 1–40.

Milne, Ida, *Stacking the Coffins: Influenza, War and Revolution in Ireland, 1918–19*, Manchester: Manchester University Press, 2018.

Ministry of Health, *Report on the Pandemic of Influenza, 1918–19*, London: HMSO, 1920.

Misra, Maria, *Vishnu's Crowded Temple: India since the Great Rebellion*, New Haven: Yale University Press, 2008.

Morens, David M., Gregory K. Folkers, and Anthony S. Fauci, 'What is a Pandemic?,' *Journal of Infectious Diseases*, 200: 7 (2009), 1018–21.

Moynan, R. N. O., and D. C. Meneses, 'The Influenza Pandemic,' *Indian Medical Gazette*, 54: 1 (1919), 14–17.

Murphey, Rhoads, 'The City in the Swamp: Aspects of the Site and Early Growth of Calcutta,' *Geographical Journal*, 130: 2 (1964), 241–56.

Murray, Christopher J., Alan D. Lopez, Brian Chin, Dennis Feehan, and Kenneth H. Hill, 'Estimation of Global Pandemic Influenza Mortality on the Basis of Vital Registration Data from the 1918–20 Pandemic: A Quantitative Analysis,' *The Lancet*, 23 December 2006, 2211–18.

Murray, John, *Report on the Attack of Cholera in the Central Prison at Agra in 1856*, Agra: Secundra Orphan Press, 1856.

Nair, Aparna, '"An Egyptian Infection": War, Plague and the Quarantines of the English East India Company at Madras and Bombay, 1802,' *Hygiea Internationalis*, 8: 1 (2009), 7–29.

Nandy, Ashis, *The Intimate Enemy: Loss and Recovery of Self under Colonialism*, New Delhi: Oxford University Press, 1983.

Nathan, R., *The Plague in Northern India, 1896, 1897*, 2 vols., Simla: Government Central Printing Office, 1898.

Nehru, Jawaharlal, *An Autobiography*, Bombay: Allied Publishers, 1962.

Nelkin, Dorothy, and Sander L. Gilman, 'Placing Blame for Devastating Disease,' *Social Research*, 55: 2 (1988), 361–78.

Neuve Chapelle: India's Memorial in France, 1914–1918, London: Hodder and Stoughton, 1928.

Newsholme, Arthur, *Epidemic Diphtheria: A Research on the Origin and Spread of the Disease from an International Standpoint*, London: Swan Sonnenschein, 1898.

Nicholas, Ralph W., 'The Goddess Sitala and Epidemic Smallpox in Bengal,' *Journal of Asian Studies*, 41: 1 (1981): 21–44.

Nichols, Christopher McKnight, Nancy Bristow, E. Thomas Ewing, Joseph M. Gabriel, Benjamin C. Montoya, and Elizabeth Outka, 'Reconsidering the 1918–19 Influenza Pandemic in the Age of Covid-19,' *Journal of the Gilded Age and Progressive Era*, 19: 4 (2020), 642–72.

Nirala, Suryakant Tripathi, *A Life Misspent*, trans. Satti Khanna, New York: HarperCollins, 2016.

Nivedita, Sister, 'The Plague,' in *The Complete Works of Sister Nivedita*, 2 vols., Calcutta, 1967, 2: 340–7.

Omissi, David, *Indian Voices of the Great War: Soldiers' Letters, 1914–1918*, London: Macmillan, 1999.

Pati, Biswamoy, 'Ordering "Disorder" in a Holy City: Colonial Health Interventions in Puri during the Nineteenth Century,' in *Health, Medicine and Empire: Perspectives on Colonial India*, ed. Biswamoy Pati and Mark Harrison, New Delhi: Orient Longman, 2001, 270–98.

Patterson, K. David, and Gerald F. Pyle, 'The Geography and Mortality of the 1918 Influenza Pandemic,' *Bulletin of the History of Medicine*, 65: 1 (1991), 4–21.

Paul, S. N., *Public Opinion and British Rule: A Study of the Influence of Indian Public Opinion on British Administration and Bureaucracy (1899–1914)*, New Delhi: Metropolitan Book Co., 1979.

Peckham, Robert, *Epidemics in Modern Asia*, Cambridge: Cambridge University Press, 2016.

———, 'Symptoms of Empire: Cholera in Southeast Asia, 1820–1850,' in *The Routledge History of Disease*, ed. Mark Jackson, London: Routledge, 2016, 183–201.

Phillips, Howard, and David Killingray, eds., *The Spanish Influenza Pandemic of 1918–19: New Perspectives*, London: Routledge, 2003.

Phipson, E. S., 'The Pandemic of Influenza in India in the Year 1918,' *Indian Medical Gazette*, 58: 11 (1923), 509–24.

Plague Advisory Committee, 'On the Seasonal Prevalence of Plague in India,' *Journal of Hygiene*, 8: 2 (1908), 266–301.

Polu, Sandhya L., *Infectious Disease in India, 1892–1940: Policy-Making and the Perception of Risk*, Basingstoke: Palgrave Macmillan, 2010.

Porter, Alexander, *The Diseases of the Madras Famine of 1877–78*, Madras: Government Press, 1889.

Prasad, Ritika, *Tracks of Change: Railways and Everyday Life in Colonial India*, Cambridge: Cambridge University Press, 2015.

Rakesh, P. S., 'The Epidemic Diseases Act of 1897: Public Health Relevance in the Current Scenario,' *Indian Journal of Medical Ethics*, 1: 3 (2016), 156–60.

Ramanna, Mridula, 'Coping with the Influenza Pandemic: The Bombay Experience,' in *The Spanish Influenza Pandemic of 1918–19: New Perspectives*, ed. Howard Phillips and David Killingray, London: Routledge, 2003, 86–98.

————, *Health Care in Bombay Presidency, 1896–1930*, Delhi: Primus, 2012.

Ramaswamy, Sumathi, and Ravinder Kaur, 'The Goddess and the Virus,' in *The Pandemic: Perspectives on Asia*, ed. Vinayak Chaturvedi, Ann Arbor: Association for Asian Studies, 2020, 75–94.

Rand, W. C., *Supplement to the Account of Plague Administration in the Bombay Presidency from September 1896 till May 1897*, Bombay: Government Central Press, 1897.

Ranking, J. L., *List of Fairs and Festivals Occurring within the Limits of the Madras Presidency*, Madras: Government Press, 1868.

Ransome, Arthur, 'On the Form of the Epidemic Wave, and Some of Its Probable Causes,' *Transactions of the Epidemiological Society of London*, 1: 1 (1883), 96–107.

Renny, C., *Medical Report on the Mahamuree in Gurhwal in 1849–50*, Agra: Secundra Orphan Press, 1851.

Richards, John F., *The Unending Frontier: An Environmental History of the Early Modern World*, Berkeley: University of California Press, 2003.

Rogers, Leonard, *The Incidence and Spread of Cholera in India: Forecasting and Control of Epidemics*, Calcutta: Thacker, Spink, 1928.

————, 'Thirty Years' Research on the Control of Cholera Epidemics,' *British Medical Journal*, 23 November 1957, 1193–7.

Rolleston, J. D., 'The Smallpox Pandemic of 1870–1874,' *Proceedings of the Royal Society of Medicine*, 27: 2 (1933), 177–92.

Rosenberg, Charles E., *Explaining Epidemics and Other Studies in the History of Medicine*, Cambridge: Cambridge University Press, 1992.

Rosenberg, I. H., W. B. Greenough, J. Lindenbaum and R. S. Gordon, 'Nutritional Studies in Cholera: The Influence of Nutritional Status on Susceptibility to Infection,' in *Proceedings of the Cholera Research Symposium, January 24–29, 1965, Honolulu, Hawaii*, ed. O. A. Bushnell and S. Brookhyser, Washington, D.C.: US Government Printing Office, 1965, 68–72.

Roy, Tirthankar, 'Water, Climate, and Economy in India from 1880 to the Present,' *Journal of Interdisciplinary History*, 51: 4 (2021), 565–94.

Russell, Patrick, *A Treatise of the Plague: Containing an Historical Journal, and Medical Account, of the Plague, at Aleppo, in the Years 1760, 1761, and 1762*, London: Robinson, 1791.

Sanghera, Sathnam, *Empireland: How Imperialism Has Shaped Modern Britain*, London: Viking, 2021.

Sarker, Subhash Chandra, 'Sarat Chandra Chatterjee: The Great Humanist,' *Indian Literature*, 20: 1 (1977), 49–77.

Satia, Priya, *Time's Monster: History, Conscience and Britain's Empire*, London: Allen Lane, 2020.

Scot, William, *Report on the Epidemic Cholera as It Has Appeared in the Territories Subject to the Presidency of Fort St George*, Madras: Asylum Press, 1824.

Seal, S. C., 'Epidemiological Studies of Plague in India,' *Bulletin of the World Health Organization*, 23: 2–3 (1969), 283–92.

Sekher, T. V., 'Influenza Pandemic of 1918: Lessons in Tackling a Public Health Catastrophe,' *Economic and Political Weekly*, 22 May 2021, 32–8.

Sellwood, Chloe, 'Brief History and Epidemiological Features of Pandemic Influenza,' in *Introduction to Pandemic Influenza*, ed. Jonathan Van-Tam and Chloe Sellwood, Wallingford: CAB International, 2010, 41–56.

Sen, A. K., 'Famine Mortality: A Study of the Bengal Famine of 1943,' in *Peasants in History: Essays in Memory of Daniel Thorner*, ed. Eric J. Hobsbawm, Witold Kula, Ashok Mitra, K. N. Raj, and Ignacy Sachs, Calcutta: Oxford University Press, 1980, 194–220.

Sen, Debendra Nath, 'Influenza Observed in the Sambhu Nath Pandit Hospital, Calcutta,' *Indian Medical Gazette*, 55: 3 (1920), 89–92.

Sen, Rajendra Kumar, *A Treatise on Influenza*, North Lakmipur: R. K. Sen, 1923.

Seventh Congress of the Far Eastern Association of Tropical Medicine, *Souvenir: The Indian Empire*, Calcutta: FEATM, 1927.

Shah, Gyanshyam, *Public Health and Urban Development: The Plague in Surat*, New Delhi: Sage, 1997.

Sharma, Jayeeta, *Empire's Garden: Assam and the Making of India*, Durham, N.C.: Duke University Press, 2011.

Sheel, Alok, 'Bubonic Plague in South Bihar: Gaya and Shahabad Districts, 1900–1924,' *Indian Economic and Social History Review*, 35: 4 (1998), 421–42.

Sherman, Irwin W., *The Power of Plagues*, Washington, D.C.: ASM Press, 2006.

Shklar, Judith N., *The Faces of Injustice*, New Haven: Yale University Press, 1990.

Siegal, Benjamin Robert, *Hungry Nation: Food, Famine, and the Making of Modern India*, Cambridge: Cambridge University Press, 2018.

Simond, Marc, Margaret L. Godley, and Pierre D. E. Mouriquand, 'Paul-Louis Simond and His Discovery of the Plague Transmission by Rat Fleas: A Centenary,' *Journal of the Royal Society of Medicine*, 91: 2 (1998), 101–4.

Simpson, W. J. R., 'Plague,' *The Lancet*, 29 June 1906, 1758.

———, 'Plague,' *The Lancet*, 13 July 1907, 73–6.

———, *A Treatise on Plague: Dealing with the Historical, Epidemiological, Clinical, Therapeutic and Preventive Aspects of the Disease*, Cambridge: Cambridge University Press, 1905.

Singh, Bhupal Singh, 'Influenza,' *Indian Medical Gazette*, 55: 1 (1920), 15–18.

Singh, Madhu, 'Bombay Fever/Spanish Flu: Public Health and Native Press in Colonial Bombay, 1918–19, *South Asia Research*, 41: 1 (2021), 35–52.

BIBLIOGRAPHY

Sivaramakrishnan, Kavita, '"Endemic Risks": Influenza Pandemics, Public Health, and Making Self-reliant Indian Citizens,' *Journal of Global History*, 15: 3 (2020), 459–77.

Smart, William R. E., 'On Cholera in Insular Position,' *The Lancet*, 14 April 1873, 522–4.

Smith, David B., *Report on Pilgrimage to Juggernauth in 1868*, Calcutta: Lewis, 1868.

Snow, P. C. H., *Report on the Outbreak of Bubonic Plague in Bombay, 1896–97*, Bombay: Times of India, 1897.

Spinney, Laura, *Pale Rider: The Spanish Flu of 1918 and How It Changed the World*, London: Jonathan Cape, 2017.

Subramaniam, Banu, *Holy Science: The Biopolitics of Hindu Nationalism*, Seattle: University of Washington Press, 2019.

Sujatha, V., 'COVID-19 Pandemic and the Politics of Risk: Perspectives on Science, State and Society in India,' *Contributions to Indian Sociology*, 55: 2 (2021), 254–67.

Suri, J. C., and M. K. Sen, 'Pandemic Influenza: Indian Experience,' *Lung India*, 28: 1 (2011), 2–4.

Sussman, George D., 'Was the Black Death in India and China?,' *Bulletin of the History of Medicine*, 85: 3 (2011), 319–55.

Swaroop, Satya, 'Endemiology of Cholera in the Madras Presidency,' *Indian Journal of Medical Research*, 39: 2 (1951), 185–96.

Tandon, Prakash, *Punjabi Century, 1857–1947*, London: Chatto and Windus, 1961.

Tharoor, Shashi, *Inglorious Empire: What the British Did to India*, London: Penguin, 2017.

Tilak, Lakshmibai, *Smritichitre: The Memoirs of a Spirited Wife*, trans. Shanta Gokhale, New Delhi: Speaking Tiger, 2017.

Tumbe, Chinmay, *The Age of Pandemics, 1817–1920: How They Shaped India and the World*, Noida: HarperCollins, 2020.

———, *Pandemics and Historical Mortality in India*, Ahmedabad: Indian Institute of Management, 2020.

Turner, J. A., and B. K. Goldsmith, *Sanitation in India*, 3rd ed., Bombay: Times of India, 1922.

Twining, William, *Clinical Illustrations of the Most Important Diseases of Bengal*, Calcutta: Baptist Mission Press, 1832.

Varlik, Nükhet, 'The Plague That Never Left: Restoring the Second Pandemic to Ottoman and Turkish History in the Time of COVID-19,' *New Perspectives on Turkey*, no. 63 (2020), 176–89.

———, 'Rethinking the History of Plague in the Time of COVID-19,' *Centaurus*, 62: 2 (2020), 285–93.

Visaria, Leela, and Pravin Visaria, 'Population (1757–1947),' in *The Cambridge Economic History of India*, vol. 2, ed. Dharma Kumar, Cambridge: Cambridge University Press, 1983, 463–532.

Wacha, D. E., *Shells from the Sands of Bombay: Being My Recollections and Reminiscences, 1860–1875*, Bombay: Indian Newspaper Co., 1920.

Wagner, Kim A., *Amritsar 1919: An Empire of Fear and the Making of a Massacre*, New Haven: Yale University Press, 2019.

Wallace, Alfred Russel, *The Wonderful Century: The Age of New Ideas in Science and Innovation*, 2nd ed., London: Swan Sonnenschein, 1903.

Wallace-Wells, David, *The Uninhabitable Earth: A Story of the Future*, London: Penguin, 2019.

Watts, Sheldon, *Epidemics and History: Disease, Power and Imperialism*, New Haven: Yale University Press, 1997.

Whitcombe, Elizabeth, 'Famine Mortality,' *Economic and Political Weekly*, 5 June 1993, 1169–79.

White, F. Norman, *A Preliminary Report on the Influenza Pandemic of 1918 in India*, Simla: Government Monotype Press, 1919.

———, 'Retrospect,' *Transactions of the Royal Society of Tropical Medicine and Hygiene*, 47: 6 (1953), 441–50.

Wilkinson, E., *Report on Plague in the Punjab from October 1st, 1901, to September 30th, 1902*, Lahore: Punjab Government Gazette, 1904.

———, *Report on Plague and Inoculation in the Punjab from October 1st, 1902, to September 30th, 1903*, Lahore: Government Press, 1904.

Williams, Raymond, *Keywords: A Vocabulary of Culture and Society*, London: Fontana, 1975.

Wolmar, Christian, *Railways and the Raj: How the Age of Steam Transformed India*, London: Atlantic Books, 2017.

Worboys, Michael, 'The Emergence of Tropical Medicine: A Study in the Establishment of a Scientific Specialty,' in *Perspectives on the Emergence of Scientific Disciplines*, ed. Gerard Lemaine, Roy Macleod, Michael Mulkay, and Peter Weingart, The Hague: Mouton, 1976, 75–98.

Zeheter, Michael, *Epidemics, Empire and Environments: Cholera in Madras and Quebec City, 1818–1910*, Pittsburgh: University of Pittsburgh Press, 2015.

Unpublished Theses

Herriot, Thomas P., 'The Influenza Pandemic, 1918, as Observed in the Punjab, India,' unpublished MD thesis, University of Edinburgh, 1920.

Prior, Katherine, 'The British Administration of Hinduism in North India, 1780–1900,' unpublished PhD, University of Cambridge, 1990.

Newspaper and Online Articles

Agarwal, Prerna, 'The Government Will Come to Its Senses,' *India Forum*, 2 May 2020, www.TheIndiaForum.in.

Alluri, Aparna, 'India's Covid Crisis Delivers a Blow to Brand Modi,' BBC News, 8 May 2021, https://www.bbc.co.uk/news/world-asia-india-56970569.

———, 'India's Covid Vaccine Shortage: The Desperate Wait Gets Longer,' BBC News, 1 May 2021, https://www.bbc.co.uk/news/world-asia-india-56912977.

BIBLIOGRAPHY

Almagro-Moreno, Salvador, and Ronald K. Taylor, 'Cholera: Environmental Reservoirs and Impact on Disease Transmission,' *Microbiology Spectrum* (2013), https://doi.org/10.1128/microbiolspec.OH-0003-2012.

Anderson, Clare, David Arnold, Juanita de Barros, Luka Bair, and Robert Peckham, 'Epidemics in the Past and Now: A Roundtable on Colonial and Postcolonial History,' *Journal of Colonialism and Colonial History*, 22 (2021), doi: 10.1353/cch.2021.0003.

Apoorvanand, 'How the Coronavirus Outbreak in India Was Blamed on Muslims,' *Al Jazeera*, 18 April 2020, https://www.aljazeera.com/indepth/opinion/coronavirus-outbreak-india-blamed-muslims-200418143252362.html.

Arabindoo, Pushpa, 'Pandemic Cities: Between Mimicry and Trickery,' *City and Society*, 32 (2020), https://doi.org/10.1111/ciso.12263.

Arafath, P. K. Yasser, 'Success of the Kerala Model,' *The Telegraph*, 23 April 2020, https://www.telegraphindia.com/opinion/coronavirus-kerala-success-with...-by -its-high-level-of-literacy-and-secular-sensibilities/cid/1767508.

Avert, 'HIV and AIDS in India,' https://www.avert.org/printpdf/node/417.

Bamzai, Kaveree, 'Between Sanitiser and Gaumutra for Covid-19,' *ThePrint*, 21 March 2020, https://theprint.in/opinion/gaumutra-for-covid-19-modis-india-made-historical-choice.

Banerjee, Argha Kumar, 'Tagore and Pandemics,' *The Statesman*, 27 December 2020, https://www.thestatesman.com/opinion/tagore-and-pandemics-1502942965.html.

Banerjee, Dwaipayan, 'Fantasies of Control,' *The Caravan*, July 2020, https://www.magzter.com/article/News/The-Caravan/Fantasies-Of-Control.

Bangash, Yaqoob Khan, 'Epidemics in South Asia-I,' *News on Sunday*, 3 May 2020, https://www.thenews.com.pk/tns/detail/652672-epidemics-in-south-asia-i.

————, 'Epidemics in South Asia,' *News on Sunday*, 6 September 2020, https://www.thenews.com.pk/tns/detail/710480-epidemiic-in-soouth-asia.

Barro, Robert J., José F. Ursúa, and Joanna Weng, 'The Coronavirus and the Great Influenza Pandemic: Lessons from the "Spanish Flu" for the Coronavirus's Potential Effects on Mortality and Economic Activity,' working paper 26866, National Bureau of Economic Research, Cambridge, MA, 2020, https://doi.org/10.3386/w26866.

Basu, Ranjini, 'Migrant Agricultural Workers in India and the COVID-19 Lockdown,' *Focus on the Global South*, 29 April 2020, https://focusweb.org/migrant-agricultural-workers-in-india-and-the-covid-19-lockdown/.

BBC News, 'Air Quality Index: Delhi Air Turns Toxic after Diwali Fireworks,' 5 November 2021, https://www.bbc.co.uk/news/world-asia-india-59172888.

BBC News, 'Coronavirus: India Enters "Total Lockdown" after Spike in Cases,' 25 March 2020, https://www.bbc.co.uk/news/world-asia-india-52024239.

BBC News, 'Coronavirus: India's PM Modi Seeks "Forgiveness" over Lockdown,' 29 March 2020, https://www.bbc.co.uk/news/world-asia-india-52081396.

BBC News, 'Coronavirus: India Temporarily Halts Oxford-AstraZeneca Vaccine Exports,' 24 March 2021, https://www.bbc.co.uk/news/world-asia-india-56513371.

BBC News, 'Coronavirus: Search for Hundreds of People after Delhi Prayer Meeting,' 31 March 2020, https://www.bbc.co.uk/news/world-asia-india-52104753.

BBC News, 'Covaxin: Concern over "Rushed" Approval for India Covid Jab,' 4 January 2021, www.bbc.co.uk/news/world-asia-india-55526123.

BBC News, 'Covid: India Launches Online Memorial to Commemorate Pandemic Victims,' 2 February 2021, https://www.bbc.co.uk/news/world-asia-india-55884038.

BBC News, 'Covid: Serious Failures in WHO and Global Response, Report Finds,' 12 May 2021, https://www.bbc.co.uk/news/world-57085505.

BBC News, 'Hydroxychloroquine: India Agrees to Release Drug after Trump Retaliation Threat,' 7 April 2020, https://www.bbc.co.uk/news/world-asia-india-52196730.

BBC News, 'India Coronavirus: Four Modi Claims Fact-Checked,' 21 October 2020, https://www.bbc.co.uk/news/world-asia-india-54615353.

BBC News, 'India Coronavirus: Patients Stranded as Delhi Struggles with Covid,' 8 June 2020, https://www.bbc.co.uk/news/world-asia-india-52961589.

BBC News, 'India Covid-19: Delhi Adds Makeshift Crematoriums as Deaths Climb,' 27 April 2021, https://www.bbc.co.uk/news/world-asia-india-56897970.

BBC News, 'India Covid-19: 'PM Modi "Did Not Consult" before Lockdown,' 29 March 2021, https://www.bbc.co.uk/news/world-asia-india-56561095.

BBC News, 'India Is Now Only "Partly Free" under Modi, Says Report,' 3 March 2021, https://www.bbc.co.uk/news/world-asia-india-56249596.

BBC News, 'India PM Modi Lays Foundation for Ayodhya Ram Temple amid Covid Surge,' 5 August 2020, https://www.bbc.co.uk/news/world-asia-india-53577942.

BBC News, 'India Surpasses 200,000 Covid Deaths amid Surge,' 28 April 2021, https://www.bbc.co.uk/news/live/world-56890174.

BBC News, 'Islamophobia Concerns after India Mosque Outbreak,' 3 April 2020, https://www.bbc.co.uk/news/world-asia-india-52147260.

BBC News, 'Maharashtra: Nagpur Becomes First Major Indian City to Return to Lockdown,' 12 March 2021, https://www.bbc.co.uk/news/world-asia-india-56369590.

BBC News, 'PM Narendra Modi Gets Covid Jab as India Scales Up Vaccination,' 1 March 2021, https://www.bbc.co.uk/news/world-asia-india-56237436.

Biswas, Soutik, 'Coronavirus: Are Indians More Immune to Covid-19?,' BBC News, 2 November 2020, https://www.bbc.co.uk/news/world-asia-india-54730290.

———, 'Coronavirus: India's Pandemic Lockdown Turns into a Human Tragedy,' BBC News, 30 March 2020, www.bbc.com/news/world-asia-india-52086274.

———, 'Coronavirus: Is the Epidemic Finally Coming to an End in India?,' BBC News, 15 February 2021, https://www.bbc.co.uk/news/world-asia-india-56037565.

———, 'Coronavirus: Is the Pandemic Slowing Down in India?,' BBC News, 6 October 2020, https://www.bbc.co.uk/news/world-asia-india-54419959.

———, 'Covaxin: What Was the Rush to Approve Homegrown Vaccine?,' BBC News, 5 January 2021, www.bbc.co.uk/news/world-asia-india-55534902.

———, 'Covid-19: India Excess Deaths Cross Four Million, Says Study,' BBC News, 20 July 2021, https://www.bbc.co.uk/news/world-asia-india-57888460.

———, 'Covid Vaccine: India Expects to "Begin Vaccination in January",' BBC News, 18 December 2020, https://www.bbc.co.uk/news/world-asia-india-55314709.

———, 'India Coronavirus: How a Group of Volunteers "Exposed" Hidden Covid-19 Deaths,' BBC News, 20 November 2020, https://www.bbc.co.uk/news/world-asia-india-54985981.

———, 'India Coronavirus: The "Mystery" of Low Covid-19 Death Rates,' BBC News, 27 April 2020, https://www.bbc.co.uk/news/world-asia-india-52435463.

———, 'India's Frightful Pandemic Projections,' BBC News, 25 March 2020, https://www.bbc.co.uk/news/live/world-52026908.

———, 'Manmohan Singh's "Three Steps" to Stem India's Economic Crisis,' BBC News, 9 August 2020, https://www.bbc.co.uk/news/world-asia-india-53675858.

———, 'Why Journalists in India Are under Attack,' BBC News, 4 February 2021, https://www.bbc.co.uk/news/world-asia-india-55906345.

Brilliant, Larry, 'The Age of Pandemics,' *Wall Street Journal*, 2 May 2009, https://www.wsj.com/articles/SB124121965740478983.

Chanda, Anirban, and Sahil Bansal, 'The 1896 Bombay Plague: Lessons in What Not to Do,' *Outlook*, 9 April 2020, https://www.outlookindia.com/website/story/opinion-colonial-experiences-from-the-bombay-plague-of-1896-no-lessons-learned/350389.

Chandra, Siddharth, and Eva Kassens-Noor, 'The Evolution of Pandemic Influenza: Evidence from India,' *BMC Infectious Diseases*, 14 (2014), https://bmcinfectdis.biomedcentral.com/articles/10.1186/1471-2334-14-510#citeas.

Chanu, Naorem Pushparani, and Gorky Chakraborty, 'A Novel Virus, A New Racial Slur,' *India Forum*, 3 July 2020, https://www.theindiaforum.in/article/novel-virus-new-racial-slur.

Chatterjee, Patralekha, 'How India Managed to Defeat Polio,' BBC News, 13 January 2014, https://www.bbc.co.uk/news/world-asia-india-25709362.

Chauhan, Chetan, 'Half of All Covid Deaths in India Took Place in April–May,' *Hindustan Times*, 25 July 2021, https://www.hindustantimes.com/india-news/half-of-all-covid-deaths-in-india-took-place-in-april-may-shows-government-data-101627204345380.html.

Chhabria, Sheetal, 'Manufacturing Epidemics: Pathogens, Poverty, and Public Health Crises in India,' *India Forum*, 5 June 2020, www.TheIndiaForum.in.

———, 'Pathogens Need Poverty: Manufacturing Epidemics in India,' https://www.platformspace.net/home/pathogens-need-poverty-manufacturing-epidemics-in-india.

Chhina, Man Aman Singh, 'When Corpses of Influenza Victims Were Dumped in Narmada River in 1918,' *Indian Express*, 6 June 2021, https://indianexpress.com/article/explained/explained-when-corpse...f-influenza-victims-were-dumped-in-narmada-river-in-1918-7310909/.

Chhun, Maura, '1918 Flu Pandemic Killed 12 Million Indians,' *The Conversation*, 17 April 2020, https://theconversation.com/1918-flu-pandem ic-killed-12-million-in..rlords-indifference-strengthened-the-anti-colonial-movement-133605.

Connolly, Catherine, 'War and the Coronavirus Pandemic,' *Third World Approaches to International Law Review* (2020), https://twailr.com/war-and-the-coronavirus-pandemic/.

Daily Mail, 'Now Chinese Scientists Claim Coronavirus Originated in India,' https://www.dailymail.co.uk/news/article-8993667/Now-Chinese-scientists-claim-coronavirus-originated-INDIA-summer-2019.html.

Das, Madhuparna, '"Never Seen Such Devastation Before,"' *ThePrint*, 21 May 2020, https://theprint.in/india/never-seen-such-devastation-before-shocked-cm-mamata-says-as-cyclone-amphan-ravages-bengal/426168/.

Debray, Bibek, 'Lessons from India's Tryst with Lockdown,' *The Mint*, 25 March 2021, https://www.livemint.com/news/india/lessons-from-india-s-tryst-with-lockdown-11616599176632.html.

Desai, Shweta, and Amarnath Amarasingam, 'Corona Jihad: COVID-19, Misinformation, and Anti-Muslim Violence in India,' https://strongcitiesnetwork.org/en/coronajihad-covid-19-misinformation-and-anti-muslim-violence-in-india/.

Dhillon, Hardeep, 'The Deadly Fever,' *India Forum*, 3 September 2021, www.TheIndiaForum.in.

Dutt, Barkha, 'India: A Broken Country, A Country in Torment,' BBC News, 23 April 2021, https://www.bbc.co.uk/news/world-asia-india.

Dutta, Prabash K., 'SARS: How India Tackled Previous Coronavirus Outbreak,' *India Today*, 29 May 2020, https://www.indiatoday.in/india/story/sars-2002-03-india-coronavirus-outbreak-1683404-2020-05-29.

Ellis-Petersen, Hannah, 'The System Has Collapsed: India's Descent into Covid Hell,' *The Guardian*, 21 April 2021, https://www.theguardian.com/world/2021/apr/21/system-has-collapsed-india-descent-into-covid-hell.

Ellis-Petersen, Hannah, and Shaik Azizur Rahman, 'Coronavirus Conspiracy Theories Targeting Muslims Spread in India,' *The Guardian*, 13 April 2020, https://www.theguardian.com/world/2020/apr/13/coronavirus-conspiracy-theories-targeting-muslims-spread-in-india.

————, 'Delhi Muslims Fear They Will Never See Justice for Religious Riot Atrocities,' *The Observer*, 28 March 2020, 24–5.

Ellis-Petersen, Hannah, and Saurabh Sharma, 'Stench of Death Pervades Rural India as Ganges Swells with Covid Victims,' *The Guardian*, 20 May 2021, https://www.theguardian.com/world/2021/may/20/stench-death-pervades-rural-india-ganges-swells-covid-victims.

Farzan, Antonia Noori, 'Amid "Heartbreaking" Coronavirus Surge in India, Government Orders Twitter to Remove Posts Critical of Response,' *Washington Post*, 26 April 2021, https://www.washingtonpost.com.world/2021/04/26/twitter-india-coronavirus/.

Financial Times, 'India and China Weaken Pledge to Phase Out Coal as COP26 Ends,' 13 November 2021, https://www.ft.com/content/471c7db9-925f-479e-ad57-09162310a21a.

Focus on the Global South, 'Statement Condemning Crackdown on Women Activists in Delhi,' 7 May 2020, https://focusweb.org/statement-condemning-crackdown-on-women-activists-in-delhi/23.

Gentleman, Jeffrey, 'Indian Billionaires Bet Big on Head Start in Coronavirus Vaccine Race,' *New York Times*, 1 August 2020, https://www.nytimes.com/2020/08/01/world/asia/coronavirus-vaccine-india-html.

Greene, Jeremy A., and Dora Vargha, 'How Epidemics End,' *Boston Review*, 30 June 2020, https://bostonreview.net/science-nature/jeremy-greene-dora-vargha-how-epidemics-end.

Guardian, Editorial, 24 April 2021, 2.

Guha, Ramachandra, 'Repeating the Past,' *The Telegraph*, 24 April 2020, https://www.telegraphindia.com/opinion/coronavirus-india-the-gover…ious-minorities-during-covid-19-lockdown-and-pandemic/cid/1767769.

————, 'Supreme Court Must Reflect on Its Calling as Defined by the Constitution,' *Indian Express*, 13 August 2020, https://indianexpress.com/article/opinion/columns/supreme-court-democracy-politicisation-judiciary-kashmir-covid-6552287/.

Gunter, Joel, and Vikas Pandey, 'Waldemar Haffkine: The Vaccine Pioneer the World Forgot,' BBC News, 11 December 2020, https://www.bbc.co.uk/world-asia-india-55050012.

Hasan, Mohammad Tareq, 'Homecoming from the City: Covid-19 and Dhaka,' *Medical Anthropology at UCL*, 15 April 2020, https://medanthucl.com/2020/04/15/homecoming-from-the-city-covid-19-dhaka/.

The Hindu, 'Coronavirus: Group Hosts "Cow Urine Party", Says COVID-19 Due to Meat-Eaters,' 14 March 2020, https://www.thehindu.com/news/national/coronavirus-group-hosts-cow-urine-party-says-covid-19-due-to-meat-eaters/article31070516.ece.

Inamdar, Nikhil, 'Three Takeaways from India's "Pandemic Budget",' BBC News, 1 February 2021, https://www.bbc.co.uk/news/world-asia-india-55884215.

Inamdar, Nikhil, and Aparna Alluri, 'How India's Vaccine Drive Went Horribly Wrong,' BBC News, 14 May 2021, https://www.bbc.co.uk/news/world-asia-india-57007004.

————, 'India Economy: Seven Years of Modi in Seven Charts,' BBC News, 22 June 2021, https://www.bbc.co.uk/news/world-asia-india-57437944.

Indian Express, 'I Don't Expect That Fatalities from Covid-19 Will Be Comparable to Those from the 1918 Influenza: Prof. Siddharth Chandra,' 23 March 2020, https://indianexpress.com/article/coronavirus/coronavirus-pandemic-covid-19-siddharth-chandra-interview-6327127/.

India Today, 'Don't Eat Non-veg Which Creates Viruses,' 14 March 2020, https://www.indiatoday.in/india/story/haryana-health-minister-anil-vij-coronavirus-non-vegetarian-food-1655591-2020-03-14.

Islam, Md Toriqul, 'Pandemic and Politics in Colonial Bengal: Lessons from History,' *Prothom Alo*, 15 April 2020, https://en.prothomalo.com/opinion/op-ed/pandemic-politics-in-colonial-bengal-lessons-for-history.

Jaffrelot, Christophe, 'Hindu Nationalism and the (Not So Easy) Art of Being Outraged: The *Ram Setu* Controversy,' *South Asia Multidisciplinary Academic Journal*, 2 (2008), https://journals.openedition.org/samaj/1372.

Jain, Sagaree, 'Anti-Asian Racism in the 1817 Cholera Pandemic,' 20 April 2020, https://daily.jstor.org/anti-asian-racism-in-the-1817-cholera-pandemic/.

Jayal, Niraja Gopal, 'Faith-Based Citizenship,' *India Forum*, 1 November 2019, https://www.theindiaforum.in/article/faith-criterion-citizenship.

Joshi, Shareen, 'Funeral Pyres Should Not Be the Symbol of India's Covid Crisis,' CNN Opinion, 2 June 2021, https://edition.cnn.com/2021/06/02/opinions/india-funeral-pyres-should-not-be-covid-symbol-joshi/index.html.

Kamat, Anilkumar, 'My Tryst with Coronavirus and Home Quarantine,' *Times of India*, 11 February 2021, https://timesofindia.indiatimes.com/readersblog/kamatsense/my-tryst-with-coronavirus-home-quarantine-29683/.

Kazmin, Amy, 'India Has Reached Coronavirus Peak, Says Government Panel,' *Financial Times*, 19 October 2020, https://app.ft.com/content/734102c3-b5f8-486a-bb65-a2ab85bffe3f.

————, 'India Unveils $10bn Plan to Boost Growth,' *Financial Times*, 13 October 2020, 8.

Khadka, Navin Singh, 'Why India and Nepal's Forest Fires Are Worrying Scientists,' BBC News, 12 April 2021, https://www.bbc.co.uk/news/world-asia-india-56671148.

Krishna, Sumi, 'I Survived a Pandemic in the Last Century. Now, I Fight One More,' *The Wire*, 3 April 2020, https://science.thewire.in/health/coronavirus-asian-flu-igk-menon-coonoor-epidemic/.

Lachenal, Guillaume, and Gaëtan Thomas, 'COVID-19: When History Has No Lessons,' History Workshop, 30 March 2020, https://www.historyworkshop.org.uk/covid-19-when-history-has-no-lessons/.

Lone, Suhail-ul-Rehman, 'What Epidemics from the Colonial Era Can Teach Us about Society's Response,' *The Wire*, 8 April 2020, https://thewire.in/history/colonial-era-epidemics-india.

McGrath, Matt, 'Climate Change: Net Zero Targets Are "Pie in the Sky",' BBC News, 1 April 2021, https://www.bbc.co.uk/news/science-environment-56596200.

BIBLIOGRAPHY

Malani, Arup, Arpit Gupta, and Reuben Abraham, 'Why Does India Have So Few Covid-19 Cases and Deaths?,' *Quartz India*, 16 April 2020, https://qz.com/india/1839018/why-does-india-have-so-few-coronavirus-covid-19-cases-and-deaths/.

Menon, Dilip M., 'Viral Histories: Will Covid-19 Help Us Generate New Thinking?,' *Scroll.in*, 7 August 2020, https://scroll.in/article/969649/viral-histories-will-covid-19-help-us-to-generate-new-thinking.

Menon, Shruti, 'Farmer Protests: India's Sedition Law Used to Muffle Dissent,' BBC News, 24 February 2021, https://www.bbc.co.uk/news/world-asia-india-56111289.

Menon, Shruti, and Jack Goodman, 'India Covid Crisis: Did Election Rallies Help Spread Virus?,' BBC News, 24 April 2021, https://www.bbc.co.uk/news/56858980.

Mohanty, Basant Kumar, 'UGC Asks Colleges to Go Back 100 Years to Rate Covid-19 Handling,' *The Telegraph*, 13 June 2020, https://www.telegraphindia.com/india/ugc-asks-colleges-to-go-back-100-years-to-rate-coronavirus-handling/cid/1780467.

Morelle, Rebecca, 'Why India's Covid Crisis Matters to the Whole World,' BBC News, 28 April 2021, https://www.bbc.co.uk/news/world-asia-india-56907007.

NDTV, 'India in "Endgame of Pandemic," Says Health Minister,' 8 March 2021, https://www.ndtv.com/india-news/coronavirus-india-in-endgame-of-pandemic-says-health-minister-2385882.

Nehru, Jawaharlal, 'A Tryst with Destiny,' 14 August 1947, https://www.files.ethz.ch/isn/125396/1154_trystnehru.pdf.

New York Times, 'India Covid Map and Case Count,' 20 October 2020, https://www.nytimes.com/interactive/2020/world/asia/india-coronavirus-cases-html.

Outlook, 'Cow Urine, Cow Dung, Can Cure Coronavirus,' 2 March 2020, https://www.outlookindia.com/website/story/india-news-cow-urine-cow-dung-can-cure-coronavirus-assam-bjp-mla-suman-haripriya/348159.

Padma, T. V., 'India: The Fight to Become a Science Superpower,' *Nature*, 521 (2015), https://www.nature.com/news/india-the-fight-to-become-a-science-superpowert-1.17518.

Pandey, Geeta, 'India Covid: Kumbh Mela Pilgrims Turn into Super-spreaders,' BBC News, 10 May 2021, https://www.bbc.co.uk/news/world-asia-india-57005563.

———, 'India's Holiest River Is Swollen with Covid Victims,' BBC News, 19 May 2021, https://www.bbc.co.uk/news/world-asia-india-57154564.

———, 'Narendra Modi: "Why Is the Indian PM's Photo on My Covid Vaccine Certificate?",' BBC News, 19 October 2021, https://www.bbc.co.uk/news/world-asia-india-58944475.

Pandey, Vikas, 'Covid 19 and Pollution: "Delhi Staring at Coronavirus Disaster",' BBC News, 20 October 2020, https://www.bbc.co.uk/news/world-asia-india-54596245.

Pandey, Vikas, and Andrew Clarance, 'Coronavirus: The Indian Children Orphaned by Covid-19,' BBC News, 31 May 2021, https://www.bbc.co.uk/news/world-asia-india-57264629.

Parkin, Benjamin, Jyotsna Singh, Stephanie Findlay, and John Burn-Murdoch, '"It Is Much Worse This Time": India's Devastating Second Wave,' *Financial Times*, 21 April 2021, https://www.ft.com/content/683914a3-134f-40b6-989b-21e0ba1dc403.

Parsons, David, and Martin Taylor, 'Coal: Why China and India Aren't the Climate Villains of COP26,' *The Conversation*, 17 November 2021, https://theconversation.com/coal-why-china-and-india-arent-the-climate-villains-of-cop26-171879.

Patel, Karishma, 'Covid-19: Fake "Immunity Booster" Found on Sale in London Shops,' BBC News, 19 December 2020, https://www.bbc.co.uk/news/uk-england-london-55318095.

Patel, Vikram, 'India's Tryst with Covid-19,' *India Forum*, https://www.theindiaforum.in/article/indi-s-tryst-covid-19

Payyappallimana, Unnikrishnan, 'Doctors at the Borders: Ayurveda's Encounter with Public Health and Epidemics,' https://culanth.org/fieldsights/doctors-at-the-borders-ayurvedas-encounter-with-public-health-and-epidemics.

Peckham, Robert, 'COVID-19 and the Anti-lessons of History,' *The Lancet*, 14 March 2020: 10.1016/S0140-6736(20)30468-2.

Pernau, Margrit, 'Introduction: Studying Emotions in South Asia,' *South Asian History and Culture* (2021), https://doi.org/10.1080/19472498.2021.1878788.

Perrigo, Billy, 'It Was Already Dangerous to Be Muslim in India. Then Came the Coronavirus,' *Time*, 3 April 2020, https://time.com/5815264/coronavirus-india-islamophobia-coronajihad/.

Pleasance, Chris, and Rachel Bunyan, 'Why Did COVID Fail to Take Off in India and Has Now Collapsed?,' *Mail Online*, 17 February 2021, https://www.dailymail.co.uk/news/article-9265495/Mystery-plunge-coronavirus-cases-India-baffles-experts-country-recorded-11m-infections.html?ito=social-twitter_mailonline.

Radhakrishnan, Sreejith, Abi Tamim Vanak, Pierre Nouvellet, and Christl A. Donnelly, 'Rabies as a Public Health Concern in India: A Statistical Perspective,' *Tropical Medicine and Infectious Disease*, 5: 4 (2020), doi: 10.3390/tropicalmed5040162.

Reuters, 'Art of the Pandemic: COVID-inspired Street Graffiti,' https://www.reuters.com/news/picture/art-of-the-pandemic-covid-inspired-stree-idUSRTXA3GSN.

Rose, Jacqueline, 'Pointing the Finger: *The Plague*,' *London Review of Books*, 7 May 2020, https://www.lrb.co.uk/the-paper/v42/n09/jacqueline-rose/pointing-the-finger.

Roy, Arundhati, 'The Pandemic Is a Portal,' *Financial Times*, 3 April 2020, https://www.ft.com/content/10d8f5e8-74eb-11ea-95fe-fcd274e920ca.

BIBLIOGRAPHY

————, 'We Are Witnessing a Crime against Humanity,' *The Guardian*, 29 April 2021, https://www.theguardian.com/news/2021/apr/28/crime-against-humanity-arundhati-roy-india-covid-catastrophe.

Safi, Michael, 'Vaccine Tensions Looming in Asia,' *The Observer*, 21 March 2021, 37.

Sajjad, Mohammad, 'When Will We Learn Our Lessons from Previous Pandemics?,' *Sabrangindia*, 1 June 2020, https://sabrangindia.in/article/when-will-we-learn-our-lessons-previous-pandemics.

Sen, Nandini C., 'Corona Mata and the Pandemic Goddesses,' *The Wire*, 25 September 2020, https://thewire.in/culture/corona-mata-and-the-pandemic-goddesses.

Sengupta, Shuddhabrata, 'Kumbh 2021: Astrology, Mortality and the Indifference to Life of Leaders and Stars,' *The Wire*, 20 April 2021, https://thewire.in/government/kumbh-2021-astrology-mortality-and-the-indifference-to-life-of-leaders-and-stars.

Singh, Prachi, Shamika Ravi, and Sikim Chakraborty, 'COVID-19: Is India's Health Infrastructure Equipped to Handle an Epidemic?,' *Brookings*, 24 March 2020, https://www.brookings.edu/blog/up-front/2020/03/24/is-indias-health-infrastructure-equipped-to-handle-an-epidemic/.

Singh, Tavleen, 'India Feels like a Ship That Is Totally Adrift,' *Indian Express*, 25 April 2021, https://indianexpress.com/article/opinion/columns/india-covid-19-crisis-oxygen-election.

Sinha, Amitabh, 'India Coronavirus Numbers Explained: A Scary Runaway Phase Begins,' *Indian Express*, 15 September 2020, https://indianexpress.com/article/explained/september-7-india-coronavirus-covid-19-cases-deaths-numbers-explained-6586353/.

Sinha, Chinki, 'Covid India: Women in Rural Bihar Hesitant to Take Vaccines,' BBC News, 1 July 2021, https://www.bbc.co.uk/news/world-asia-india-57551345.

Sontag, Susan, 'AIDS and Its Metaphors,' *New York Review of Books*, 27 October 1988, https://www.nybooks.com/articles/1988/10/27/aids-and-its-metaphors/.

Sriraman, Tarangini, 'Plague Passport to Detention: Epidemic Act Was a Surveillance Tool in British India,' *ThePrint*, 22 March 2020, https://theprint.in/opinion/plague-passport-to-detention-epidemic-act-was-a-medical-surveillance-tool-in-british-india/385121/.

Sundararaman, T., and Alok Ranjan, 'Challenges to India's Rural Healthcare System in the Context of Covid-19,' *Review of Agrarian Studies*, 10: 1 (2020), http://ras.org.in/79332f54f12620b88534aa93a142dc1f.

Swami, Praveen, 'Covid-19 in India: Leaders Are Accountable for Near-Collapse of the State,' *Firstpost*, 4 May 2021, https://www.firstpost.com/india/covid-19-in-india-leaders-are-accou...for-near-collapse-of-the-state-apocalypse-must-matter-9589821.html.

Tanwar, Pranav, and Saurabh Pandey, 'Epidemic Diseases Act, 1897: 123 Year Old Weapon against Coronavirus,' https://ijlpp.com/epidemic-disease-act-1897-123-year-old-weapon-against-corona/.

Times of India, '12-Year-Old Dies after Walking for 3 Days from Telangana to Reach Her Home in Chhattisgarh,' 21 April 2020, https://timesofindia.indiatimes. com/india/12-year-old-dies-after-w...langana-to-reach-her-home-in-chhattisgarh/articleshow/75278563.cms.

Tisdall, Simon, 'Amnesty Specialises in Hard Truths. No Wonder India's Modi Froze It Out,' *The Observer*, 4 October 2020, 25.

Tomar, Konya, 'Ayurveda in the (Mis)Information Age,' *Society for Cultural Anthropology*, 23 June 2020, https://culanth.org/fieldsights/ayurveda-in-the-misinformation-age.

Wallen, Joe, 'India's Covid Excess Death Toll Nearly 10 Times Higher Than Official Estimates,' *The Telegraph*, 20 July 2021, https://www.telegraph.co.uk/global-health/science-and-disease/indias-covid-excess-death-toll-nearly-10-times-higher-official/.

Weber, Thomas, and Dennis Dalton, 'Gandhi and the Pandemic,' *Economic and Political Weekly*, 20 June 2020, https://www.epw.in/joiurnal/2020/25/perspectives/gandhi-and-pandemic.html.

The Week, 'Delhi's Tryst with the Third Wave of Covid-19 Infections,' 22 November 2020, https://www.theweek.in/news/india/2020/11/22/delhi-tryst-with-the-third-wave-of-covid-19-infections-what-numbers-tell-us.html.

Wikipedia, 'COVID-19 Vaccination in India,' https://en.wikipedia.org/wiki/COVID-19_vaccination_in_India.

Wikipedia, 'HIV/AIDS in India,' https://en.wikipedia.org/wiki/HIV/AIDS_in_india.

World Health Organization, 'WHO Director-General's Remarks at the Media Briefing on 2019-nCOV on 11 February 2020,' https://www.who.int/dg/speeches/detail/who-director-general-s-remarks-at-the-media-briefing-on-2019-ncov-on-11-february-2020.

World Health Organization, 'WHO Director-General's Opening Remarks at the Media Briefing on COVID-19 – 11 March 2020,' https://www.who.int/director-general/speeches/detail/who-director-general-s-opening-remarks-at-the-media-briefing-on-covid-19---11-march-2020.

INDEX